## Praise for *Parents Need to Eat Too*

"**If only this book came with every box of newborn diapers or baby blanket!** New and seasoned parents alike will find delicious and simple recipes. Debbie Koenig's food feeds not only sleepy parents with little time to spare in the kitchen, but families, too—from first nibbles to toddler tastes and full-grown meals enjoyed together."

—Emily Franklin, author of *Too Many Cooks: Kitchen Adventures with 1 Mom, 4 Kids, and 102 New Recipes* and founder of wellcookedlife.com

"**Finally, a book that reminds new moms: yes, your life may be totally wrapped up in feeding your baby right now, but you need—and deserve!—to eat well, too.** And with wit, wisdom, and empathy, author Debbie Koenig shows us how it can be done. Packed with crucial information (for example, which foods belong in a new mom's pantry), meal-saving tips (such as how to prep dinner during nap time), and delicious recipes (for everyone from "non-cooks" to nursing moms who are eating with one hand)—*Parents Need to Eat Too* will help new moms and dads get the nutrition and nourishment they need as they adjust to parenthood. I'm recommending it to every expecting mom I know!"

—Meagan Francis, author of *The Happiest Mom: 10 Secrets to Enjoying Motherhood*

"**I laughed, I learned, I dreamed up a hundred fantastic meals while reading** *Parents Need to Eat Too*. Whether you're looking for advice on feeding your family healthy food in a flash, making sure your own needs don't fall by the wayside when you have a new baby in the house, or just wanting to make an incredible batch of chocolate chip cookies, this is the book for you. As the mother of two young children, I only wish I'd had it sooner. As a person who loves to eat, I suspect I'll be cooking from it long after my sons have grown up, as much for Debbie Koenig's intelligent, entertaining company as for her delicious recipes."

—Melanie Rehak, author of *Eating for Beginners*

"Put your kids' leftover chicken nuggets down and pick up Debbie Koenig's cookbook. It's filled with simple yet tasty recipes. *Parents Need to Eat Too* **should be on every baby shower registry.**"

—Jen Singer, author of the *Stop Second-Guessing Yourself* guides to parenting

"**Debbie Koenig's new book promises and delivers the plan you need for the whole family to eat well.** In a clear, comforting tone Debbie explains how to create the New Mom's Pantry, stocked with all the basic ingredients you will need to make her delicious recipes. She even tells you how to turn grown-up food into baby food, which is both good for baby and efficient for the cook. With more than 150 recipes, dozens of intelligent health tips, and comments throughout from real moms just like you, *Parents Need to Eat Too* will be your go-to resource and make you the confident parent you want to be."

—Eileen Behan, RD, family nutritionist and author of
*The Baby Food Bible* and *Eat Well, Lose Weight, While Breastfeeding*

"**You don't have to be a parent to learn from Debbie Koenig's eminently sensible book.** Long work hours often leave me and my husband with little energy for making tasty, wholesome meals—and we don't even have a newborn around! *Parents Need to Eat Too* is full of smart tips and tools for reclaiming our time in the kitchen. And I have no doubt that, as our family grows, we'll be returning to it again and again for recipes and reassurance."

—Molly Wizenberg, author of *A Homemade Life*

"**This book is a must-have for new parents who enjoy eating good food with real flavor.** It's loaded with helpful tips for fitting cooking into a busy new-mom schedule (yes, it can be done!) and sneaking in needed nutrients, and Debbie is a great writer who includes lots of hilarious anecdotes from her own life. Plus, the recipes are all tested by real moms so you know you can trust them!"

—Leah McLaughlin, editor in chief, *Edible Communities/Edible Queens*

"Though my daughters are now teenagers, it feels like just yesterday when I was one of those parents attempting to take care of baby and feed my family. **If only Debbie Koenig's *Parents Need to Eat Too* had existed back then. Every new parent should ask for Debbie's book as a baby shower gift!**"

—Leah Ingram, author of *Suddenly Frugal: How to Live Happier and Healthier for Less* and founder of the blog *Suddenly Frugal* (www.suddenlyfrugal.com)

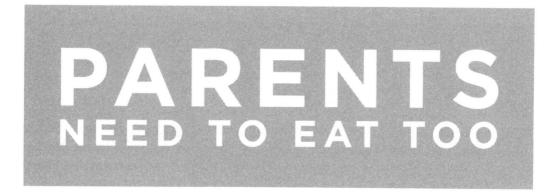

# PARENTS
## NEED TO EAT TOO

Nap-Friendly Cooking, One-Handed Meals, and
Time-Saving Kitchen Tricks for New Parents

## DEBBIE KOENIG
Foreword by Lara Field, MS, RD, CSP, LDN

*wm*

WILLIAM MORROW
*An Imprint of HarperCollinsPublishers*

Parents should consult with their pediatrician about all issues that bear on their children's health.

HarperCollins books may be purchased for educational, business, or sales promotional use.
For information please write: Special Markets Department, HarperCollins Publishers,
10 East 53rd Street, New York, NY 10022.

FIRST EDITION

Designed by Lisa Stokes

Library of Congress Cataloging-in-Publication Data is available upon request.

ISBN 978-0-06-200594-6

12  13  14  15  16  DIX / RRD  0  9  8  7  6  5  4  3  2  1

*To Stephen, whose love, humor, and willingness to taste anything (and tell me when it sucks) encourage me every day.*

*To Harry, my favorite little boy in the whole world. Being your mom has made me a better person, or at least I hope it has.*

*To my Ponies, without whom this whole motherhood gig would be much, much less fun.*

# CONTENTS

# FOREWORD

BY LARA FIELD, MS, RD, CSP, LDN

Having gone through the wonderful journey of pregnancy twice, in addition to my professional background as a registered dietitian and certified specialist in pediatrics, I've had first-hand experience with the difficulties of making smart eating decisions while tackling the responsibility of feeding a new member of the family. Both may be equally daunting. A 2011 study in *Pediatrics* compared the dietary intake and weight status of parents with and without children. The results indicated that parents, especially mothers, ate more calories and had a higher Body Mass Index than women without children.

If constant feedings aren't enough to get a new parent off track in the kitchen, there are two added inconveniences when a new baby is in the picture that research has proven affect our eating decisions: 1) lack of sleep—which over time can cause appetite-stimulating hormones to rise, leading us to overeat; and 2) lack of time—more like no time, for many—which usually translates into no time to exercise or make healthy food choices, both of which make it more difficult to lose the baby weight. Think of it this way: When you're completely exhausted and hungry, you may have a "see it and eat it" approach.

It's important to be realistic in the postpartum period; no one should expect to be back to her pre-pregnancy size in a matter of weeks. As many say, it takes nine months to put it on; it may take nine months to take it off. Really, with any weight loss, a healthy rate of loss is approximately 1 pound per week. Further, those who are breastfeeding need to focus on the task at hand. Current nutritional recommendations state that lactation requires an additional 500 calories per day—you'll find more detail about what foods to include in Chapter 9. Reducing calories too drastically or not consuming the *right* calories during the immediate postpartum period may affect lactation negatively, in terms of milk quality and composition.

Healthy eating starts with proper meal planning, and this book is a fantastic tool to get you through a challenging time. Here are a few key tips:

1) **Sit down for meals.** Having a new baby around keeps many of us so busy we forget the importance of actually sitting down to eat. Sitting at the table for meals helps us concentrate on the task at hand; without this, we have a tendency to not pay attention to what goes into our mouths, leading us to overeat. Now, keep in mind these don't have to be, and most likely won't be, four-course dinners; just taking a break from the routine to sit down and eat is valuable and worth it.

2) **Make time for three meals per day.** Research is abundant in the consequences of skipping meals and overeating, leading to weight gain. Again, it doesn't have to be a large meal, but taking time out for breakfast, lunch, and dinner is the key to healthy weight management.

3) **Don't drink your calories.** This is key for anyone, not just postpartum moms. Choosing zero-calorie beverages most often will assist with weight control. Further, many times we are actually thirsty when we think we're hungry, so drink 8 ounces of water, wait 10 minutes, and reassess if you really need to indulge.

4) **Incorporate fiber- and calcium-rich foods.** These two nutrients are vital for healthy weight loss. Fiber will assist in appetite control, making you feel fuller for longer, and research has shown calcium may be a key mineral in assisting with weight loss. Don't skimp on either. Fiber is found in whole grains, fresh fruits, vegetables, and legumes. Keep fresh fruit and vegetables cut up and on hand, so you'll be less inclined to grab the sweets your friends brought over to welcome your new baby.

5) **Make time to exercise.** This doesn't have to be taxing or strenuous. Get out of the house for at least 45 minutes each day and go for a walk. If you're able to do it alone, even better! If not, bring that baby out for a stroll. It will feel good to get your body moving. And don't use the weather as an excuse—fortunately or unfortunately, there are plenty of shopping malls convenient for a walk. Use them!

Use the recipes and tips in this book to help you find the will and the way to make healthy and delicious meals, not just for yourself but for your little one, too. Each recipe includes a section on how to make a baby-friendly version. There is nothing more satisfying than making a delicious recipe that you and your family can all enjoy.

As our new babies grow, the question of when to start solids comes up. Most research indicates it's appropriate to start at around four to six months—however, I always recommend not to rush this. Starting at four months won't make babies sleep through the night, and they won't earn higher test scores by eating rice cereal for two additional months. It's important to focus on your baby's developmental cues to determine if he or she is ready for solids:

1) Make sure he has adequate head control; he should be able to sit up without assistance.

2) He needs to have moved past the extrusion reflex—the tongue-thrust movement that will push against food rather than allowing him to swallow it. When this is gone, usually at some point between four and six months, infants are ready to eat.

3) He must actually be interested in eating solids: grabbing your spoon, reaching for food on your plate.

The process of eating should be fun and not stressful for anyone involved, so start at a time when you and your infant are ready. Don't succumb to any pressure from those around you. Remember, your child will eat solids for the rest of his life; there's no rush!

The transition from a liquid diet to solids is a delicate balancing act, which can be stressful for parents. In general, as solids are introduced, formula/breastmilk consumption should decrease a bit as more calories come from foods. See the chart on the following page for guidelines on portions for infants.

## SOLID FEEDING GUIDELINES

### 6 TO 8 MONTHS

Breastmilk (BM)/Formula = 6 to 8 ounces per feeding (24 to 32 ounces/day)

Baby Cereal/Soft Breads/Noodles = 2 to 3 servings/day (1 to 2 tablespoons/serving)

Fruits/Vegetables = 2 to 3 times/day, begin to offer soft cooked/mashed baby foods, Stage 1 to 2 (1 to 2 tablespoons/serving)

### 8 TO 10 MONTHS

Breastmilk/Formula = 7 to 8 ounces per feeding (24 to 32 ounces/day)

Baby Cereal/Soft Breads/Noodles = 2 to 3 servings/day (1 to 2 tablespoons/serving)

Fruits/Vegetables = 2 to 3 servings/day (1 to 3 tablespoons/serving); soft, cut up, mashed Stage 2 to 3 foods

Meat/Protein = Begin to offer soft, finely cut or pureed meats, cheeses, and casseroles

### 10 TO 12 MONTHS

Breastmilk/Formula = 7 to 8 ounces per feeding (24 to 32 ounces/day)

Baby Cereal/Breads/Other starches = 4 servings/day (1 to 2 tablespoons/serving)

Fruits/Vegetables = 4 servings/day (1 to 3 tablespoons/serving)

Meats/Protein = 1 to 2 ounces/day; soft, finely cut, chopped meat, beans, or other protein foods

## SAMPLE DAY

|  | 6 TO 8 MONTHS | 8 TO 10 MONTHS | 10 TO 12 MONTHS |
|---|---|---|---|
| BREAKFAST | Baby Cereal (¼ c)*<br>½ jar Stage 1 or 2 Fruit<br>6 to 8 oz BM/formula | Baby Cereal (¼ c)*<br>1 jar Stage 2 Fruit or<br>baby yogurt (4 oz)<br>6 to 8 oz BM/formula | Pancakes (2 mini)<br>2 Tbsp banana<br>1 to 3 Tbsp yogurt<br>6 to 8 oz BM/formula |
| LUNCH | Baby Cereal (¼ c)<br>1 jar Stage 1 or 2 Veggie<br>6 to 8 oz BM/formula | 6 to 8 oz BM/formula<br>2 Tbsp cooked noodles<br>1 jar Stage 2 Meat &<br>Veggie<br>6 to 8 oz BM/formula | 2 Tbsp turkey<br>2 to 3 Tbsp avocado<br>1 to 2 Tbsp applesauce<br>¼ slice cut-up bread<br>6 to 8 oz BM/formula |
| DINNER | 1 jar Stage 1 or 2 Fruit<br>1 jar Stage 1 or 2 Veggie<br>6 to 8 oz BM/formula | 1 jar Stage 2 Fruit<br>1 jar Stage 2 Veggie or 1<br>jar Stage 3 Meat/Veggie<br>6 to 8 oz BM/formula | 2 Tbsp cooked rice<br>2 Tbsp canned beans<br>2 Tbsp squash<br>6 to 8 oz BM/formula |
| SNACK | None | Finger puffs or other<br>easy-to-dissolve cereal<br>(2 Tbsp) | ¼ c dry cereal |
| BEDTIME | 6 to 8 oz BM/formula | 6 to 8 oz BM/formula | 6 to 8 oz BM/formula |

*after preparation with breastmilk/formula

Many of the parents I work with ask about what foods to avoid during infancy, and new research states that there is more of a risk in waiting to introduce foods than in starting early. Unless there are food allergies in your immediate family, most allergists recommend not avoiding any food within the first 12 months—so it's safe to introduce foods that used to be taboo for the youngest eaters, like eggs, fish, and peanut butter. Keep in mind that peanut butter can be a choking hazard; including it as an ingredient is safe, but you should wait until he's older to give your child a peanut butter sand-wich. The exception to this anything-goes rule is honey and corn syrup; these should be avoided in the first year due to the risk of botulism, a deadly food-borne illness.

The American Academy of Pediatrics recommends that, at least in the beginning, parents wait three to five days after introducing each new food before moving on to the next one. The idea is that if, say, you introduce chicken, carrots, and potatoes at the same time and your baby reacts negatively, you won't know which food is the cause. But most of us find it difficult to wait to introduce every single food—there are so many! Instead, I suggest waiting a few days between introducing the following due to potential allergy concerns: milk or milk products (yogurt, cheese), soy, wheat (including oats, due to potential cross-contamination with wheat in manufacturing), eggs, peanuts and tree nuts, and fish and shellfish. It's also a good idea to introduce fruits and vegetables relatively slowly. Once you have a sense for your baby's tolerance of solids, you'll be able to offer foods in combination.

Remember, infancy is when you start your child on the road to making good eating decisions. Try to take the time to enjoy the process and set a good example for your baby by making healthy food choices a priority in your life too. Spend a little time in the kitchen, even if you feel you aren't good at it. Use this book to explore your inner chef, while setting a good example for your children.

# INTRODUCTION

If you're holding this book, odds are congratulations are in order. Either you're a new parent yourself, or you know someone who is. Mazel tovs all around! Or perhaps you're shopping for a shower gift—in which case you deserve a pat on the back for being so thoughtful.

I became a cookbook author almost by accident. I'm not a big believer in Destiny with a capital D, but in some ways it seems as if everything in my life led me here. As far back as I can remember, writing and food were my twin comforts. (Picture a chubby, curly-haired little girl, wiping the cookie crumbs off her notebook.) A career in book marketing introduced me to such single-name food luminaries as Martha, Ina, and Mario, as well as many of New York's finest restaurants. Classes at the renowned Institute of Culinary Education taught me how to cook without a recipe. And a sustained stint in Weight Watchers, during which I lost 100 pounds, led me to learn about nutrition. In 2002 I left my cushy job, intending to open a gourmet shop, but after six months of learning the business alongside my mentor, herself a successful restaurateur and caterer, I realized my calling was slightly different: I wanted to *write* about food. To get my feet wet, I started a food blog, *Words to Eat By*, which led to actual, paid food-writing assignments. But sharing my food through words wasn't enough—I wanted a family of my own to nurture.

By then I'd met Stephen, a man who will eat anything from sea urchin to chili cheese dogs, the man I'd marry. Together we endured seventeen months of trying to conceive before I finally got pregnant on the eve of my fortieth birthday. (How's that for a party?) With Harry growing inside me, *Words to Eat By* became a slow stream of pregnancy-food posts, comforting things like mushroom risotto and chocolate Amazon cake. As my due date neared, I planned to cook and freeze things for us to eat later: turkey meatloaf, Little Gram's meatballs, big pots of chili, not even thinking to blog about them. I had an inkling that there wouldn't be time for much cooking once the baby was born, but I assumed I'd be back in the swing within a week or two. *Wrong.*

*Parents Need to Eat Too* began gestating, in a sense, soon after my son came home from the hospital in September 2006. Picture this: It's Day Six of Harry's life. My boy, teeny and perfect and miraculous, is nursing, again. For him, eating is a relatively simple thing: All he has to do is open wide and suck. For Stephen and me it's a more challenging proposition. Since Harry came home, we've eaten nothing but family-supplied meals, fried egg sandwiches, Clif bars, and takeout. I wonder what the readers of my food blog would think if they could see me. A hard truth is sinking in: Cooking—and by that I mean cooking healthy, nourishing, yum-I-want-more dishes—while caring for a newborn is a very tall order, even for a food writer like me. And too much takeout is as hard on the waistline as it is on the wallet.

Several months passed before I regained my kitchen legs—months during which Stephen and I ate jar after jar of spaghetti sauce over angel hair (the fastest-cooking pasta), telling ourselves, "Hey, at least we're eating tomatoes—they're healthy!" A turkey sandwich was a treat, since it required the forethought to buy both rye bread *and* turkey breast. Green vegetables? Not so much.

During that time, I learned a new way to cook—taking advantage of Harry's morning nap to chop and roast vegetables, knowing that during his afternoon nap I'd layer them with no-boil noodles, sauce, and cheese for a lasagna to bake later. I created healthy, filling, crave-worthy meals I could eat with one hand, so the other would be free to hold the baby (and which wouldn't drip on Harry's sweet little head, either!). My mom's contribution: a slow cooker. Until necessity kicked in, I'd been too much of a food snob to consider using such a thing. With the help of a fantastic lactation consultant, I discovered galactagogues—foods like oatmeal, which would help my meager breast-milk supply—and incorporated them into recipes. In other words, I cracked the code. I figured out how to take care of Stephen and myself with as much love as I poured into Harry, but with far less energy than he required. It was almost enough to make me want to get pregnant again, just so I could put it all into use!

Instead, I found another way to use that hard-earned knowledge: teaching other new mothers. It started with a single presentation to the moms' group from Harry's preschool, and soon grew into a series of classes I teach informally in my home. Each time I offer the class, four moms and their babies crowd around my kitchen table, peeling and chopping and comparing notes and coming to realize that yes, things will go back to normal. It might be a different normal, but everything will turn out fine. Even dinner.

Which brings us to this cookbook. *Parents Need to Eat Too* is not about locavore cooking, organic food, or any other of-the-moment rages (although I do encourage you to eat organic as much as you can afford to; see the sidebar on page 4 for more info). It's about kitchen triage, plain and simple: getting dinner on the table for the grownups while there's an infant—or heck, even a toddler—attached to your body. Trust me, you can do this. You just need to change your expectations a bit. While before you may have sought authenticity and even perfection in your cooking, now you'll be seeking deliciousness and doability. Repeat after me: authenticity, shmauthenticity—we just want to *eat*.

Each of the recipes in this book is constructed with an eye to nutrition as well as time-management, since those are the two biggest challenges most new parents face when it comes to their own eating. And every single recipe has been tested by a group of more than 100 new moms, all of whom volunteered to spend a year with me making sure these recipes really work. These amazing women (plus quite a few of their husbands) let me know if a flavor was off, or I'd underestimated the cooking time, or the directions confused a bleary-eyed cook. When a recipe didn't get enough feedback—or enough positive feedback—I didn't include it in the book.

And did I mention that every recipe tastes fantastic? Bursting with robust flavors and interesting combinations, these dishes are simple enough for the most sleep-deprived mom—and many are elegant enough to serve to company (because let's face it, after the first few weeks, most visitors don't think to cook for you. They want to hold the baby, and if they bring some sort of food with them, it's a bonus). Comforting and nourishing, exciting and homey, these are the kinds of foods you'll want to eat. And for those times when your I-can't-cook partner wants to pitch in, there's an entire chapter full of what I call "un-recipes"—things so simple even your baby can make them. Almost.

Sooner than you can imagine, your baby's going to start eating solids, so each recipe also includes a section at the end, "Make Baby Food," which does exactly what you think: It tells you how to use the very food you've prepared for yourselves to feed the newest eater. You'll save a bundle by not buying jarred food, and hopefully you'll wind up with a kid who enjoys food as much as you do.

More than just recipes, this cookbook will provide you with something all new parents need: *reassurance*. Reassurance that this little creature won't rule your lives forever (well, not entirely, anyway). Reassurance that it's possible to take care of yourself *and* a baby. Reassurance that life will resume something approaching normalcy, and sooner than you think.

So, dig in. Enjoy. And know that you can do it. Really, you can. You don't need to please anyone but yourself.

### A FEW WORDS ON ORGANICS

If I could afford it, I'd only use organic food. But my finances don't allow that, so I'll assume yours don't, either. If you need to pick and choose your organics, here's a little guidance:

- Check out the Environmental Working Group's "Dirty Dozen" list—it's the twelve fruits and vegetables that their testing has found to be the highest in pesticide residue. Those, you should always buy organic. The list is updated annually, so go to their site, www.foodnews.org, for this year's, um, winners. EWG provides both an iPhone app and a downloadable wallet-sized card. Carrying it with you is much easier than trying to remember the whole list!

- Another option for produce is the farmers' market, where you can ask the farmer about his growing practices. At my local market there's only one stand that's certified organic, but the other farmers use many of the same methods.

- If your family goes through a lot of milk, stick to organic—especially once your baby turns one and begins to drink it. Yogurt and cheese are often a big portion of an early eater's diet, so go organic there too.

- A good rule of thumb is this: Think proportionally, in terms of your child's body weight. If she can down an entire package of, say, frozen peaches and peaches aren't on EWG's list, buy organic anyway. Twelve ounces of peaches is a lot when you weigh less than 20 pounds!

- Is yours a family of hard-core carnivores? Try to buy organic meats. Which, given the expense, may force you to reconsider your carnivorous ways . . .

- For the most part, you can skip organic processed foods like breakfast cereal and packaged snacks. The further removed something is from the way it came out of the ground, the less likely it is to have a lot of pesticide residue remaining. Who knew, all that processing is actually good for something!

- If you'd like to dig deeper into all this, I recommend the book *To Buy or Not to Buy Organic* by Cindy Burke. I interviewed her once for a story I wrote, and found her research solid and her advice sensible.

## THE NEW MOM'S KITCHEN EQUIPMENT

I realize you may not have a fully outfitted gourmet kitchen at your disposal (I created these recipes in a Brooklyn rental, with a stove that's circa 1990), so I've tried to ensure that my recipes don't require anything fancy. Here's a basic list of what you'll need to make almost anything in the book; hopefully, you've already got just about all of it:

- Kitchen timer (no joke, this just might be the most important tool in a sleep-deprived parent's kitchen—make sure it's loud enough to wake you if you doze off while the soup's simmering)
- Three knives: chef's, paring, and serrated
- Cutting board, ideally separate ones for meat and produce
- Vegetable peeler
- Microplane or other hand-held grater
- Measuring cups (both dry and liquid) and spoons
- Wooden spoon with a nice long handle
- Slotted spoon, again with a nice long handle
- Spatula
- Whisk
- Rolling pin
- Two mixing bowls: one large, one small
- Five or six small bowls or custard cups
- Two saucepans: one large, one small, both with lids
- Stock pot, ideally with a lid
- Slow cooker or Dutch oven
- Large nonstick skillet, ideally with a lid
- Colander
- 2 baking sheets with rimmed edges
- Cooling rack
- Large rectangular baking dish (9 x 13-inch is standard)
- Square baking dish (8-inch is standard)
- Blender, hand-held blender, or food processor (ideally a blender and a food processor, if you've got room, for ultimate flexibility)
- Electric mixer, if you intend to bake

**NOTE:** You'll hear a lot about the notion of mise-en-place in this book. It simply means you do all your prep work before you start cooking, and put each ingredient into its own bowl, in order of use. It makes for more cleanup, yes, but it also means you won't discover halfway through a recipe that you forgot to pick up carrots.

# CHAPTER 1
# THE NEW MOM'S PANTRY

Harry was almost two weeks old before I set foot outside our apartment without him. We were having major breastfeeding issues (more about that in Chapter 9) and if Harry wasn't attached to my boob, I was essentially chained to a hospital-grade pump. And then one day my husband, Stephen, whose idea of a good time does not involve bringing items to a cash register, came home from a trip to the baby store (*more* burp cloths), the drugstore (antibiotics for me), and the medical supply store (pump parts) with a gift for me.

"How about *you* hit the supermarket today," he offered. "Would you be up for it?"

Would I like to take over an errand in his place? I know what you're thinking. Some gift. You were expecting jewelry.

But see, I really do enjoy food shopping. And the chance to unhook myself from pump and baby to venture into one of my favorite places was as sweet a present my husband could ever give me. Who needs Tiffany when you have Trader Joe's?

When I travel, a foreign supermarket is a tourist attraction. Picking out food, and daydreaming about how to use it, is a cherished pastime. There's inspiration in every aisle—I veer off-list every time I walk through those automated doors.

Stephen and I consulted our very complicated feeding/pumping schedule to pinpoint a 90-minute window, and off I went.

At the store, bounteous displays of late-summer produce beckoned. I swear the tomatoes were flirting with me with their seductively full curves. Into the cart went crisp romaine lettuce, sweet corn, perfectly smooth eggplant. Look at that zucchini! And the herbs, oh the herbs! I went bonkers. The cart overflowed with freshness and my pulse raced at the thought of all the things I'd cook.

Of course, I forgot to take into account that whole chained-to-the-pump thing. Ten days later, much of my luscious produce was still sitting in the fridge, only now the greens were slimy, the eggplant was squishy, and my kitchen dreams were dashed. It would be weeks before I became a good enough juggler to really *cook*, to plan a meal, shop for ingredients, and find time to use them.

In the meantime, I learned to depend on my pantry. And now, when I begin a new round of cooking classes, our first session is always dedicated to the humble, but well-stocked, pantry. It's a shelf-stable Garden of Eden.

With a cabinet full of staple goods, there's *always* something for dinner. A humble can of chickpeas mixed with onion, garlic, and ginger, dried spices, and canned tomato becomes Cheater's Chana Masala. Yes, I do consider onions, garlic, and ginger to be part of the pantry. Potatoes, too. If stored properly, they all last for quite some time: Onion, garlic, and potatoes actually thrive in the pantry proper—they love cool and dark. Ginger needs cold, not cool, but it'll last for a good 6 to 8 weeks in a resealable bag in the fridge, even longer in the freezer. And while we're talking about my loose definition of *pantry items*, I'll point out that I also include a handful of staples straight from the freezer aisle.

The list that follows is the foundation of this cookbook. Just about every single thing on it is used in at least one recipe. In several cases I mention specific brands, because I've found them to be full of flavor as well as nutrients. If you use my list as your guide before you go shopping, you'll never be hungry again. No wait, that's Scarlett O'Hara. I mean, you'll never give up and order greasy takeout again.

## PASTA, RICE, GRAINS

- **Barilla Plus pasta** (the yellow box): It's full of protein, fiber, and omega-3s, making it exceptionally healthy pasta. And it doesn't have the musty flavor and mushy texture of many whole-wheat varieties. In general, look for whole-grain pasta with at least 3 grams of dietary fiber per serving.

- **Orzo or other small-shaped pasta:** Keep some on hand to add to soups or quick pasta salads. Note: Barilla Plus doesn't come in smaller sizes, so go with whole-wheat or regular for this.

- **No-boil lasagna noodles:** Did you catch the "no-boil" part? Nuf said. There are several brands on the market—I've used Ronzoni, Barilla, and Trader Joe's with good results.

- **Success Brown Rice** (the boil-in bag): This is a godsend to new parents. Nutritionally, Success Brown is nearly identical to plain brown rice, but instead of taking more than half an hour to cook it's ready in just ten minutes and—here's the best part—it can sit in hot water, off the heat, for up to half an hour without turning mushy. Other good options are Trader Joe's frozen brown rice and Uncle Ben's 90-second microwave pack (which, while super-convenient, does have added fat).

- **Long-grain brown rice:** For times when you *do* have the wherewithal. And it's vital for Lentil and Brown Rice Soup (page 25).

- **Arborio rice:** Yes, it *is* possible to make risotto with a baby in the house! You'll learn two different methods in Chapter 2, "Nap-Friendly Cooking" and Chapter 4, "The Slow Cooker."

- **Shelf-stable polenta rolls:** If you can find shelf-stable polenta rather than the refrigerated kind, go for it. It'll last longer.

- **Quinoa:** Not technically a grain (though it behaves like one), quinoa is full of protein, fiber, magnesium, and iron, and it's gluten-free. Cooks quickly too!

- **Steel-cut oats:** Oatmeal has long been recommended to nursing mothers as a galactagogue—something that increases breastmilk supply—and making steel-cut oats overnight in the slow cooker is about the easiest thing in the world. (There's a "recipe" on page 136.) Oatmeal in general—not just the steel-cut variety—is also a great source of soluble fiber, which helps control your blood sugar and keeps you feeling fuller for longer (super-helpful for losing the baby weight).

- **Cornmeal:** Oh, how I love thee, cornmeal. Cornbread is a quick and easy accompaniment for chili, soups, etc., and can be thrown together during baby's nap. Also, cornmeal makes a wonderfully crisp (whole-grain) coating for baked fish and chicken.

- **Couscous,** whole wheat if you can find it: Boil a little salted water, dump it in, turn off the heat, and it's ready in five minutes. Ain't nothing faster.

- **Whole-grain bread:** Can't make a sandwich without bread, people. To be sure you're getting all the health benefits of whole grains, read labels carefully, and be certain that the first ingredient listed includes the word "whole."

## CANS AND BPA

Unless you live under a rock, you've probably heard about Bisphenol A (BPA), the toxic substance that's in all sorts of plastic. Well, it's also used to line cans. And it makes its way into breastmilk, which brings things to a whole 'nother level of scary. The jury's still out on exactly how harmful BPA is, but I do my best to avoid it. Aseptic packaging—foods packed in oversized juiceboxes—are BPA-free but still shelf-stable, as are glass jars. Today several companies, including Eden Organic and Trader Joe's, are making many of their products available in BPA-free cans.

## CANNED AND JARRED GOODS

- **Oils:** I'm not going to recommend that you stock a variety of oils, each with its own uses. For the purposes of this cookbook, all you need is an inexpensive, mild-flavored olive oil for cooking, and a good-quality, fruity extra-virgin olive oil for salads and other places where flavor really counts.

- **Nonstick cooking spray:** If you're looking to keep calories down, this is a helpful product—it applies a very fine mist of oil to pans.

- **Vinegars:** Balsamic and red wine are musts, as is rice (also labeled rice wine) vinegar, which adds a light Asian flavor to salads, sauces, and marinades. I'm also a big fan of sherry vinegar, but that's optional.

- **Toasted sesame oil:** for the same reason as rice vinegar. (Yes, it's another oil, but I consider it almost a condiment.)

- **Canned beans, beans, beans:** Black, white (cannellini), chickpeas, red kidney . . . beans are a great source of protein, fiber, iron, folate, magnesium, and manganese, they're low in fat, and for all that nutritional punch they're inexpensive. Trader Joe's and Eden Organics' canned beans are BPA-free (see sidebar, page 10). And unlike virtually every other brand, Eden's have no salt added, either.

- **Broth:** chicken, beef, vegetable. My cabinet always has small juicebox- and quart-sized boxes. Look for reduced-sodium varieties.

- **Tomatoes:** chopped or diced (without added seasonings like basil or garlic), sauce, puree. Don't bother with whole unless you like squishing them in your hands—chopping is just another step you don't need! I'm a huge fan of Pomi brand tomatoes. They're imported from Italy, they're wonderfully fresh-tasting, and they come in aseptic boxes, not cans, so they're BPA-free.

- **Tomato paste** in a tube is a must-have—very few recipes call for an entire can of paste, but with a tube you squeeze out what you need and refrigerate the rest. In the fridge, it stays good practically forever.

- **Anchovy paste** in a tube is necessary for similar reasons, even if you think you don't like anchovies (and I don't!). The paste dissolves into the dish and leaves a depth of flavor that's subtle but important.

- **Artichoke hearts:** Use marinated ones to liven up salads (add some olive oil to the marinade itself to make a quick salad dressing), and plain ones in recipes.

- **Chipotles in adobo:** Use one with seeds scraped out and discarded for moderate heat (don't forget to include some adobo sauce!), transfer the rest to an airtight container, and refrigerate indefinitely. Adds depth and spice to tomato-based dishes, beans, etc. Note: Always wash your hands well after handling a chipotle—it's a smoked jalepeño chile, and you don't want to touch your eyes (or your baby) with those oils on your fingers.

- **Tuna:** I always buy light tuna in olive oil, imported from Italy—it's in most supermarkets. Light tuna has fewer mercury worries, and the Italian stuff is very good quality. Imported tuna packed in jars is more expensive, but it's pretty fantastic in terms of flavor. And again, no BPA in jars. Just drain it well, since the olive oil does add fat and calories.

- **Jarred pasta sauce:** Hey, I'm a realist. Sometimes the best you can do—really—is spaghetti with jarred sauce. All I ask is that you make sure you buy the good stuff. My favorite is Rao's. It costs more, but a look at the ingredients list will show you why: It's made from what you'd use if you *did* have time to cook. Tomatoes, garlic, olive oil, salt, maybe basil. It'll set you back $8 a jar, but it's still cheaper and healthier than takeout. Plus it's useful for a quick lasagna or baked ziti.

- **Barbecue sauce:** Just like with pasta sauce, look for as few ingredients as possible, and ones that you recognize. Try to avoid high-fructose corn syrup. One brand I really like is Dinosaur.

- **Reduced-sodium soy sauce:** A dash of this adds flavor (and salt, of course) to everything from salad dressings to marinades. Not just for stir-fries.

- **Worcestershire sauce:** Its uses are practically limitless, especially in meat- or mushroom-based dishes.

- **Mustard:** for sandwiches, salad dressings, and recipes. Dijon is most often used in cooking.

- **Peanut butter:** Look for "natural" peanut butter—the only ingredients should be peanuts and salt. It's the kind with the oil floating on top; that oil is a pain to stir back in the first time, but if you keep it in the fridge it won't re-separate.

- **Dry vermouth:** I use this as a substitute for white wine in risotto and just about any other recipe that calls for it. It's shelf-stable when opened, so I never have to worry about wasting a good bottle of wine. (Since Harry was born, my wine consumption has dwindled to embarrassingly low levels.) Of course if you drink white wine regularly, you don't have such worries—you can skip this one with my blessing and respect.

- **Dry sherry:** Like vermouth, an open bottle lasts a good long while. It can transform a mushroom dish from fine to fantastic.

### 10 PROCESSED FOODS IT'S ACTUALLY OK TO EAT

"Processed food" has become a catch-all phrase to describe everything that's wrong with the way America eats—but if you've eaten canned beans or baby carrots, you've eaten processed food. The idea is to find processed foods that are prepared as closely as possible to homemade. Here are the ten ready-to-use products I find most helpful in a new parent's kitchen:

1. Boil-in bag, parboiled, or frozen brown rice
2. Chicken sausages (look for ones that are antibiotic- and nitrate-free, with a short, recognizable list of ingredients)
3. Soup and broth (with two caveats: seek out low-sodium versions, and try to purchase in aseptic boxes or jars)
4. Jarred pasta and barbecue sauce
5. Vacuum-packed gnocchi
6. Polenta rolls
7. Hummus
8. Salsa
9. Frozen waffles
10. Frozen products from Amy's, Kashi, Dr. Praeger's, or Morningstar Farms (Again, with a caveat that you must read labels—many frozen meals, even from organic companies, are extremely high in sodium and saturated fat. Look for a short, recognizable list of ingredients.)

## DRY GOODS

- **Split peas, red lentils, green (or brown) lentils, and black lentils (sometimes labeled "Beluga lentils"):** None need pre-soaking and all cook quickly, so they're perfect for healthy, no-planning-needed meals.

- **Dried black beans:** I know, I know, you can't think straight enough to pre-soak dried beans. But there's a recipe in this very chapter for Frijoles Negros that's ready 90 minutes after you open the bag, no soaking necessary. NOTE: Cooking time for dried legumes can vary widely, depending on things like age of the beans and altitude. Shop in stores with a fast turnover to ensure freshness.

- **All-purpose flour and whole-wheat flour:** for baking, of course, but also for thickening the occasional sauce and coating meat pre-browning. If you've got whole-wheat resistant family members, look for "white whole wheat," which is a whole-grain variety that looks like white flour.

- **Cocoa powder:** Sometimes you just need to bake. Or make pudding. Or hot cocoa.

- **Sugar and vanilla:** See cocoa, above.

- **Breadcrumbs:** Sauté a half-cup in olive oil for a quick, crunchy topping to liven up spaghetti and jarred sauce. It's even better when you add some grated Parmesan cheese. And check out the recipe for Angel Hair with Lemon-Parmesan Breadcrumbs on page 40.

- **Sun-dried tomatoes:** I prefer the kind that's not packed in oil, for calorie-watching reasons. But if you're not concerned with that, the oil-packed ones are deeelicious.

- **Nuts:** Pine nuts, pecans, almonds (whole, slivered, sliced, Marcona)—whatever kinds of nuts you like, keep some on hand. Toss into salads, pasta dishes, and oatmeal, or grab a small handful for a healthy snack.

- **Dried fruit:** Whatever kinds you like, to use in salads and for snacks, on top of oatmeal or in desserts. I always have raisins, cherries, blueberries, cranberries, papaya (Harry's favorite), and figs. Trader Joe's has an especially good selection. Try to buy dried fruit without added sugar.

- **Dried herbs and spices:** Over the course of the cookbook, you'll primarily use cinnamon, basil, oregano, thyme, red pepper flakes, cayenne, ground cumin, ground coriander, ground ginger, bay leaves, garam masala, turmeric, paprika, chili powder, salt, and pepper. Experts will tell you that spices stay fresh for six months to a year if stored tightly closed in a cool, dry place, but I've got a confession: I've used two-year-old cinnamon and been just fine. As long as it doesn't smell musty, there's no need to throw it away—though you may want to use a little bit more than the recipe calls for if the spice's smell is relatively faint.

### PEOPLE *WILL* DROP IN. BE PREPARED.

There's something about having a new baby in the house that redefines gravity, with your home suddenly being at the center. Just when you wish people would most respect your privacy, your need to bond as a family, or even the notoriously unpredictable schedule you're now living with, that's when Aunt Judgy will "happen to be in the neighborhood." If you're lucky she'll call first, but even then, you probably won't have time to run out and buy those little nibbly things that lend you the air of competence Aunt Judgy's looking for. Arrange some of these on that tray she gave you as a wedding present, and I'll bet she won't even notice the spitup in your hair.

- Nuts (Marcona almonds are especially swanky, if you ask me)
- Jarred olives
- Cheese
- Dry-cured sausage
- Jarred roasted or pickled peppers
- Tapenade or other jarred spreads
- Baby carrots
- Fruit: When refrigerated, grapes, apples, and citrus fruits like clementines all have a relatively long life-span
- Whole-grain crackers or breadsticks

## PRODUCE

OK, so technically these aren't "pantry" items, but if you keep these greens (and oranges and yellows and reds) around you'll almost always have what you need to make a good, healthy, quick dinner. They're my staples, listed below in approximate order of how long they stay fresh. In many cases, you can buy vegetables pre-cut, either in the produce section or from the salad bar. Normally I don't recommend such things—after several days, cut vegetables may begin to lose some nutrients—but when it's a choice between shortcuts and takeout, you go right ahead and buy the pre-cut vegs. It may raise the odds of contracting a food-borne illness, though, so wash *everything* with soapy water or a vegetable rinse. This won't protect you 100 percent (nothing can!), but it will lower the chances considerably. (If you're wondering what to buy organic, see the sidebar in the Introduction, on page 4.)

**NOTE:** Do not store potatoes with onions. Each emits a gas that hastens spoilage of the other.

- Potatoes: I keep Yukon gold and sweet potatoes on hand. Yukon golds are versatile—mashed, roasted, in stews—and sweet potatoes are super-healthy thanks to beta-carotene, which gives them that rust-orange hue. Even plain ol' russets are good: a stuffed baked potato can be a perfect easy dinner.
- Garlic
- Onions
- Carrots
- Celery
- Lemons
- Broccoli
- Zucchini
- Eggplant
- Red peppers
- Baby spinach
- Flat-leaf parsley
- Grape tomatoes

## WHERE DOES IT ALL GO?

It's all well and good to have a perfectly stocked pantry, but if you can't find that jar of capers, you can't use them. It's probably insane to consider a top-to-bottom reorganization with a new baby in the house, so here are some simple, basic guidelines:

- Group like with like, and keep your everyday items front and center. In my pantry, there's a carbs shelf for pasta, rice, couscous, and other bits of starchy goodness. This is my most-visited shelf, so it's easy to access. Another shelf holds oils, vinegars, and other liquid seasonings, and there's a designated space for baking items too. You get the idea.

- Store heavier items, like bottles of juice, on lower shelves. You do *not* want that dropping on your foot while you're holding a baby.

- Most packaging will have a date stamped on it. "Best by," "best if used by," and "use by" all refer to the quality of the product—go beyond that date and the food's still safe to eat, but it may not taste as good as you'd expect. "Sell by" tells the store when to remove it from the shelf—don't buy food that's approaching that date unless you'll be using or freezing it right away.

- A word about formula and baby food: Federal regulations require a "use by" date, which should ensure both safety and nutritional quality. Beyond that date formula may separate and clog the nipple, and baby food may lose nutrients—don't buy or use it.

- In general, higher-acid canned foods like tomatoes and pineapple are good for 12 to 18 months on the shelf; low-acid foods like animal proteins and most vegetables can stay there for two to five years.

- As long as a food remains frozen until use, it's safe indefinitely. You may notice a decline in flavor with prepared foods, but safety is not an issue. For more information about freezing food, check out Chapter 5, "Big Batch Bonanza."

- Not sure if an open package is safe to use? Check out Still Tasty, stilltasty.com, a food database packed with clear, useful information about storage times.

## HOW TO SHOP WITH A BABY

Ridiculous as it seems in retrospect, figuring this out was one of the biggest challenges I faced when Harry was tiny. My best advice: Go early on weekday mornings. Stores tend to be less crowded then, which means you'll get in and out that much faster. It will take some trial and error to determine what works best for you and your baby, but here are some mom-tested tips and techniques for handling a baby *and* a shopping cart:

- Wear your baby in a sling or carrier. This is my preferred method—it leaves the entire cart for groceries, it encourages baby to nap, and it discourages well-meaning strangers from touching your infant.

- When you just need a few things, use your stroller instead of a shopping cart. Many of the models that work with infant car seats have sizable baskets underneath.

- Set the car seat inside the main body of the cart, and put your items all around it and in the front section of the cart. Obviously, this won't work for a huge haul.

- Make grocery shopping a family outing—one of you pushes the cart with the car seat set inside the main section, while the other pushes the cart for groceries.

- If you're lucky, your supermarket offers carts with built-in infant seats. I was not so lucky, and every time I see one I still get a little bit jealous.

- Consider doing your grocery shopping online. Here in New York City, Fresh Direct is well-known as a friend to parents.

- Leave the baby at home! Seriously, food shopping was a great escape for me, 90 minutes when I didn't have to worry about Harry's well-being. And it's good practice for your partner—the more often you go out solo, the more comfortable s/he'll become with babywrangling.

- **NOTE:** Please *don't* put your car seat into the front section of the cart, where older babies sit. Even if it latches on, it's not necessarily safe: Infant carriers tend to weigh quite a lot, which makes a shopping cart, especially an empty one, top-heavy. Go over an unexpected bump, and the whole cart might tip.

## REFRIGERATOR

This is the shortest list by far, since refrigerated items are the most perishable.

- Eggs
- Milk
- Parmesan cheese: Splurge on the good stuff, a wedge of Parmigiano-Reggiano. A small amount, freshly grated, adds tons of flavor, and you can freeze the rinds to use in soups and stews.
- Butter
- Plain, nonfat Greek yogurt: It's packed with protein, and the tangy flavor makes it a good substitute for sour cream.

## FREEZER

I try to buy all my frozen fruits and vegs in bags, never boxes—that way I can use as much or as little as I need, without having to defrost a block.

- Chopped spinach
- Mixed vegetables (corn, green beans, peas, and carrots) make Chicken Pot Pie (page 50) and Cottage Pie (page 71) incredibly easy.
- Peas
- Corn
- Artichoke hearts
- Butternut squash, either pureed or chopped
- Mixed berries and/or strawberries, blueberries, and raspberries
- Sliced peaches
- Mango
- Prepared pie crust (I buy Pillsbury from the refrigerated section—just pop it in the freezer. Trader Joe's also makes a good frozen variety.)
- Whole-wheat pizza dough (I use Trader Joe's, again from the refrigerated section.)
- Empanada shells (You'll need these for several recipes in Chapter 6—you'll find them in the supermarket wherever there's a Hispanic community.)
- Ground turkey breast

- Ground beef (Look for extra-lean—it's got less fat and cholesterol than regular ground turkey.)
- Veggie burgers (I like Morningstar Farms Garden Veggie Patties.)
- Ice cream: Every new parent *needs* ice cream. And ice cream sandwiches can be eaten with one hand!

**CRIB NOTES**

- Without a well-stocked pantry, the odds that you'll be able to put together a delicious, healthy meal are slimmer than Posh Spice. This may just be the most important chapter in the book.

- If grocery shopping isn't your thing, delegate. In the early days of a baby's life, you'll likely have friends and family just itching to help. Stick a grocery list on the fridge and keep track of what's running low, so you're ready to take advantage—and get the ingredients you need, not what a volunteer guesses you might like—whenever an offer comes in.

- No friends or family nearby? Look online for a grocery service. Many local supermarkets now allow you to create your shopping list online, which they'll fulfill for you. All you need to do is pick it up! If you're really lucky, they deliver.

- Extend your definition of the word "pantry" to include the freezer. When stored properly (tightly wrapped, frozen solid), most foods will stay safe to eat indefinitely—your only concern will be flavor, which may lessen after several months. If you've got a spare fridge or chest freezer in the basement, keep it stocked with fruits, vegetables, meat, poultry, and fish. Because they contain oils that can go rancid relatively quickly, whole-grain flours, nuts, and seeds also benefit from freezer storage. (You'll find more about freezing cooked food in Chapter 5.)

# CHIPOTLE TORTILLA SOUP

**Serves 6 to 8**

**Cooking time: 35 minutes to 1 hour (20 minutes active)**

Here's a pantry-based soup that's endlessly flexible. Most tortilla soups have shredded chicken in them—but since we sometimes think we've got chicken in the freezer and, um, we don't, this version uses canned beans instead. Don't sweat it if you don't have an avocado or cilantro, either. If you're a vegetarian, swap in vegetable broth for the chicken and you'll be just fine. And if you're a nursing mom whose baby is affected when you eat spicy food, use less of the chipotle.

One 28-ounce can whole tomatoes, with juice

1 chipotle in adobo, plus 1 tablespoon sauce
*Scrape the seeds out of the chipotle pepper for milder heat, or add a second pepper if you like things really spicy.*

1 small onion, roughly chopped

2 garlic cloves, peeled and smashed

1½ teaspoons chili powder

1 teaspoon ground cumin

1 teaspoon dried oregano

6 cups low-sodium chicken broth

One 15- to 16-ounce can black or pinto beans, drained and rinsed

2 cups frozen corn kernels

Salt and pepper

6 to 8 small corn tortillas

Olive oil, for brushing

1 avocado, peeled and cut into chunks

½ cup cilantro leaves, roughly chopped

Grated sharp Cheddar or Jack cheese, sour cream, and lime, for serving

**Preheat oven to 350°F.**

1. Puree the tomatoes and their juices, along with the chipotle with sauce, onion, garlic, chili powder, cumin, and oregano in a blender. Transfer to a large, heavy pot or Dutch oven and cook over medium heat, stirring, until mixture thickens and color darkens, 5 to 7 minutes. If it spatters, put a lid on partway to catch at least some of it.

2. Add the broth, beans, and corn, and bring to a boil. Lower heat and simmer, covered, for at least 15 minutes and up to an hour. Add salt and pepper to taste.

3. While the soup simmers, brush each tortilla lightly with olive oil. Stack the tortillas and cut into ½-inch-wide strips, then cut the longer strips in half. Scatter the tortilla

strips in a single layer on a baking sheet and bake for 10 minutes, or until lightly browned and crisp.

4. Divide the tortilla strips, avocado chunks, and cilantro among six to eight bowls. Top with the soup, and serve with cheese, sour cream, and lime wedges.

*The quickest way I know to clean a blender: Rinse the jar and fill partway with hot tap water. Add a drop or two of dish detergent and set it back on the base. Turn on the blender for a few seconds and voilà! Clean blender. Rinse it out after, of course.*

> MAKE BABY FOOD: Folks, I'm not sure I'd feed this one to a baby—unless you already know your baby likes spice. What you *can* do is reserve some of the canned beans, corn, tortilla strips, avocado, cheese, and sour cream, and serve those to junior separately.

**MAMA SAID**
**"We really loved this one, surprisingly filling too. Definitely a meal more than a soup. My husband said it reminded him of his favorite tortilla soup from one of our favorite gourmet Mexican restaurants. Delicious." —Amber D., mom of two, Los Angeles, CA**

• • • • • • • • • • • • • • • • • • • • • • • • • • • • • • • • • • •

# QUICK PASTA E FAGIOLI

**Serves 4 to 6**
**Cooking time: 25 minutes**

OK, *maybe* this will take you 30 minutes. But if you use a food processor to chop the vegetables, it will be closer to 20. In deepest, darkest winter, when the mere thought of running to the supermarket in predawn darkness gets me down, I turn to this simple, filling soup. Don't stress if you don't have a Parmesan rind, though it does add a lovely deep flavor. And if your partner can swing a trip to the bakery on the way home, oh boy does fresh Italian bread go well here.

**NOTE:** This makes terrific leftovers, but you'll likely find that it's thickened up considerably. If so, add a little water or broth when reheating.

One 15- to 16-ounce can cannellini beans, drained and rinsed

2 tablespoons olive oil

1 small onion, finely chopped

1 medium carrot, chopped

1 celery rib, chopped

3 garlic cloves, minced

Pinch of red pepper flakes, optional (leave out if serving to infants)

2 tablespoons tomato paste

One 28-ounce can crushed or chopped tomatoes, with juice

4 cups low-sodium chicken or vegetable broth

1 bay leaf

1 teaspoon dried oregano

1 Parmesan rind (approximately 2 inches long), optional

1½ cups small pasta (ditalini, elbows, small shells, broken-up spaghetti—whatever you've got)

Salt and pepper

Good-quality extra-virgin olive oil, grated Parmesan, and crusty bread, for serving

1. Combine roughly half of the cannellini beans in a blender or food processor with 3 tablespoons water. Puree, and set aside.

2. Heat the olive oil in a large Dutch oven or heavy pot over medium heat. When it shimmers, add the onion and cook, stirring occasionally, until translucent, about 3 minutes. Add the carrot and celery and cook just until they begin to soften, 1 to 2 minutes. Add the garlic and red pepper flakes, if using, and cook, stirring, until fragrant, about 30 seconds. Reduce heat to low and add the tomato paste. Cook, stirring, until the paste darkens and seems to melt into the vegetables, 2 to 3 minutes. Add the tomatoes, broth, bay leaf, oregano, and Parmesan rind, if using. Raise the heat to high and bring to a boil. Add the pasta and whole beans and simmer, covered, over low heat until the pasta is barely cooked, 8 to 10 minutes. Stir frequently, especially in the first few minutes, to keep pasta from sticking to the pot.

3. Stir in the reserved pureed beans and simmer, uncovered, until the pasta is fully cooked but not mushy, 1 to 2 minutes more. Season with salt and pepper to taste— if you used low-sodium beans and broth, you may need as much as 1 teaspoon.

4. Remove bay leaf and Parmesan rind before serving. Drizzle each bowl with olive oil, and pass the grated Parmesan and bread.

MAKE BABY FOOD: The texture of this thick soup should be just right to serve as finger food, or if you're not there yet, puree it.

**MAMA SAID**

"I married an Italian, so I have had lots of pasta dishes. I have to say that this is now one of my favorites! So quick and easy, with a flavor that tastes like it cooked all day. My husband and I both had seconds, and my father-in-law asked for the leftovers." —Jane B., mom of one, Pleasanton, CA

"Another success! I did not add the Parmesan rind because I am too cheap to buy the block. I just added some grated Parm in the serving bowls. The pasta cooking time gave me a chance to clean up the kitchen from the prep, which was nice." —Mary T., mom of one, Ankeny, IA

· · · · · · · · · · · · · · · · · · · · · · · · · · · · · · · · · · · · · · · · · · · · ·

# DRIED MUSHROOM AND BARLEY SOUP

**Serves 4 to 6**

**Cooking time: 2½ hours (20 minutes active)**

My mom made this thick, hearty soup at least twice a month all winter long when I was a child, and for me it's true comfort food. She prefers to use dried button mushrooms, which are usually found in the kosher foods section of the grocery store, but it's delicious with just about any variety. If your mushrooms are fairly large, break them up a bit with your hands before adding to the pot. Unless you're already a fan of its uniquely sweet, mellow flavor, rutabaga (sometimes labeled "swede") probably isn't a staple in your kitchen. If you don't have one on hand, just add another carrot, but if you've got time, it's worth seeking out.

1 tablespoon vegetable or olive oil

1 medium onion, finely chopped

1 large carrot, chopped

1 celery rib, chopped (include some leaves, if you have them)

Half of a small rutabaga, peeled and chopped

Salt and pepper

4 cups low-sodium chicken broth

1 cup water

¼ ounce dried mushrooms (roughly ½ cup)

¼ cup pearl barley

Crusty bread, for serving

1. Heat the oil over medium-low heat in a large, heavy pot or Dutch oven. When it shimmers, add the onion, carrot, celery, and rutabaga and cook gently, stirring occasionally, until the vegetables soften, 8 to 10 minutes. Season with salt and pepper to taste.

2. Add the broth, water, mushrooms, and barley, raise the heat to high, and bring to a boil. Reduce the heat to low and simmer, covered, until barley is tender and soup has thickened, about 2 hours. Season with salt and pepper to taste.

3. Serve with bread.

MAKE BABY FOOD: This was one of Harry's favorite soups when he was tiny, either pureed or as is. If the mushrooms seem a little tough for the very youngest eaters, just fish them out before serving.

**MAMA SAID**
"We just ate this soup for dinner and my husband told me I should 'start making it a lot.' If that ain't success, I don't know what is. I drizzled some olive oil on top of each bowl of soup and then cracked some sea salt on top. *Yum.*" —Jesse Z., mom of two, Los Angeles, CA

• • • • • • • • • • • • • • • • • • • • • • • • • • • • • • • • • • • • • • • • • • •

# LENTIL AND BROWN RICE SOUP

**Serves 6 to 8**
**Cooking time: 1 hour (10 minutes active)**

This recipe is adapted from one that ran in a long-ago issue of the late *Gourmet* magazine. Basically, you cut up some ingredients (in the food processor, even!) and throw it in a pot with lentils and brown rice. About an hour later, you've got a richly satisfying dinner. What could be better?

Two things to note: First, lentils, like all dried beans, vary in their cooking time depending on several factors, including age. Yours may take longer to become tender, but it shouldn't take much more than an hour. Hard water can also affect the cooking time—if your water is hard, use bottled water. And second, as it stands, this thickens something fierce. Overnight, leftovers turn virtually solid. Add water to turn it back into soup, plus a little more salt, and it's just as wonderful.

4 cups low-sodium chicken or vegetable
broth

4 cups water

1½ cups brown or green lentils, picked over
and rinsed

1 cup brown rice

One 28-ounce can diced tomatoes, with their
juices

3 carrots, chopped

1 onion, chopped

1 celery rib, chopped

3 garlic cloves, minced

1 teaspoon dried basil

1 teaspoon dried oregano

½ teaspoon dried thyme

2 bay leaves

1 pound of smoked sausage, chopped,
optional

½ cup minced flat-leaf parsley

2 tablespoons cider vinegar, or to taste

Salt and pepper

*To get the most flavor from dried herbs, crumble them in your hands before adding to the pot.*

1. Combine the broth, water, lentils, rice, tomatoes with juice, carrots, onion,
   celery, garlic, and dried herbs in a large, heavy pot or Dutch oven. Bring to a boil
   over medium-high heat, then reduce heat to low and simmer, covered, stirring
   occasionally, until the lentils and rice are tender, 45 to 55 minutes. The soup should
   be quite thick, but if it seems too thick, add a little more water. If you're using the
   sausage, add it and cook just until heated through.

2. Remove from heat and stir in the parsley, vinegar, and salt and pepper to taste.
   Discard bay leaves before serving.

MAKE BABY FOOD: This one's great, pureed or as is.

**MAMA SAID**
**"I had my husband play with our daughter while I was putting the ingredients into the
pot, and then it was basically set it and forget it. I used vegetable broth and didn't have
the parsley, but it was still really good! Bonus: It made a ton. I'm going to freeze some."
—Kristy P., mom of one, Utica, NY**

## SMOKY SPLIT PEA SOUP

**Serves 6 to 8**

**Cooking time: 1½ hours (20 minutes active)**

Here's another toss-together-and-walk-away soup, with a velvety, smoky result. For a vegetarian version, substituting smoked paprika for the turkey bacon provides a nice level of smokiness. Please don't use regular bacon for this—the cooked-off grease will overwhelm the dish.

2 tablespoons olive oil

2 large onions, finely chopped

4 celery ribs with leaves, chopped small

4 large carrots, chopped small

2 medium parsnips, peeled, tough center removed, and chopped small, optional

4 slices turkey bacon, chopped, or 1 teaspoon smoked paprika

3 sprigs fresh marjoram, or 1 tablespoon dried

3 sprigs fresh thyme, or 1 tablespoon dried

3 cups green split peas

4 quarts water

2 bay leaves

Salt and pepper

1.  Heat the oil in a large, heavy pot or Dutch oven over medium heat. When it shimmers, add the onions, celery, carrots, and parsnips, if using. Cook, stirring occasionally, until the vegetables begin to soften, about 8 minutes.

2.  Add the turkey bacon or smoked paprika and herbs, and cook until the bacon is lightly browned, about 2 minutes.

3.  Add the split peas, water, and bay leaves. Raise the heat and bring to a boil. Reduce the heat to medium-low and simmer, partially covered and stirring often, until the vegetables are tender and the peas are falling apart, about 1 hour and 10 minutes.

4.  Season with salt and pepper, and remove the bay leaves before serving.

> MAKE BABY FOOD: Do I need to say it? Split pea soup is perfect for babies. You can fish out the bacon from baby's portion, if you've included it.

**MAMA SAID**
**"This soup has a nice smoky flavor, and you don't have to deal with a ham hock. Big improvement! I love split pea soup and it generally takes a lot more work than this recipe—really great time savings. At the end, I pureed it smooth with an immersion blender."**
**—Jane B., mom of one, Pleasanton, CA**

# QUINOA SALAD WITH CHICKPEAS, DRIED FRUIT, AND ALMONDS

**Serves 6**

**Cooking time: 20 minutes**

Quinoa is a fantastic food for new parents: It acts like a grain, but it's really a protein-packed relative of leafy greens like Swiss chard, and its mild, slightly nutty flavor mixes well with all kinds of seasonings. Best of all, quinoa cooks in a jiff, making it perfect for last-minute meals. This salad is almost entirely pantry-based; if you shopped off my list at the beginning of the chapter, dinner is just 20 minutes away.

1½ cups quinoa, rinsed

One 15- to 16-ounce can chickpeas, rinsed
   and drained

½ cup dried cranberries or cherries

½ cup almond slivers, toasted
   *An easy way to toast nuts: Use the toaster
   oven! 3 minutes at 350°F usually does it, but
   watch carefully so they don't burn.*

½ shallot, minced

Handful of chopped fresh herbs, such as
   parsley, basil, and mint, optional

¼ cup good-quality extra-virgin olive oil

2 tablespoons sherry or red wine vinegar

1 teaspoon honey

½ teaspoon Dijon mustard

Salt and pepper

½ cup shaved Parmesan cheese (use a
   vegetable peeler)

1. Bring a medium pot of salted water to a boil over high heat. Add quinoa and boil until it is translucent but not mushy, about 10 minutes. Drain and spread out on a baking sheet to cool.

2. Combine the quinoa, chickpeas, dried fruit, almonds, shallot, and chopped herbs, if using, in a large serving bowl.

3. Combine the oil, vinegar, honey, mustard, and salt and pepper to taste in a small air-tight container. Cover and shake well. Pour the dressing over the salad and toss, adding more salt and pepper, if necessary.

4. Top with the cheese just before serving.

MAKE BABY FOOD: Babies under a year old can't have honey, due to botulism concerns. If you plan to serve this to an infant, swap maple syrup or agave nectar for the honey. Also, because of their size, chickpeas, dried cranberries or cherries, and toasted almonds can be a choking hazard. Either puree the salad with a little water or broth (skip the nuts if there are food allergies in your immediate family), or reserve some plain quinoa and toss with fork-smashed chickpeas and a bit of the dressing.

**MAMA SAID**
"Wearing my eight-month-old on my back in our Ergo, I prepared everything for this dish in the time it took to boil the water and cook the quinoa. I even had some time to start cleaning up the kitchen!" —Sarah T., mom of one, Calgary, AB

· · · · · · · · · · · · · · · · · · · · · · · · · · · · · · · · · · · · · · · · · ·

# TUNA AND WHITE BEAN SALAD

**Serves 4 to 6**

**Cooking time: 15 minutes**

This is one of the easiest recipes in the book, with one of the biggest payoffs in flavor. Seriously, you'll be sitting down to eat approximately 20 minutes after you decide to make it.

Two 6-ounce cans light tuna in olive oil

Two 15- to 16-ounce cans cannellini beans, drained and rinsed

1 shallot, finely chopped

¼ cup capers, rinsed and drained

¼ cup roughly chopped pitted Kalamata or Gaeta olives

2 celery ribs, chopped

2 teaspoons grated lemon zest (about 1 lemon's worth)

Salt and pepper

Fresh lemon juice

Good-quality extra-virgin olive oil

4 to 6 cups salad greens, such as arugula, lettuce, spinach, or mesclun mix, torn by hand

1.  Drain some of the olive oil from the cans of tuna, then flake the tuna into a large bowl and toss with the beans, shallot, capers, olives, celery, lemon zest, and salt pepper to taste.

2.  Add lemon juice and olive oil to taste, and toss. Serve over the greens.

*Spooned into a baguette, leftovers make a mighty fine lunch.*

MAKE BABY FOOD: Puree with a bit more olive oil for the youngest eaters. Most older babies can handle the texture of everything but the celery, which may be too crunchy to chew—add that at the very end, after you've reserved a portion for baby.

MAMA SAID

"I really appreciated the ease of preparation, tastiness, and healthiness of this dish. It was so quick that I had no problem leaving my daughter to play while I threw it together."
—Karissa J., mom of one, Vancouver, BC

# BAKED FALAFEL

**Serves 2 to 3**

**Cooking time: 35 minutes (15 minutes active)**

This takeout favorite is traditionally made with dried chickpeas that have been soaked and ground. To speed things up, I use canned beans and whir everything together in a food processor. Baking the falafel does away with the mess (and fat) of frying. If you don't have a food processor, mash the chickpeas with a potato masher, and finely chop the garlic and parsley before combining everything.

One 15- to 16-ounce can chickpeas, drained and rinsed

1 small onion or 2 scallions (white and light green parts), roughly chopped

2 garlic cloves, smashed

3 tablespoons roughly chopped flat-leaf parsley

1 teaspoon ground coriander

1 teaspoon ground cumin

¼ teaspoon cayenne

2 tablespoons all-purpose flour

1 teaspoon baking powder

Juice of 1 lemon, divided (3 tablespoons)

3 tablespoons olive oil, divided

Salt and pepper

A mixture of salad vegetables, such as romaine, cucumber, and grape tomatoes

Whole-wheat pitas

Store-bought hummus (or use the quick homemade version on page 344), tzatziki, tahini, etc.

**Preheat oven to 450°F, and set racks in upper and lower thirds of oven. Grease or line 2 baking sheets.**

1.  Combine the chickpeas, onion, garlic, parsley, spices, flour, baking powder, half of the lemon juice, 1 tablespoon olive oil, and salt and pepper to taste in a food processor. Pulse until well combined but mixture is still relatively coarse. You do *not* want a puree.

2.  Using your hands or a small cookie scoop, shape the mixture into about 24 balls (roughly 1½ inches in diameter) and arrange on the prepared baking sheets. Flatten each slightly, and brush the tops with 1 tablespoon of the remaining olive oil.

3.  Bake for 10 to 12 minutes, then turn patties (rotating the trays when you take them out) and bake for another 10 to 12 minutes. You may find it easiest to turn them using two forks.

4. Toss the salad vegetables with the remaining lemon juice and olive oil and salt and pepper to taste. Serve with hummus or other condiments, as sandwiches or as a platter.

> MAKE BABY FOOD: If your baby likes well-seasoned food, there's nothing in the falafel he can't eat. If you're concerned about the crunchy outside, pull a few out of the oven before they get too well done. Hummus and pita are both fine for young'ns.

**MAMA SAID**

"I took the lazy way out and whizzed the onion, garlic, and parsley together in the food processor before adding the chickpeas, and it worked out fine. The lemony salad on top of the creamy hummus with the crispy falafel was a very satisfying combo. My husband really enjoyed it, despite normally being suspicious of things that aren't Italian or Mexican or a steak." —Alana D., mom of one, Providence, RI

"I tried freezing half the mixture in little flattened balls. It worked well (with slightly longer cooking times, of course), and being able to make a big batch to freeze is a HUGE bonus to me. I did not have high hopes for a baked falafel, but they were great, and far better than the home-fried ones I've tried. This is going to be my new lunch standard!" —Darcy G., mom of two, Pleasant Prairie, WI

· · · · · · · · · · · · · · · · · · · · · · · · · · · · · · · · · · · · · · · · · · ·

# MUJADARA

**Serves 4 to 6**

**Cooking time: 1 to 1½ hours (45 minutes active)**

Lentils, rice, olive oil, and onions—this Middle Eastern standard is the ultimate pantry recipe. It's also the classic example of a dish that's greater than the sum of its parts. There are literally dozens of recipes for mujadara out there—each country, possibly even each family, seems to have its own version. The one I like best is adapted from Claudia Roden's *Book of Jewish Food.* The crispy onion topping is the best part, so go ahead and make a lot.

**NOTE:** Lentils, like all dried beans, vary in their cooking time depending on several factors, including age. Yours may take longer to become tender, but they shouldn't take much more than an hour. Hard water can also affect the cooking time—if your water is hard, use bottled water.

⅓ cup olive oil

4 or 5 large onions, halved and thinly sliced (use the slicing blade on your food processor, or a mandoline if you have one)

Salt and pepper

1½ cups brown or green lentils, sorted and rinsed

1¼ cups long-grain white rice

Plain yogurt or sour cream, optional, for serving

1. Heat the olive oil in a very large nonstick skillet over low heat (if you only have smaller skillets, divide the oil and onions between two). When the oil shimmers, add the onions and cook, stirring frequently, until golden, 15 to 20 minutes. Season with salt and pepper to taste.

2. Meanwhile, bring 4½ cups water to a boil in a large saucepan or small stockpot and add the lentils. Simmer, uncovered, for 20 minutes, then add the rice and half the cooked onions. Season with salt and pepper to taste. Simmer, covered, over very low heat until the lentils and rice are tender, about 20 minutes more. You may need to add more water toward the end; check after 15 minutes. Remove from the heat and let rest, covered, for 5 minutes.

3. While the rice and lentils are cooking, cook the onions remaining in the skillet over low heat, stirring often, until dark brown and nearly crisp, 15 to 20 minutes.

4. Serve hot or at room temperature, with browned onions sprinkled on top. Add a dollop of the yogurt or sour cream if desired.

> MAKE BABY FOOD: Puree the entire thing with an additional splash of water. For finger food, skip the browned onion topping, which may be challenging to young eaters.

**MAMA SAID**

"It's nice to have a dinner in the pantry that doesn't involve powdered cheese. We have mixed the leftover mujadara with spinach and Parm and a beaten egg, which we fried up like a pancake." —Beth P., mom of one, Los Angeles, CA

"This dish is the paragon of efficiency. Very little prep time (just onion slicing) and almost no downtime while cooking. I had a skillet going for the onions and a pot for the lentils, and the timing was exquisite. And there's nothing like having two pots side-by-side on the stovetop to feel like you are cooking again after too many days in a row of scrambled eggs." —Jenn C., mom of one, Boston, MA

· · · · · · · · · · · · · · · · · · · · · · · · · · · · · · · · · · · · · · ·

# CHEATER'S CHANA MASALA

**Serves 4**

**Cooking time: 25 minutes (15 minutes active)**

Traditional chana masala—a spiced chickpea stew you'll find on the menu of almost any Indian restaurant—is a complicated affair, with an ingredient list as long as your arm. We're not going there. Remember my mantra: New parents don't have time for authenticity! Instead, I've simplified things to make this a quick and easy dish based almost exclusively on pantry items. It still tastes warm and comforting, but you'll have dinner on the table in no time.

2 tablespoons vegetable oil

1 medium onion, finely chopped

One 1-inch piece of fresh ginger, peeled and
   grated, or ½ teaspoon ground ginger

2 garlic cloves, minced

2 teaspoons ground coriander

2 teaspoons ground cumin

⅛ teaspoon cayenne

Two 15- to 16-ounce cans chickpeas,
   rinsed and drained

¾ cup water

One 14.5-ounce can diced tomatoes, drained

Salt

2 tablespoons chopped cilantro

1 teaspoon garam masala

Juice of ½ lemon (about 1½ tablespoons)

Cooked brown rice, plain yogurt, and
   prepared chutney, optional, for serving

1.  Heat the oil in a large saucepan over medium-low heat. When it shimmers, add the onion, fresh ginger, if using, and garlic and cook, stirring occasionally, until the onion is translucent but not browned, about 5 minutes.

2.  Add the coriander, cumin, cayenne, and ground ginger (if not using fresh) and cook for 1 minute.

3.  Add the chickpeas, water, diced tomatoes, and salt to taste and raise heat to medium. Simmer uncovered (if it spatters too much, cover it partially) until the sauce has thickened, 5 to 10 minutes.

4.  Remove from heat, then stir in the chopped cilantro, garam masala, lemon juice, and salt to taste.

5.  Serve over brown rice and top with a spoonful of yogurt and chutney, if desired.

MAKE BABY FOOD: Leave out the cayenne if you're nervous about spicy foods, and if you're wary of the acidity in citrus add the lemon juice after reserving baby's portion. This'll puree nicely (make sure to include some of the liquid), or you can serve it as finger food—just smash the chickpeas with a fork, to prevent a choking hazard.

**MAMA SAID**

"I went into this recipe both excited and skeptical, because chana masala is one of my absolute favorite dishes. Since we have yet to find a kid-friendly Indian restaurant in our neighborhood, I rarely get my fix. I really didn't think there was any way I could approximate that yummy spiciness at home, let alone from pantry ingredients without advance planning and a special trip to the store. But the proof was totally in the pudding—a fabulous success that I will make again and again." —Jenn C., mom of one, Boston, MA

"Everyone liked this—even my picky three-year-old ate three chickpeas!—and the adults (me, my husband, mother-in-law) all had seconds. I used a few shakes of cayenne pepper, and that seemed like enough to make it interesting for the adults and not too spicy for the kids." —Jennifer S., mom of three, San Diego, CA

# VEGETARIAN FRIJOLES NEGROS

**Serves 6 as a main course, 10 to 12 as a side**
**Cooking time: 1½ hours (15 minutes active)**

If you think cooking dried beans means planning a day ahead, think again. These babies go from bag to bowl in 90 minutes flat, and most of that time, you don't even have to be in the kitchen.

Some shopping notes: Sofrito is a Latin-American cooking base, most often comprised of pureed tomatoes, onion, garlic, cilantro, and bell peppers. Look for prepared sofrito in the Latin-American section of your supermarket (Goya is a widely available brand). If you can't find it, substitute a straightforward salsa, but if the salsa is hot, you may want to use less chipotle.

**NOTE:** Dried beans vary in their cooking time depending on several factors, including age. Yours may take longer than expected to become tender, but not much more than 90 minutes. Hard water can also affect the cooking time—if your water is hard, use bottled water.

Two or three cups of these beans would be terrific in the Southwestern Polenta Lasagna on page 38, or you can mash them to make refried beans. They also freeze well.

One 1-pound package dried black beans,
   sorted and rinsed
   *When sorting black beans, I find it easier*
   *to spot small pebbles against a white*
   *background—line a baking sheet with*
   *paper towels.*

1 medium onion, peeled and quartered
3 garlic cloves, peeled and smashed
1 chipotle in adobo, seeded and minced

1 teaspoon ground cumin
1 bay leaf
½ cup prepared sofrito
Salt and pepper
Cooked brown or white rice (Success boil-in
   bags come in handy here)
Chopped avocado, sour cream, shredded
   Cheddar or Monterey Jack cheese, lime
   wedges, cilantro, and hot sauce, for serving

**Preheat oven to 250°F.**

1. Combine the beans, onion, garlic, chipotle, cumin, bay leaf, and sofrito in a Dutch oven with a tight-fitting lid. Add salt and pepper to taste and water to cover by 1 inch. Bring to a boil, uncovered, over high heat.

2. Cover pot, and transfer to the oven. Cook until beans are tender, about 1 hour and 15 minutes (check around the 45-minute mark and add more water if necessary). If beans are not tender by that time, continue to cook for another 15 minutes.

2. Season with salt and pepper. Before serving, remove large pieces of onion, garlic cloves, and bay leaf.

3. Serve over rice with suggested toppings.

*If you're making this ahead of time and the beans are just a bit too firm at the end of the suggested cooking time, turn off the oven and let them sit, covered, for 1 to 2 hours. The residual heat will finish cooking them.*

> MAKE BABY FOOD: If your baby's eaten food with a bit of spice in it and been OK, these minimally spicy black beans are wonderful finger food—and they puree well too.

**MAMA SAID**
"I was pleasantly surprised to discover that there was very little chopping involved. Quartering an onion and peeling some garlic is so much easier than chopping an entire onion. I actually ended up preparing the beans in two- to three-minute intervals while entertaining my three-month-old daughter, so that made me really like this recipe. I could swing by the kitchen and throw a few things in the pot while in the midst of doing other things and actually have a meal as a result!" —Melissa K., mom of one, Seattle, WA

• • • • • • • • • • • • • • • • • • • • • • • • • • • • • • • • • • • • •

# SOUTHWESTERN POLENTA LASAGNA

**Serves 4**

**Cooking time: 40 to 50 minutes (15 minutes active)**

Great news for the knife skills–challenged: There is almost no chopping involved here. Most of the work is simply layering. Slightly-less-great news: Sliced polenta gets mighty slippery. Take care when serving, or the layers will slide apart—this won't affect the taste, but your plate might not win any beauty contests.

**NOTE:** This is a terrific way to use about 1½ cups of leftover Vegetarian Frijoles Negros (page 36). If you do, omit the canned black beans entirely, and swap a 14.5-ounce can of diced tomatoes for the tomatoes with green chiles or salsa.

One 15- to 16-ounce can black beans, drained and rinsed

One 10-ounce can diced tomatoes and green chiles (such as Ro-Tel), or 1 generous cup of your favorite salsa, drained
*Once you've drained and rinsed the black beans, just pour this on top and drain again.*

1 cup frozen corn kernels, not thawed

1 whole roasted red pepper from a jar, chopped, optional
*I like piquillo peppers for this, but bell peppers are fine too.*

Handful of cilantro leaves, chopped, optional

1½ cups shredded Cheddar, Monterey Jack cheese, or a combination, divided

One 1-pound roll ready-made polenta

Sour cream, for serving

**Preheat oven to 400°F. Grease an 8-inch square baking dish.**

1. Combine the black beans, tomatoes and chiles, corn, roasted pepper, cilantro, and 1 cup of the shredded cheese in a large bowl.

2. Cut the polenta log lengthwise into ¼-inch slices. Arrange half the slices in the prepared baking dish, covering the bottom of the dish (if necessary, trim slices to fit).

3. Spoon about two-thirds of the tomato-bean mixture over the polenta. Arrange the remaining polenta slices on top. Press down gently, and cover with the remaining tomato-bean mixture, then the remaining cheese.

4. Bake, uncovered, until the cheese is bubbly and beginning to brown, 25 to 30 minutes. Cool for 10 minutes before serving, and top each serving with sour cream.

MAKE BABY FOOD: If you're concerned about the chiles, set aside a crosswise slice of polenta, as well as some of the beans, corn, and cheese before cooking. Each of these items works as finger food—just cut the polenta into bite-sized pieces. Otherwise, serve the finished dish, either in small pieces or pureed with a splash of water or broth.

**MAMA SAID**

"The polenta lasagna was fantastic! In short: ridiculously good and absurdly easy to make. I prepped and assembled it while the girls napped in the morning (and still had plenty of time to relax and unwind before they woke up). It was so nice to go through the rest of the day knowing that all I'd have to do dinner-wise was pop the pan in the oven." —Tracy A., mom of twins, Portland, OR

# ANGEL HAIR PASTA WITH GARLIC AND LEMON-PARMESAN BREADCRUMBS

**Serves 4**

**Cooking time: 25 minutes**

This easy, satisfying, and super-fast dish was born out of exhaustion. One night, after flirting with the idea of serving jarred sauce on pasta yet again, I decided it would be just as easy to make a quick sauce of garlic and oil. Stephen suggested adding some toasted breadcrumbs for contrast, and I was off and running. A little lemon, some Parmesan, fresh parsley, and whaddya know? It's a fantastic little dinner! The brightness of the lemon is what makes this more than just a bowl of garlicky pasta (which I admit is, in itself, quite a satisfying meal).

While you're waiting for the water to boil, mince the garlic, zest the lemon, and chop the parsley; you'll be done cooking by the time the pasta timer goes off.

⅓ cup olive oil, divided

⅔ cup dried breadcrumbs

1 tablespoon lemon zest (from about 1 lemon)

3 tablespoons chopped flat-leaf parsley, divided

Salt and pepper

¼ cup grated Parmesan cheese, plus more for serving

One 12- to 14.5-ounce box whole-wheat or whole-grain angel hair pasta (I use Barilla Plus)

3 large garlic cloves, minced

Juice of 1 lemon (about 3 tablespoons)

1.  Bring a large pot of salted water to a boil (covered to speed things up).

2.  Heat about half the olive oil in a large nonstick skillet over medium heat. When it shimmers, add the breadcrumbs and stir to combine. Cook, stirring occasionally, until the breadcrumbs are lightly toasted, 3 to 4 minutes.

3.  Add the lemon zest, half the parsley, and salt and pepper to taste and cook 1 minute more, taking care so the crumbs don't get too dark. Sprinkle the Parmesan over the mixture, remove from heat, and stir. (The cheese will melt a bit and form some clumps. This is perfectly fine and ridiculously tasty. Try not to eat them all while you do the next steps.) Transfer the breadcrumbs to a bowl and wipe out the pan.

4. Add the pasta to boiling water.

5. Meanwhile, heat the remaining oil in the skillet over medium heat. When it shimmers, add the garlic. Cook, stirring, until barely golden, about 1 minute, then turn off heat.

6. Scoop out about 1 cup of the pasta cooking water and set aside. When pasta is ready, drain and stir it plus the lemon juice into the skillet with the garlic, and turn the heat to medium-low. If pasta seems dry, add the reserved cooking water as needed. The sauce will thicken slightly but remain quite light.

7. Divide pasta between big bowls. Sprinkle some of the breadcrumb mixture and some of the reserved parsley over each bowl, and serve with the additional grated Parmesan cheese.

> MAKE BABY FOOD: Babies love pasta—it's so much fun for them to play with. If you're concerned that the lemon makes this too acidic for your infant, reserve some pasta before adding the sauce. To serve as finger food, cut up the long strands and toss with some olive oil, Parmesan, and maybe some defrosted frozen peas, and you're golden. If you're still on purees, whir the pasta with a bit of olive oil and Parm.

**MAMA SAID**
*"Yum!* It was great! I spent probably 20 minutes prepping all of the ingredients first—I wasn't sure when my husband would be done working or when the baby would wake up from his nap, so I wanted to have everything ready to throw together quickly when it was time. Because of this prep, I had dinner on the table 15 minutes after turning the water on to boil. That was a pleasant surprise!" —Mary T., mom of one, Ankeny, IA

## SPAGHETTI ALLA PUTTANESCA

**Serves 4**

**Cooking time: 30 minutes (15 minutes active)**

I'll let you in on a secret: My husband knows his way around a kitchen. (Maybe your partner does, too, but if not please don't hate me for this; it's pure dumb luck that I snapped Stephen up before you had the chance to meet him.) This zesty pasta is one of his signature dishes. I hereby award him bonus points for producing such complex flavor with so little effort.

One 12- to 14.5-ounce box whole-wheat or whole-grain spaghetti

2 tablespoons olive oil

2 garlic cloves, minced

½ teaspoon red pepper flakes, or to taste

1 scant tablespoon anchovy paste

One 28-ounce can diced tomatoes, drained

1 tablespoon tomato paste

¾ cup pitted Gaeta or Kalamata olives, roughly chopped

3 tablespoons capers, rinsed and drained

1. Bring a large pot of salted water to a boil (covered to speed thing up), and cook the spaghetti according to package directions.

2. While the spaghetti cooks, heat the olive oil in a large nonstick skillet over medium heat. When it shimmers, add the garlic and red pepper flakes and cook until the garlic softens, about 1 minute; don't let it brown.

3. Add the anchovy paste and cook until it melts into the garlic, about 2 minutes.

4. Add the tomatoes and tomato paste. Raise heat to medium-high and bring to a rapid boil. Cook until the sauce thickens and deepens in color, about 5 minutes.

5. Stir in the olives and capers and remove from heat.

6. Drain the pasta and toss with the sauce.

MAKE BABY FOOD: Plain spaghetti (cut up for safety) is fine for babies, and oh boy, did Harry love olives and capers from an early age. I'd skip the spicy tomato sauce, though—if a red pepper flake hits baby's tongue, he probably won't be terribly happy. Instead, serve the pasta, olives, and capers as finger foods.

**MAMA SAID**

"We've used this recipe again and again AND again. It is one of the few recipes I actually follow exactly, partly because it is so easy. This is a favorite *'oh no, I haven't gone shopping, have no time, don't want to cook, but too broke to eat out meal'* for us, which means it gets a turn on the dining room table at least every other week." —Rachel M., mom of one, Tucson, AZ

• • • • • • • • • • • • • • • • • • • • • • • • • • • • • • • • • • • • • • • • • • •

# PASTA WITH PORCINI MUSHROOMS

**Serves 4 to 6**

**Cooking time: 1 hour (20 minutes active)**

Don't let the one-hour cooking time prevent you from trying this cozy, richly flavored vegetarian dish. Most of that hour is spent softening up the dried mushrooms, which requires nothing more than pouring some boiling water over them and walking away. This sauce is also wonderful with filled pasta like tortellini.

1½ ounces dried porcini mushrooms

1½ cups boiling water

One 12- to 14.5-ounce box whole-wheat or
   whole-grain spaghetti

2 tablespoons olive oil

1 large shallot, minced, or half a large onion,
   finely chopped

⅓ cup dry sherry

2 teaspoons fresh thyme leaves, or
   1 teaspoon dried thyme

Salt and pepper

1 tablespoon tomato paste

Grated Parmesan cheese, for serving

1. Place the dried mushrooms in a measuring cup (or bowl with a pouring spout) and add boiling water. Set aside for at least 30 minutes and up to 1 hour.

2. Bring a large pot of salted water to a boil (covered to speed things up).

3. Remove the reconstituted mushrooms from the water and finely chop. Reserve soaking water.

4. When the water comes to a boil, add the pasta and set a timer for 2 minutes less than the suggested cooking time.

5. While the pasta cooks, heat the oil in a large nonstick skillet (it should be big enough to hold the pasta later) over medium heat. When it shimmers, add the shallot and cook, stirring occasionally, until softened, about 3 minutes.

6. Add the chopped mushrooms, sherry, thyme, and salt and pepper to taste, and increase heat to medium-high. Cook until most of the liquid has evaporated, then add about half of the reserved soaking water. Boil for 1 to 2 minutes, then stir in the tomato paste.

7. By now the pasta timer should be ready to beep. Scoop out about 1 cup of pasta cooking water and set aside. Drain the pasta and add it to the skillet with almost all of the remaining reserved mushroom-soaking water (be careful not to pour in any grit that may have accumulated at the bottom of the measuring cup). Cook, stirring frequently, until the pasta is al dente and coated in a thin sauce, adding some of the reserved pasta water if needed.

8. Serve with the grated Parmesan cheese.

MAKE BABY FOOD: If you're at all worried about the alcohol, much of which will have cooked off, reserve some plain pasta and toss with olive oil or butter. But if you're comfortable with it (as I was), the texture of the sauce is perfect for babies. Serve pureed (with a splash of water or oil, if needed) or as finger food.

**MAMA SAID**
"This is a great dish for parents of young children, because it's quick to prepare, but is a gourmet treat that made me feel like an adult! My husband has been raving about the combination of the sauce and the Parmesan cheese. My not-quite-one-year-old also really liked it, and the leftovers have provided a quick and easy snack to give her whenever she needs one." —Heather M., mom of one, Los Gatos, CA

# CHAPTER 2
# NAP-FRIENDLY COOKING

Experts tell us to sleep when the baby sleeps. Most moms learn pretty quickly that that's a load of hooey—there's too much else to do. When Harry was a baby, I only pulled off a concurrent nap when my exhausted body made the decision for me. As long as my brain had enough energy to race through the endless list of Things to Be Accomplished, sleep was an unattainable fantasy. I was vertical, and itching to get things done.

But once I gave up on catching forty winks and decided to aim for half that, Nap-Friendly Cooking was born.

The basic idea here is to take a recipe that has multiple steps, perhaps something you think is too complicated to accomplish in the hour before dinner time, and divide up the steps so you're only doing one part of the recipe during each nap. This frees you up to do something else—like, say, *catch twenty winks*—while still getting a rewarding dinner on the table. Trust me, it's possible to get a delicious meal such as my Roasted Vegetable Lasagna prepared over the course of a few naps.

It's pretty simple and works something like this: During Junior's morning nap, you chop and roast the zucchini, eggplant, and other vegetables. (Skip the salting and rinsing of eggplant; new moms don't have time for such luxuries!)

During the day's second nap, you assemble the lasagna, using top-quality jarred pasta sauce, shredded cheese, and no-boil lasagna noodles, then refrigerate.

Third nap: Pop it in the oven. (Don't worry if your baby's already down to two naps a day—these recipes are flexible.)

It's amazing how little steps spread throughout the day can yield a comforting, nutritious, and plate-licking meal. With leftovers!

Right about now you might be saying something like, "This is all well and good, but my baby won't nap unless I'm holding him." That means your baby is still practically a larva. This is where babywearing comes in handy—pop Junior into a sling and go about your business. (You'll hear more about babywearing in Chapter 6, "One-Handed Meals.") And remember: With a newborn things change so fast that in practical terms, you've got an entirely different baby every few weeks. By the time Harry was two months old, he was snoozing regularly without being held—in his swing, his vibrating rocker, his stroller, and sometimes even in his crib.

### TRICKS FOR HANDS-FREE BABY NAPS

Having trouble getting baby to sleep anywhere but on top of you? Give some of these a shot— I guarantee, you'll eventually find a way to move her off your body.

- **A swing or vibrating rocker:** One reason your baby loves to sleep attached to you is that you're constantly moving (much as you might wish you weren't). She's used to being jostled quite a bit in utero, so movement is comforting to her. Find a mechanized way to keep her in motion, and she should snooze happily.

- **Swaddling:** Do you wrap her up like a burrito each night? Try it during the day too—it took me a good six weeks to realize that swaddling might be the key to upgrading Harry's naps. Sure enough, when he was snuggled inside his Miracle Blanket (which, yes, was miraculously effective), he'd fall asleep faster and stay asleep longer.

- **Room-darkening shades:** Harry's naps improved immeasurably when we did everything we could to recreate nighttime during the day. Pulling down those shades and turning on the white noise machine helped convince him it was time to nod off.

- **Go for a walk:** Bundle your baby into the stroller, with the seat fully reclined, and hit the street. I know, I know, you're exhausted. You don't want to go for a walk. But keep moving for about ten minutes after baby dozes, and you should be able to sneak her back inside and cook or put your feet up. No need to attempt a transfer from stroller to crib, either—she's just fine where she is, as long as she's nearly horizontal.

- - - - - - - - - - - - - - - - - - - - - - - - - - - - - - - - - - - - - - - - - - - - - - - -

Of course, we don't all have infants in our lives. Harry's now a very active and sometimes, ahem, *not-so-charming* preschooler, and since I work from home, I still use the Nap-Friendly Cooking technique several times a week. I'll chop the ingredients for Vegetable Couscous while I'm getting my lunch ready, or whisk together the marinade for Lime-Oregano Fajitas before I sit down to work. Really, it's about time management: We've got so little of it, and grabbing a few minutes here and there is the best we can hope for some days.

**MAMA SAID**
"I totally, totally loved this method. I would otherwise certainly have read a recipe, seen that there was about 40 minutes of work, plus 30 minutes of cooking, and determined that it would have to be done on a weekend. This really opens up possibilities for cooking while watching the kids." —Rebecca N., mother of two, San Francisco, CA

## A FEW WORDS ABOUT FOOD SAFETY

In order to ensure that my Nap-Friendly Cooking technique follows all current food safety guidelines, I spoke to an expert: Catherine Strohbehn, PhD, RD, CP-FS, and HRIM Extension Specialist at Iowa State University. (I'll translate that alphabet soup: RD = Registered Dietitian; CP-FS = Certified Professional-Food Safety; HRIM = Hotel, Restaurant, and Institution Management.)

Here's Dr. Strohbehn's advice:

- In general, cover and refrigerate semi-prepared foods that will wait more than two hours between stages. There are two exceptions:

  - Since bacteria need moisture to thrive, vegetables with dry surfaces (like carrots, sweet potatoes, and winter squash) are considered safe at room temperature.

  - And once cooked, just about any vegetable should be fine at room temperature for a couple of hours, as long as it hasn't touched protein—especially if you'll be cooking it again in later stages, when heat above 165°F will kill off much of the bacteria.

- The temperature "danger zone" for cooked foods is between 40° and 135°F—foods should stay in this range for no more than two hours.

- *Any* protein that will be at room temperature for more than two hours must be refrigerated. This includes pan drippings.

- For this reason, be extremely careful about cross-contamination. Use a separate cutting board and knife for animal proteins. If any vegetables or other ingredients come in contact with the meat, the board, the knife, or even drippings, those ingredients must be refrigerated too. After browning meats, don't return them to the original packaging—use a clean container.

- Is all this making you a wee bit nervous? Don't be! Each recipe in this chapter takes these guidelines into account. Follow them as written and you'll be just fine.

## CRIB NOTES

- Nap-Friendly Cooking = breaking down a complicated recipe into separate, small steps, each to be dispatched relatively quickly during progressive naps.

- The recipes in this chapter are among the most ambitious in the entire book— if, pre-baby, you considered cooking to be a pleasure and now yearn to attack a recipe with gusto, this is the chapter for you.

- Generally, you'll be measuring spices, prepping, and sometimes pre-cooking the vegetables during Stage 1; browning any meat and/or sautéing vegetables during Stage 2; and doing the final work during Stage 3. See the sidebar on page 75 for tips on breaking down your own recipes.

- Often, Stage 3 takes the longest (because it's when most of the actual cooking happens) but requires the least effort.

- If your baby is on a two-nap schedule, you can accomplish Stages 1 and 2 during the morning nap—I've noted the exceptions, for which you'd combine Stages 2 and 3, in the recipes. Use your noodle here: If a step (like refrigeration) seems unnecessary when you're combining stages, it probably is. Which means that combined cooking times will be slightly shorter.

- I've said it before, and I'll say it again: for foggy-brained, sleep-deprived new parents, having a well-organized mise-en-place (French for "everything in place") is essential. Assemble and measure out your ingredients before you ever go near the stove. Arrange them in order of use on your countertop. Sounds like too much work? Once you accidentally add a tablespoon of salt when the recipe called for a teaspoon, you'll come around.

• • • • • • • • • • • • • • • • • • • • • • • • • • • • • • • • • • • • • •

# (RELATIVELY) LOW-FAT CHICKEN POT PIE

**Serves 6**

Many chicken pot pie recipes call for half-and-half or cream to achieve a velvety sauce. I grew up in a kosher household, so mixing meat and dairy wasn't possible. I confess: Bacon enticed me to abandon kashrut long ago (sorry Mom), but I'm still uneasy about pairing creamy foods with meat. Plus, thanks to cholesterol issues in our family, the fridge is stocked with low-fat dairy products. Cooking the potatoes in broth, and then combining the potato starch–thickened broth with a roux, provides the consistency we crave without adding fat- and cholesterol-filled dairy.

1 large potato, peeled and chopped into ½-inch pieces

4 cups low-sodium chicken broth

1 bay leaf

3 sprigs fresh thyme or 2 teaspoons dried thyme

2 large or 3 small carrots, chopped into ½-inch pieces (or use frozen, see below)

1 medium onion, chopped

2 celery ribs, chopped

3 tablespoons olive oil

3 tablespoons all-purpose flour, plus more for rolling out dough

Frozen peas *or* peas and carrots, about 1 cup, not thawed

2 cups cooked chicken, chopped
*If you don't have any cooked chicken, poach some boneless, skinless pieces in the broth you'll be using for the potatoes and carrots. Five to six minutes should do it—it will finish cooking in the oven with the pie.*

1 unbaked pie crust, either store-bought or homemade (not pie shells)

1 egg, beaten

## STAGE 1 (25 minutes)

1. Peel and chop the potato and combine it with the broth, bay leaf, and thyme in a large saucepan. Bring to a boil, then lower the heat and simmer until potato is barely cooked, 10 to 15 minutes.

2. While potato simmers, prepare all the remaining vegetables. Combine onion and celery in a bowl and refrigerate, covered; if you're using fresh carrots, set them aside.

3. Using a slotted spoon, transfer potatoes to a small bowl (don't worry if some of the thyme comes out too).

4. Add the fresh carrots, if using, to the broth and simmer until barely cooked, about 8 minutes. Using a slotted spoon, transfer carrots to the bowl with the potatoes. Cover, and refrigerate.

5. Cool broth slightly, transfer to a measuring cup or bowl with a pouring spout, discard bay leaf, cover, and refrigerate.

## STAGE 2 (15 minutes)

1. Grease a 9 x 13-inch baking dish and set aside.

2. Heat the olive oil in a very large skillet over medium heat. When it shimmers, add the onion and celery and cook until softened but not browned, 5 to 6 minutes. Sprinkle the flour over the vegetables and cook, stirring, until the flour turns golden, 2 to 3 minutes.

3. Stir the reserved broth to incorporate the potato starch, then add it to the skillet and simmer until thickened, another minute or 2.

4. Add the reserved potato and carrots, frozen vegetables, and cooked chicken, and cook just until heated through, 2 to 3 minutes.

5. Pour mixture into the prepared baking dish. Cool slightly, cover, and refrigerate.

## STAGE 3 (1½ hours, 10 minutes active)

1. About 20 minutes before you're ready to cook, preheat oven to 425°F.

2. Remove pie crust and prepared baking dish from the refrigerator.

3. Roll out dough on a lightly floured work surface until it's an inch wider on all sides than your baking dish, and drape it over the dish. Tuck edges under, and score the top with a sharp knife so steam can escape. Brush dough with the beaten egg.

4. Bake until the crust begins to brown, about 20 minutes, then lower heat to 350°F and bake until filling is bubbling and crust is golden brown, another 25 to 30 minutes. Let rest 5 to 10 minutes before serving.

MAKE BABY FOOD: If you're on purees, give the entire thing a whir; for older babies serve as finger food, with the crust cut up.

**MAMA SAID**

"I always enjoy doing pot pies in individual bowls or ramekins, especially when there are kids involved who might be more prone to eat something if it looks cute and enticing. Sometimes I prep six bowls and then only cook three, saving the rest for dinner the next night."
—Jesse Z., mom of two, Woodland Hills, CA

• • • • • • • • • • • • • • • • • • • • • • • • • • • • • • • • • • • • • • • • • •

# PROVENÇAL BRAISED CHICKEN

**Serves 4**

Sophisticated, flavorful, and guaranteed to impress, this is a company's-coming dish. Nobody will guess how easy it really is—just sit back and let them think you've got this new-parent gig *down.* If you don't have herbes de Provence, a simple, relatively authentic substitute is equal amounts of dried thyme, rosemary, and marjoram.

1 medium onion, chopped

1 carrot, chopped

2 garlic cloves, minced

8 ounces cremini or white button
   mushrooms, sliced

15 to 20 black olives (like Kalamata), pitted
   and roughly chopped

3 tablespoons olive oil, divided

2 to 3 tablespoons all-purpose flour

Salt and pepper

4 bone-in chicken breast halves with skin
   (about 8 ounces each)

½ cup dry vermouth

¾ cup low-sodium chicken broth

2 cups tomato puree, or ⅔ cup tomato paste
   mixed with 1⅓ cups water

1 teaspoon herbes de Provence

Cooked pasta or rice, for serving

## STAGE 1 (15 minutes)

1.  Chop the onion and carrot, mince the garlic, slice the mushrooms, and chop the olives.

2.  Combine onion, carrot, and garlic in one bowl. Put mushrooms and olives in separate bowls.

3.  Cover all bowls and refrigerate.

## STAGE 2 (25 minutes; if doing in two sessions combine with Stage 3)

1. Combine the flour with about ½ teaspoon of salt and ⅛ teaspoon of pepper in a resealable bag. Add the chicken and toss to coat. Remove the chicken from the bag and pat to remove excess flour.

2. Heat 2 tablespoons oil in a large, heavy nonstick skillet (one you can cover) over medium-high heat. When it shimmers, arrange chicken, skin side down, and cook until browned, about 5 minutes. Turn chicken over and cook 3 more minutes. Transfer to a bowl.

3. Add the remaining tablespoon of oil to the skillet. When it shimmers, add the mushrooms and cook until just beginning to brown, about 10 minutes. Add the onion, garlic, and carrots and cook 2 minutes.

4. Remove skillet from the heat and cool 10 to 15 minutes, then cover and refrigerate. Cover chicken and refrigerate.

## STAGE 3 (35 minutes)

1. Remove chicken from refrigerator to take off some of the chill.

2. Return skillet with cooked vegetables to stove and cook over low heat.

3. Add vermouth, broth, and tomato puree, raise heat to medium-high, and boil until sauce has thickened slightly, about 10 minutes.

4. Arrange chicken, skin side up, in the sauce and sprinkle with herbes de Provence. Reduce heat to medium-low, and simmer, covered, until chicken is cooked through and tender, 15 to 20 minutes.

5. Stir in the olives and cook until heated through, about 30 seconds.

6. Serve chicken and sauce with pasta or rice.

*A note on leftovers: I remove the chicken from the bones and roughly chop it, add it to the sauce, and combine it with leftover pasta or rice. Tomorrow's lunch—or dinner—will only need a zap in the microwave.*

MAKE BABY FOOD: Thanks to the vermouth, there is a bit of alcohol in here. Most, but not all, will cook off—the amount that remains is minuscule enough that I didn't worry about feeding this to Harry, but that's your call. Other than that, you're good to go. Puree it with some of the sauce, or serve cut-up bits as finger food.

**MAMA SAID**

"I tasted the sauce midway through and thought 'wow, I *made* this?' I think the olives really made the recipe. Naps ended up being super-wonky the day I prepared this, but even so, it went together fairly easily." —Heather B., mom of two, Westmont, IL

· · · · · · · · · · · · · · · · · · · · · · · · · · · · · · · · · · · ·

# ARROZ CON POLLO

**Serves 4**

Arroz con pollo means, simply, "chicken with rice." It's a traditional dish all over Latin America and much of the Caribbean. This version is—surprise—not particularly authentic. (Heck, it uses brown rice, definitely not what you'll find in a recipe handed down by *abuelita*.) But this book isn't about authenticity, is it? We're going for healthy, delicious, and doable, and this recipe meets both those requirements and then some.

**NOTE:** This recipe calls for smoked paprika, which I realize you may not have on hand. If that's the case, go ahead and use regular sweet paprika. You'll lose the smoky undertone but it'll still taste great.

1 green bell pepper, chopped

1 red bell pepper, chopped

½ cup finely chopped red onion (about half a large red onion)

2 garlic cloves, minced

One 14- to 15-ounce can whole tomatoes, with juice

5 teaspoons dried oregano, divided

1 teaspoon salt, plus more to taste

½ teaspoon black pepper, plus more to taste

2 teaspoons ground cumin

2 teaspoons ancho chile powder

1 teaspoon smoked or sweet paprika

4 bone-in skinless chicken breast halves, each breast cut in half crosswise (to make 8 small pieces)

3 to 4 tablespoons olive oil, divided

1½ cups brown rice, rinsed

3 cups low-sodium chicken broth

1 cup frozen peas, not thawed

## STAGE 1 (10 minutes)

1.  Chop the peppers, red onion, and garlic. Put the peppers in a bowl and set aside.

2.  Combine onion and garlic in a blender with the canned tomatoes and puree until very smooth. Refrigerate the blender jar and its contents.

## STAGE 2 (20 minutes; if doing in two sessions combine with Stage 3)

1. Combine 4 teaspoons of the oregano, 1 teaspoon of the salt, ½ teaspoon of the black pepper, plus the cumin, chile powder, and paprika in a large resealable bag. Add the chicken, seal, and toss to coat. Remove chicken from bag, and pat to remove excess spice mixture.

2. Heat 2 tablespoons olive oil in a large Dutch oven or heavy pot over medium-high heat. When oil is almost smoking, arrange chicken pieces in 1 layer and cook each side until browned, 3 to 5 minutes per side (you may need to do this in 2 batches, adding more oil for the second batch).

3. Transfer chicken to a plate, cover, and refrigerate.

4. Add another tablespoon olive oil to the pot. When it shimmers, add the chopped peppers, lower the heat to medium, and cook until softened, 4 to 5 minutes.

5. Allow to cool slightly, then cover pot and refrigerate.


## STAGE 3 (55 minutes, 15 active)

1. Preheat oven to 375°F.

2. Return pot with cooked peppers to the stove and cook over low heat. Add a glug of oil if peppers look dry.

3. When peppers have warmed, add rice, increase heat to medium, and cook, stirring, until rice colors a bit, 2 to 3 minutes.

4. Add the reserved tomato mixture and cook, stirring frequently, until liquid has been mostly absorbed.

5. Stir in the broth, remaining teaspoon oregano, and salt and pepper to taste, then add the chicken, along with any accumulated juices, and the frozen peas. Raise heat to high and bring to a boil.

6. Cover, and transfer pot to the oven. Bake until chicken is cooked through, rice is tender, and liquid has been absorbed, 35 to 40 minutes.

> MAKE BABY FOOD: This recipe has several spices, but none of them are hot-spicy (even that ancho chile powder is pretty mild). It should be fine for most babies, either pureed with a bit of broth or water, or as finger food.

**MAMA SAID**

"Delicious! I was surprised that the brown rice turned out so tender. I am such a convert to your way of cooking, in stages. I abhor chopping, so it made a big difference to me to be able to chop the veggies the night before and refrigerate, then just leave everything else until the next stage. Oh, and I used, um, a whole head of garlic rather than two cloves. It turned out great, not too garlicky at all." —Anita J., mom of two, San Ramon, CA

· · · · · · · · · · · · · · · · · · · · · · · · · · · · · · · · · · · · · · ·

# CHICKEN CHILI

**Serves 6**

Chili is a new parent-friendly dish: It's nutritious, it's filling, it's got tons of flavor, and it's hard to mess up. Maybe that's why I've included three different chili recipes in this cookbook? This first one, for Chicken Chili, combines a fairly spicy broth with bite-sized chunks of tender white meat and mild white beans. It has a long Stage 3, but most of that time the chili is simmering away, unattended. I recommend using that loud kitchen timer I mentioned in the Introduction (you do have one, don't you?), just in case you get distracted. Because let's face it, sleep-deprived people get distracted pretty easily.

2 chipotles in adobo (scrape out the ribs and
    seeds for a milder chili)

1 cup water

2 large onions, chopped

4 celery ribs, chopped

4 tablespoons minced garlic, divided
    (approximately half a head)

2 tablespoons ground cumin

2 tablespoons chili powder

2 bay leaves

1½ teaspoons dried oregano,

Salt

1 tablespoon cornmeal

1 tablespoon vegetable oil

2 pounds boneless, skinless chicken breasts,
    chopped into ¼-inch pieces

One 28-ounce can whole tomatoes, chopped

1½ to 2 cups low-sodium chicken broth

One 19-ounce can white beans, drained and
    rinsed

Cooked brown rice, shredded Cheddar
    cheese, sour cream, and chopped onion,
    for serving

## STAGE 1 (10 minutes)

1. Puree the chipotles with the water in a blender and refrigerate.

2. Chop the onions, celery, and garlic. Put the onions, celery, and half of the garlic in one bowl and cover. Put the remaining garlic in a separate bowl and cover. Refrigerate both bowls.

3. Combine cumin and chili powder in a small bowl. Combine bay leaves, oregano, and 1 teaspoon salt in another small bowl. Measure cornmeal into a third small bowl.

*I have a set of tiny glass bowls that are perfect for holding small amounts of spices. You could also use shot glasses—my guess is they're not seeing much action these days, anyway. One drawback to Nap-Friendly Cooking is that you use a lot of bowls. This is why God gave us dishwashers, and spouses.*

## STAGE 2 (10 minutes)

1. Heat the oil in a large, heavy pot or Dutch oven over medium heat. When it shimmers, add the onion mixture and cook, stirring occasionally, until softened, about 10 minutes.

2. Add the cumin and chili powder and cook, stirring, for 30 seconds.

3. Remove from heat; cool slightly, cover, and refrigerate.

## STAGE 3 (1½ hours, 30 minutes active)

1. Return the pot to the stove over low heat. When mixture has warmed, increase heat to medium, add chicken, and cook, stirring, until chicken is no longer pink, about 8 minutes.

2. Add the chipotle puree, chopped tomatoes, broth, bay leaves, oregano, and salt, and simmer, uncovered, adding more water if necessary to keep the chicken barely covered, 1 hour.

3. Add the cornmeal and simmer, stirring occasionally, 15 minutes.

4. Stir in the white beans and remaining garlic and simmer until the beans are heated through, 3 to 5 minutes.

5. Adjust salt to taste, and discard bay leaves before serving over brown rice with cheese, sour cream, and chopped onion.

MAKE BABY FOOD: I'm not gonna lie: This is spicy. Some babies are fine with that—seriously, some really do like heat—but you know your own child. If he enjoys spicy food there's no reason not to let him try this, either pureed or as finger food. If not, reserve some of the rinsed beans, rice, sour cream, and cheese for him.

**MAMA SAID**

"My 11-month-old woke up while we were on Stage 1 so I tossed her in the Moby, gave her a measuring spoon, and continued on my way. I measured the spices out into empty baby food jars, and that worked pretty nicely. My husband really liked the 'bite' of the finished dish. In fact, he plays league hockey and told me that he didn't grab a snack at the concession stand after the game because he wanted to come home and have some of the leftover chili instead. I was a bit worried about it being too spicy for my daughter, but she didn't mind. I guess she's more like her dad than I know." —Monica W., mom of one, St. Louis, MO

### WILL MY BREASTMILK BE SPICY?

If you eat spicy food, yes, your breastmilk will taste different to your baby. But that's not a bad thing! Unless you notice that your baby is fussy or seems unhappy after nursing, there's no reason for you to abstain from any kind of food. In fact, some experts believe that exposing your baby to spice via breastmilk (and even in utero) will make him more open to new flavors once he starts eating real foods.

# BRAISED CHICKEN WITH ARTICHOKE HEARTS, MUSHROOMS, AND PEPPADEW PEPPERS

**Serves 6**

Peppadew peppers, a unique variety grown in South Africa, are relatively new on the market. They're sold pickled, and can be found either in jars or in the olive bar at supermarkets and specialty stores. I love their sweet, spicy flavor. Toss them into salads, and layer them in sandwiches. Set them out in small bowls alongside olives and Marcona almonds—they're the perfect nibble for unexpected guests (new parents have *plenty* of those; see the sidebar on page 15 for more ideas). If you can't find Peppadews, substitute 8 to 10 pepperoncini or pickled cherry peppers. They won't provide any sweetness, but they'll give this a nice bite.

1 large onion, finely chopped

4 garlic cloves, minced

12 Peppadew peppers, minced

1 red bell pepper, thinly sliced

8 to 10 ounces cremini or white button
   mushrooms, sliced

3 tablespoons minced flat-leaf parsley

6 bone-in chicken breast halves with skin

Salt and pepper

2 tablespoons olive oil

1½ cups dry white wine

1 cup low-sodium chicken broth

Two 6-ounce jars marinated artichoke hearts,
   mostly drained

Cooked noodles or rice, for serving

## STAGE 1 (15 minutes)

1. Prepare all the vegetables, including the parsley.

2. Put the onions, garlic, and Peppadew peppers into one bowl, the bell pepper and mushrooms into another, and the parsley into a third. Cover all and refrigerate.

## STAGE 2 (30 minutes; if doing in two sessions combine with Stage 3)

1. Pat dry the chicken breasts and season with salt and pepper. Heat oil in a large, heavy pot or Dutch oven over medium-high heat until hot but not smoking. Arrange chicken skin side down, in 1 layer, and cook until browned, 4 to 5 minutes per side, and transfer to a plate. (You may need to do this in two batches, adding more oil for the second batch.)

2. Cover the browned chicken and refrigerate.

3. In the fat remaining in the pot, cook the onion, garlic, and Peppadews over medium-low heat, stirring, until onion is softened. Add the bell pepper, mushrooms, and salt and pepper to taste, and cook over medium heat, stirring, until bell pepper is softened, 5 to 8 minutes.

4. Remove from heat and cool slightly, then cover pot and refrigerate.

### STAGE 3 (45 minutes)

1. Remove the chicken from the refrigerator and let it sit out for 10 minutes, to take off some of the chill.

2. Return the pot to low heat. When it's warmed, add the wine, broth, artichoke hearts, and chicken with any accumulated juices, and bring to a boil. Reduce heat and simmer, covered, until the chicken is cooked through, 20 to 25 minutes.

3. Transfer chicken to a platter. Using a slotted spoon, transfer the vegetables to the platter, raise heat to high, and cook sauce until reduced and thickened, 5 to 10 minutes.

4. Stir in the parsley and return the chicken and vegetables to the pot and stir to coat with sauce.

5. Serve over noodles or rice.

MAKE BABY FOOD: I served this to Harry with no worries, but there are two factors to weigh before doing the same with your own baby: 1) Most of the alcohol from the wine will cook off, but not all of it. 2) Sometimes those pickled peppers can be surprisingly spicy. Taste them before serving to your baby. OK with all that? Puree with some sauce, or serve as finger food. Not OK? Serve the chicken naked, no sauce—it should be just fine.

**MAMA SAID**
"I would make this for guests. It's really good and something a little bit different, plus it seems fancier and more complicated than it is. Also, it would be a nice thing to bring over to someone with a new baby —it tastes even better reheated." —Ann S., mom of two, Lebanon, NH

# VEGETABLE COUSCOUS, WITH OR WITHOUT CHICKEN

**Serves 6 to 8**

This is one of the first recipes I learned when I started living on my own, and I still turn to it several times a year. It's terrific for busy parents: filling, flexible, and extremely comforting, thanks to the spicy-but-not-hot seasoning—plus it makes enough to qualify for my chapter on big-batch cooking. There are quite a few ingredients, but if you don't have all the vegetables called for that's just fine—substitute almost anything you like. Just add the aromatics like onion, garlic, celery, and fennel first, the hard, longer-cooking vegetables next, and the softer ones like zucchini last.

1 large onion, chopped

4 garlic cloves, minced

3 celery ribs, chopped

1 fennel bulb, tops and tough outer layers discarded, sliced

½ medium butternut squash, peeled and cut into 1-inch pieces (packaged pre-cut is fine)

1 sweet potato, peeled and chopped into 1-inch pieces

2 large carrots, chopped into 1-inch pieces

2 medium zucchini, halved lengthwise and sliced

2 tablespoons curry powder

¼ teaspoon turmeric

½ teaspoon paprika

½ cup sliced almonds

2 tablespoons olive oil

Salt

1 to 1½ cups low-sodium vegetable or chicken broth

One 28-ounce can diced tomatoes, with juices

½ cup raisins

¼ cup pomegranate juice, optional

1 cup diced, cooked chicken breast, or one 15-ounce can chickpeas, rinsed and drained

Cooked couscous, for serving

## STAGE 1 (25 minutes)

1. Prepare all of the vegetables.

2. Put the onion, garlic, and zucchini in separate bowls. Combine the celery and fennel in one bowl. Combine butternut squash, sweet potato, and carrots in another. Cover all. Refrigerate onion and garlic; the rest will be fine at room temperature for several hours.

3. Measure all the spices into a small bowl, cover, and set aside.

4. Toast the almonds (either in a toaster oven at 350°F for 4 to 5 minutes—watch closely so they don't burn—or in a dry skillet for a similar length of time) and transfer to a small bowl to cool. Cover and set aside.

## STAGE 2 (10 minutes)

1. Heat the olive oil over medium-low heat in a large, heavy pot or Dutch oven. When it shimmers, add onions and cook until translucent, 3 to 5 minutes. Add garlic and cook until fragrant, about 30 seconds.

2. Add spices to onions and garlic, stir, and cook for a few seconds. Add celery and fennel, stir, and cook just until they start to soften, about 3 minutes.

3. Remove pot from the heat, cover, and refrigerate.

## STAGE 3 (45 minutes)

1. Return pot to medium-low heat. When it's warmed, add the hard vegetables (butternut squash, sweet potato, and carrots), plus 1 cup of the broth, tomatoes, and raisins. Reduce heat to low and simmer, covered, until vegetables are tender, 15 to 20 minutes (a fork should pierce the hardest vegetables with minimal resistance). Check mixture occasionally to make sure it's not sticking; if it is, stir in a little more broth.

3. Add the zucchini, pomegranate juice, if using, and the chicken or beans, and cook 5 to 10 minutes more, until zucchini is tender and the stew is mellow and rich-looking. Season with salt to taste.

4. Serve over couscous, topped with the toasted almonds.

MAKE BABY FOOD: If you use a mild curry powder, this is ideal for babies—the vegetables get quite squishy (if you know your baby likes spice, go ahead and use a hot variety). You can either puree the stew, or serve chunks as finger food. Babies like couscous too! Break the almond slices into small pieces to avoid a choking hazard—but if you have a family history of food allergies, skip them altogether until your pediatrician says it's OK.

**MAMA SAID**
**"Loved it! Also loved that it would be vegan if made with vegetable broth and no chicken."**
**—Beth P., mom of one, Los Angeles, CA**

# A GREEKISH ORZO-TOMATO SALAD

**Serves 4**

Before I moved in with Stephen, I lived for 12 years in Astoria, Queens, New York's largest Greek neighborhood. Lord, it was heaven: I was surrounded by grilled whole fish, garlicky potato dip, and all manner of phyllo-based goodies. But the thing I ate most often was a simple Greek salad, the most perfect combination of fresh, vibrant flavors I can think of. This homage adds a few unorthodox ingredients (chicken sausage, almonds, marinated artichoke hearts) to create a dinner salad substantial enough for the burliest of men.

It's best made with beautifully ripe summer tomatoes, but if it's the off-season, use grape tomatoes or Campari, a small, sweet variety that's sold in clamshell boxes in the produce section.

2 large, ripe tomatoes, seeded and diced

1 large cucumber, quartered lengthwise and chopped into small pieces

12 Kalamata olives, pitted and roughly chopped

One 6-ounce jar marinated artichoke hearts, drained and halved

Half a small red onion, finely chopped

½ pound orzo

1 package (about 12 ounces) chicken sausages (choose one with Mediterranean flavors)

Handful of Marcona almonds, halved, or lightly toasted sliced or slivered regular almonds

4 ounces feta or ricotta salata, crumbled

Juice of 1 lemon

1 tablespoon red wine vinegar

4 tablespoons flavorful extra-virgin olive oil

½ teaspoon dried oregano

## STAGE 1 (15 minutes)

1. Prepare all of the vegetables.

2. Toss everything but the onion into a large salad bowl, cover, and refrigerate.

3. Put the onion into a small bowl of ice water to take off some of the raw-onion bite, cover, and refrigerate.

## STAGE 2 (25 minutes)

1. Cook orzo according to package directions, drain in a colander and rinse under cold water until cool, drain well again and add to the salad bowl. Drain onions and add to the bowl.

2. Cover bowl and refrigerate.

## STAGE 3 (15 minutes)

1. Prepare sausages according to package directions (I cook mine whole in a nonstick frying pan with a little olive oil for about five minutes per side, then slice them and brown for another 30 seconds or so. I like things well browned, but there's no need to do that second part if you don't want to). Set aside to cool slightly.

2. When cool, add the sausage plus all remaining ingredients to the bowl, toss, and serve.

> MAKE BABY FOOD: I'd give a finger-food-eating infant everything in this salad except the whole almonds and artichokes, both of which are too challenging to eat. Raw tomatoes may be too acidic for your baby—give her a taste and see how she responds. Still on purees? Whir up the whole thing! Leave out the nuts if you have a family history of food allergies.

### NOTES FROM THE RECIPE TESTERS

- Several of my mom-testers reported that they prepared this recipe in one straight shot, no stages, and that it took well under an hour.

- One mom swapped shrimp for the chicken sausage and was thrilled with the result.

- Vegetarian moms left out the sausage altogether and just added more cheese.

• • • • • • • • • • • • • • • • • • • • • • • • • • • • • • • • • • • • • • • • • • • • • • • •

# ROASTED VEGETABLE BEEF BARLEY SOUP

**Serves 6 to 8**

I realize this ingredient list might look intimidating, but each element adds a particular flavor and together, they make a rich soup that will get you excited for cold weather. And like the Vegetable Couscous, the recipe makes enough for leftovers and then some—freeze a quart, if you like, following the instructions in Chapter 5, "Big Batch Bonanza."

This recipe's a good one to pull out when your sister's over and asks what she can do to help. Hand her a knife and let her start chopping.

¾ pound beef chuck, cut into bite-size pieces
*Save time by asking the butcher to do this for you.*

2 carrots, quartered lengthwise and chopped into ¼-inch pieces

2 celery ribs, halved lengthwise and chopped into ¼-inch pieces

1 zucchini, quartered lengthwise and chopped into ½-inch pieces

1 red bell pepper, chopped into ½-inch pieces

4 ounces cremini or white button mushrooms, thickly sliced

3 garlic cloves, unpeeled

2 large shallots, peeled, bulbs halved

3 tablespoons olive oil, divided

Salt and pepper

½ ounce dried porcini mushrooms

½ cup reduced-sodium soy sauce

1 cup pearl barley

8 sun-dried tomato halves, slivered

1½ tablespoons chili powder

4 cups low-sodium beef broth

4 to 6 cups water

2 bay leaves

2 to 4 tablespoons tomato paste, optional

## STAGE 1 (15 minutes)

1. If the beef isn't already cut into small pieces, do that now, cover, and return to the refrigerator.

2. Prepare the carrots, celery, zucchini, red pepper, mushrooms, garlic, and shallots and combine in a large bowl. Toss with 2 tablespoons olive oil and salt and pepper to taste. Cover and refrigerate.

## STAGE 2 (30 minutes)

1. Preheat oven to 425°F. Grease or line two baking sheets.

2. Divide prepared vegetables between the two sheets and roast for 25 minutes, stirring halfway through. Set aside (no need to refrigerate).

3. While vegetables are roasting, put dried mushrooms in a small bowl, cover with boiling water, and set aside.

4. Heat remaining tablespoon olive oil in a large, heavy pot or Dutch oven over medium-high heat. Add the beef, sprinkle lightly with salt and pepper, and brown on all sides, 6 to 8 minutes. If there seems to be a lot of fat, remove it and discard. Cover the pot and refrigerate.

## STAGE 3 (1 hour to 1 hour 15 minutes, 20 minutes active)

1. Remove the pot from the refrigerator to take off some of the chill. Slip peels off the roasted garlic and roughly chop with the roasted shallots.

2. Return pot to the stove over medium heat and add all of the roasted vegetables.

3. While vegetables are heating, pluck the dried mushrooms from the bowl (don't pour the liquid over them, as there might be gritty sediment at the bottom), roughly chop them, and add them to the pot, reserving the liquid.

4. Add the soy sauce to the pot and cook until almost evaporated, 5 to 10 minutes, then add the barley and the sun-dried tomatoes, sprinkle with the chili powder, and cook briefly, stirring.

5. Add the browned beef, broth, water, reserved mushroom soaking liquid (but be careful not to pour in the sediment, if there is any), and bay leaves, and bring to a boil. Lower the heat and simmer gently, covered, 45 minutes.

6. If the soup seems too thin after this time, either uncover partially or add tomato paste, 2 tablespoons at a time, and simmer for another 10 to 15 minutes.

7. Remove the bay leaves and season with salt and pepper to taste before serving.

> MAKE BABY FOOD: This makes a beautiful puree. Or you can separate the solids and treat it like finger food—the texture of the vegetables is perfect for young eaters, and picking up grains of barley helps to build small motor skills.

**MAMA SAID**
"If I owned a restaurant, I would put this soup on the menu. Seriously. That is how much I love it. It was a bit labor intensive but not overly so, and making this dish made me feel like a cook. Roasting the vegetables, rehydrating the mushrooms, and just simply creating this yummy-smelling and -tasting soup from scratch, made me feel like I'm finally starting to learn my way around the kitchen and I may even be kind of decent at this cooking thing."
—Lee P., mom of two, Pittsburgh, PA

• • • • • • • • • • • • • • • • • • • • • • • • • • • • • • • • • • •

# LIME-OREGANO FAJITAS

**Serves 6**

The marinade for this dish works equally well with chicken or beef. I like to combine skinless, boneless chicken breasts and flank steak.

3 bell peppers, any color, thinly sliced

1 large onion, halved vertically then thinly sliced

1 avocado, peeled and sliced

1½ tablespoons lemon juice (from about ½ lemon)

¼ cup lime juice (from 3 to 4 limes)

3 garlic cloves, minced

⅓ cup olive oil, plus more for cooking

½ teaspoon ground cumin

1 tablespoon dried oregano

¾ teaspoon salt

2 pounds meat, cut into strips: you can use boneless, skinless chicken (thighs or breasts), flank steak, skirt steak, or a combination

12 to 15 tortillas (choose ones with whole-grain corn or wheat as the first ingredient)

Sour cream and your favorite jarred salsa, for serving

## STAGE 1 (10 minutes)

1. Prepare all of the vegetables.

2. Put the sliced pepper into a bowl and cover (no need to refrigerate). Put the onion into an airtight container (to contain the smell!) and refrigerate. Put the avocado into a bowl, toss with the lemon juice, and cover with plastic wrap, letting the plastic touch the avocado (the less air the avocado is exposed to, the less likely it is to turn brown). Refrigerate.

3. To make the marinade, juice the limes and combine with the garlic, ⅓ cup oil, cumin, oregano, and salt in a resealable bag or glass or stainless-steel bowl large enough to hold the meat. Seal tightly (no need to refrigerate).

## STAGE 2 (10 minutes)

1. Stir the marinade briefly.

2. Cut the meat into thin strips and add to the marinade. Seal and refrigerate.

## STAGE 3 (15 to 30 minutes)

**You have several options for cooking the fajitas, which I've listed in order of my preference. In each case, discard the marinade once you remove the meat:**

**NOTE:** I use the microwave to warm tortillas: stack the tortillas together and wrap loosely in damp paper towels, then cook on high for 15 to 30 seconds.

### Use a stovetop grill pan:

1. Coat the pan lightly with about 1 tablespoon of oil and heat over medium-high heat.

2. Grill the beef until it's cooked to your desired level of doneness, turning halfway through, and grill the chicken until it's no longer pink, about 4 minutes per side.

3. Transfer meat to a platter and cover with foil.

4. Add the peppers and onions to the pan and cook until softened and lightly charred.

### Use a large nonstick skillet:

1. Put about 1 tablespoon oil into the pan and heat over medium-high heat.

2. When the oil shimmers, add the peppers and onions. Cook, stirring occasionally, until softened and barely browned.

3. Transfer peppers and onions to a platter and cover with foil.

4. Add meat to the pan and cook, stirring occasionally, until cooked through, 8 to 10 minutes.

### Use your broiler:

1. Preheat broiler for about 15 minutes.

2. Place the peppers and onions on a baking sheet that will fit inside the broiler and slide it on top of the broiler pan. Cook, checking once or twice, until softened and lightly charred, 5 to 10 minutes.

3. Remove the baking sheet and cover peppers and onions with foil.

4. Place the meat on the broiler pan. Broil, turning halfway through, until beef reaches your desired level of doneness, 3 to 4 minutes per side, and chicken is no longer pink, about 4 minutes per side.

**Serve the fajita meat, peppers, and onions with warmed tortillas, avocado slices, salsa, and sour cream.**

MAKE BABY FOOD: Puree the meat and some of the vegetables with a splash of broth or water. As for finger food, beef is often too tough for babies to chew, but Harry ate bits of chicken from quite a young age. Tear a tortilla into small pieces. If your peppers are charred, remove the skin before serving. Avocados are also fantastic for babies—mash them with a fork if you're still on purees.

**MAMA SAID**
**"The taste was great—I really enjoyed it. This is one of those meals whose leftovers won't end up being thrown out—we both wanted to take it to work with us the next day."**
**—Monica W., mom of one, St. Louis, MO**

# COTTAGE PIE

**Serves 6**

While shepherd's pie is typically made with lamb (get it: "shepherd"?), Cottage Pie is the same idea made with beef. This recipe doubles well. Before pouring in the filling, line the second baking dish with heavy-duty foil. Bake the pies together, then cool the spare and freeze it. Once it is frozen, you'll be able to slip the whole pie out of the baking dish—wrap it well and return to the freezer. To reheat, remove the wrapping and slide the pie back into the baking dish. Bake at 350°F for about an hour, straight from the freezer.

6 medium or 4 large Yukon gold potatoes, peeled and chopped into 1-inch pieces

2 cups low-sodium beef or chicken broth

1 large onion, chopped

One 16-ounce package mixed frozen vegetables (carrots, peas, corn, green beans), or 2 cups fresh vegetables, chopped

½ to ¾ cup milk (I use 1 percent)

Salt and pepper

1 tablespoon olive oil

1 pound extra-lean ground beef (I use 85 percent lean, which has less fat and cholesterol than regular ground turkey!)

1 tablespoon Worcestershire sauce

1 tablespoon reduced-sodium soy sauce

½ tablespoon pomegranate molasses, optional

2 tablespoons tomato paste

## STAGE 1 (25 minutes)

1. Peel and chop the potatoes, then combine them with broth in a large saucepan (the broth should just cover the potatoes) and bring to a boil. Lower heat and simmer, covered, until fork-tender, about 15 minutes.

2. While the potatoes are simmering, chop the onions and, if you're not using frozen, the fresh carrots, corn, and green beans. Put the onions and fresh carrots, if using, into one bowl and cover; place the other vegetables into a separate bowl and cover. If using frozen vegetables, leave them in the freezer for now.

3. Drain potatoes, reserving broth in a liquid measuring cup. Return potatoes to pot and mash well, adding as much reserved broth as needed to hold together. Stir in enough milk to make a creamy mixture, and season with salt and pepper to taste.

4. Refrigerate the potatoes, fresh vegetables, and remaining potato-broth in separate, covered containers.

## STAGE 2 (25 minutes; if doing in two sessions combine with Stage 3)

1. Heat the olive oil in a large nonstick skillet over medium heat. When it shimmers, add the onion (and carrots, if you're using fresh) and cook, stirring occasionally, until just tender, 3 to 5 minutes.

2. Add the ground beef and cook, breaking the meat up with the back of a spoon, until it's no longer pink, 5 to 8 minutes.

3. Add the remaining vegetables, fresh or frozen. Add the Worcestershire sauce, soy sauce, pomegranate molasses if using, and tomato paste.

4. Stir the reserved potato-broth and add enough to the pan to keep things moist. Simmer until the mixture has thickened slightly, 5 to 10 minutes. Cool slightly and refrigerate, covered.

## STAGE 3 (45 minutes to 1 hour, 15 minutes active)

1. Preheat oven to 400°F, and put the refrigerated items on the counter to take off the chill. Grease a 9 x 13-inch baking dish.

2. When the oven's warmed up, transfer the beef and vegetable mixture to the baking dish, and top with the mashed potatoes. The potatoes should reach no higher than a quarter-inch below the top of the baking dish, otherwise the juices will bubble over. (If you have too many mashed potatoes, refrigerate the excess and serve as a side dish another day.) Spread the potatoes out with the back of a spoon, then draw a fork back and forth across the potatoes to make a pattern (these ridges will make the top crustier). Bake until the top is golden-brown and the juices are bubbling, 30 to 45 minutes.

> MAKE BABY FOOD: I can't think of a better baby food than mashed potatoes, and the filling is ideal for pureeing or serving as finger food.

**MAMA SAID**
"The taste is really classic, exactly as I remembered it from childhood. Not too dry or wet, it had the perfect texture. My three-year-old had seconds—he loved it too!" —Amber D., mom of two, Woodland Hills, CA

# ASIAN FISH EN PAPILLOTE

**Serves 2, and doubles or triples easily**

Don't be intimidated by the French. "En papillote" simply means it's folded inside a little pouch and baked.

Half a large red bell pepper, thinly sliced

10 to 12 snow peas, cut diagonally into ¼-inch pieces

4 mushrooms, such as shiitake or cremini, sliced

2 scallions (white and light green parts), thinly sliced

One 1-inch piece of fresh ginger, peeled and julienned

2 handfuls baby spinach

Two 6-ounce fillets mild whitefish (tilapia, scrod, cod, pollock, snapper—whatever fish you like as long as it's not too thin)

3 tablespoons reduced-sodium soy sauce

2 tablespoons rice vinegar

1 teaspoon toasted sesame oil

1 teaspoon sugar

Cooked rice, for serving

## STAGE 1 (15 to 20 minutes)

1. Prepare all of the vegetables.

2. Combine the bell pepper, snow peas, and mushrooms in one bowl and put the scallions and ginger in another. Cover and refrigerate.

## STAGE 2 (15 minutes)

1. Tear off 2 sheets of aluminum foil, each 12 to 14 inches long. Lay the sheets next to each other on a baking sheet or cutting board that will fit in the refrigerator.

2. Place one handful of the baby spinach on each piece of foil, keeping the spinach an inch or two to the right of center, since you'll be folding the foil up and over. On top of each pile of spinach, place half of the peppers, snow peas, and mushrooms, then lay a fish fillet on top. Scatter the scallions and ginger over the fish.

3. Combine the soy sauce, vinegar, sesame oil, and sugar in a small bowl, and stir until sugar dissolves. Drizzle mixture evenly over each packet of fish and vegetables (fold the edges of the foil upward first to keep it from spilling off).

4. Loosely fold the empty half of the foil over the top of the fish and crimp the three edges closed. Leave some air in the packet, and take care not to tear the foil. The packets definitely need to be sealed, but you'll want to have easy access on one side to test for doneness.

5. Refrigerate the prepared packets on the baking sheet.

## STAGE 3 (30 minutes, 10 minutes active)

1. Preheat oven to 450°F. While the oven is heating, remove packets from refrigerator and leave at room temperature.

2. Bake packets on baking sheet for 12 to 15 minutes if fish is on the thin side, 15 to 20 minutes if fish is an inch thick or greater. Check doneness by carefully opening one packet (there will be lots of steam), sticking a fork into the thickest part of the fish, and twisting slightly. The fish is done when it's no longer translucent.

3. Place the packets directly onto dinner plates and open immediately or the fish will overcook. Again, be mindful of the steam.

4. Serve with rice, to soak up all the sauce.

MAKE BABY FOOD: Fish is a wonderful early food, either pureed with some of the vegetables, rice, and a splash of broth, or as finger food. Even with reduced-sodium soy sauce, the sauce may be too salty for babies, so leave that on your own plate.

**MAMA SAID**
"It was delicious and the house had this lovely, toasted sesame scent from the baking—not fishy! The nice thing about having the ingredients separate is that it was very easy to accommodate my preschooler's insistence to not have mushrooms. I was able to scale back on the ginger and scallions as well, since she's been known to call cereal 'spicy.' (Really.) The sauce was terrific and simple." —Anita J., mom of two, San Ramon, CA

## MAKE YOUR OWN RECIPES NAP-FRIENDLY

If you've got a favorite recipe that seems too complex to pull off with a baby in the house, adapt it for Nap-Friendly Cooking:

First, review the Food Safety guidelines on page 48.

Stage 1 is generally devoted to prep:

1. Measure out any spices and put into small bowls.
2. Wash, peel, and chop vegetables and herbs—one of the few I'd recommend leaving for later is fresh basil, which turns black after being chopped.
3. Once cut, firm, dry vegetables can remain at room temperature for hours. If it will be more than two hours before you move on to Stage 2, prepared vegetables that are moist or juicy (including sprouts and washed and cut tomatoes, leafy greens, fresh herbs, and onions) should be refrigerated. Refrigerate cut onions in an airtight container, or the odor might infiltrate all your other food! Acid deters the growth of bacteria, so naturally acidic items like citrus fruits are considered safe at room temperature.
4. All proteins must be refrigerated.

If you're using three stages, Stage 2 is for intermediate preparation: browning or marinating meat, and preliminary cooking of vegetables.

1. All protein must go back in the fridge in a clean container.
2. If you're softening vegetables in the pan drippings the whole pot should be cooled slightly, then refrigerated.
3. Roasted or sauteed vegetables that haven't touched protein are fine at room temperature; just remove from the heat and set aside.

Stage 3 is for the final cooking—assembling, baking, simmering on the stove, and tossing with the remaining ingredients.

1. If you're baking, remember to preheat your oven about 20 minutes before you plan to start.
2. If you've refrigerated the pot, remove it from the fridge at least ten minutes before you start cooking, and be sure to reheat gently, over a low flame, before resuming the recipe.

Having trouble breaking down the recipe for Aunt Bessie's Famous Meatloaf? Drop me a line at parentsneedtoeattoo@gmail.com and I'll help you sort it out.

· · · · · · · · · · · · · · · · · · · · · · · · · · · · · · · · · · · ·

# MINESTRONE WITH PARMESAN GREMOLATA

**Serves 6–8**

Hearty, hearty, hearty. The addition of gremolata, a finely minced combination of garlic, parsley, lemon peel, and in this case Parmesan, adds a bright, fresh flavor to this substantial soup. There are a lot of ingredients in this recipe, but it makes a *ton* of soup—you should have enough left over to freeze a quart, maybe more.

1 medium onion, chopped small

2 large garlic cloves, minced, divided

2 medium carrots, chopped small

2 celery ribs, chopped small

Half a large red bell pepper, chopped small

1 medium zucchini, chopped small

Half a small head of Savoy cabbage, about ½ pound, shredded

Salt and pepper

1 tablespoon olive oil

2 sprigs flat-leaf parsley, plus ¼ cup leaves, divided

One 2- to 3-inch piece Parmesan rind, optional (I save these in the freezer)

4 cups low-sodium chicken broth

One 28-ounce can crushed or chopped tomatoes and their juice

One 15-ounce can cannellini or red kidney beans, drained and rinsed

½ cup Arborio rice

1 tablespoon lemon zest (from about 1 lemon)

2 tablespoons grated Parmesan

1 tablespoon flavorful extra-virgin olive oil, plus more for serving

Crusty bread, for serving

## STAGE 1 (20 minutes)

1.  Prepare all of the vegetables.

2.  Put the onion and garlic into separate airtight containers. Place the carrots and celery into one covered bowl, the bell pepper and zucchini in another, and the cabbage in a third.

3.  Refrigerate the onions, garlic, and cabbage; the rest is fine at room temperature.

## STAGE 2 (1 hour 15 minutes, 20 minutes active)

1. Heat the olive oil in a large, heavy pot or Dutch oven over medium heat. When it shimmers, add the onion and cook, stirring occasionally, until translucent, about 3 minutes.

2. Reserve 1 teaspoon garlic and stir in the rest. Cook until fragrant, about 30 seconds. Add the carrots and celery and cook until just softened, about 3 minutes. Add the pepper and zucchini and cook, stirring occasionally, 3 minutes more. Season with salt and pepper to taste.

3. Add the cabbage, parsley sprigs, Parmesan rind, if using, broth, and tomatoes. Bring to a boil, then lower the heat and cover. Simmer 30 minutes, stirring occasionally.

4. Add the beans and rice, and cook until rice is mostly cooked but still firm in the center, 20 to 25 minutes (rice will continue to cook as it sits).

5. Remove from heat. Cool at least 30 minutes (but no more than two hours), then refrigerate, covered.

## STAGE 3 (10 to 15 minutes)

1. Remove the parsley sprigs and parmesan rind, and reheat the soup over low heat. It will have thickened; stir in some water if it seems too thick.

2. While soup is heating, make the gremolata: Chop the reserved parsley leaves. Add the lemon zest and reserved teaspoon garlic and finely chop everything together. Transfer to a small bowl and stir in the grated Parmesan and extra-virgin olive oil.

3. Serve the soup, and top each bowl with about a teaspoon of gremolata. Add a drizzle of olive oil, if you like, and serve with crusty bread!

> MAKE BABY FOOD: If you haven't already guessed, long-simmering soups and stews are ideal for babies. In this recipe the solids get so wonderfully soft, you may not even need to puree. I'd skip the gremolata, though.

**MAMA SAID**
**"I did the bulk of the cooking on this one the night before. My three-month-old wakes up every hour or so after going down for the night so there were a few times I needed to stop and start up again, but that really wasn't a big deal. This recipe is very forgiving in that respect. The taste was great—hearty and delicious." —Monica W., mom of one, St. Louis, MO**

# ZUCCHINI AND SPINACH RISOTTO

**Serves 4 to 6**

Yes, you *can* make risotto with a baby in the house! Here's a little secret: Risotto doesn't actually need to be attended to like, well, a baby, with you hovering over the stove, adding liquid in stages, and stirring, stirring, stirring. Heresy, perhaps, but wouldn't you rather eat a creamy, satisfying bowl of inauthentic risotto than yet another frozen pizza?

1 shallot or small onion, finely chopped

2 garlic cloves, minced

2 medium zucchini, shredded

Half a 5-ounce bag of baby spinach, roughly chopped

2 tablespoons olive oil

Salt

2 cups Arborio rice

4 to 5 cups low-sodium chicken broth, vegetable broth, water, or a combination

1 cup white wine or vermouth

2 tablespoons chopped basil

1 tablespoon butter

1 cup grated Parmesan cheese

## STAGE 1 (10 minutes)

1. Prepare the shallot, garlic, zucchini, and spinach.

2. Put each in a separate bowl, cover, and refrigerate.

## STAGE 2 (15 minutes)

1. Heat the olive oil in a large saucepan over medium heat. When it shimmers, add the shallot and cook, stirring occasionally, until translucent, about 3 minutes.

2. Add the garlic and cook until fragrant, about 30 seconds, then add the zucchini and a pinch of salt. Cook, stirring frequently, until zucchini has released most of its liquid and almost all liquid has evaporated, 8 to 10 minutes.

3. If it will be more than two hours before you cook again, cover pan and refrigerate. If not, it's OK to keep at room temperature, covered.

## STAGE 3 (25 to 30 minutes)

1.  Heat the broth or water until nearly boiling (I usually do this in the microwave).

2.  Return pan with the zucchini mixture to the stove, and heat over low heat. If mixture looks dry, add a glug of olive oil.

3.  When mixture is heated through, raise heat to medium and add the rice. Cook, stirring frequently, until each grain is coated with oil and rice begins to make a clacking sound.

4.  Add the wine and cook, stirring frequently, until most of the liquid has been absorbed, 3 to 5 minutes. Add 4 cups of the broth or water all at once, and bring to a boil. If you're using plain water, add ½ teaspoon salt; if using broth, don't salt at this point.

5.  Lower the heat and simmer, covered, stirring occasionally, until rice is almost tender, 15 to 17 minutes. Toward the end of this time, chop the basil (it will turn black if chopped too early). When the rice looks moist and creamy but not soupy, add the basil and the chopped spinach (a handful at a time) and stir until spinach is just cooked.

6.  You want to maintain that creamy-not-soupy consistency, with rice that is just slightly firm in the center, so add some of the remaining broth or water if needed.

7.  Remove from heat, stir in the butter and Parmesan, and season with salt if desired.

> MAKE BABY FOOD: Texturally this one's ideal, just as it is. There is alcohol in the recipe but most of it will have cooked off. I did feed this to Harry when he was a baby, but that's a decision each family must make on its own.

**MAMA SAID**
"We *love* this recipe and have already made it twice. It's pretty easy to put together and amenable to a number of different things. The second time around we added the zucchini and then raided our fridge for other veggies to add—mushrooms and chard worked really well. It's a great side and a filling dinner all by itself. Our four-year-old loved it and I can easily see the baby eating this soon too." —Alexandra S., mom of two, Baltimore, MD

# CORN, PEACH, TOMATO OVER GRILLED POLENTA

**Serves 4**

I think this may be the most delicious salad I have ever eaten. During the late summer, when corn, peaches, and tomatoes are at their peak, we have this for dinner at least once a week, and it's always a refreshing treat.

Since this recipe depends entirely on the freshness of the main ingredients, I'd save it for summertime only. The rest of the year, you'll just have something to look forward to!

5 ears corn, shucked

2 large or 3 small peaches, peeled, pitted, and chopped

2 medium-large tomatoes, chopped

1 small red onion, finely chopped

3 tablespoons flavorful extra-virgin olive oil

1 to 2 tablespoons sherry vinegar (depending on how tart you like your dressing—I use 2)

16 to 20 bocconcini (small fresh mozzarella balls)

Salt and pepper

1 tablespoon olive oil

One 1-pound roll ready-made polenta

15 to 20 large basil leaves

## STAGE 1 (15 minutes)

1. Microwave or steam corn until crisp-tender, 3 to 5 minutes. Set aside to cool.

2. Meanwhile, peel and chop the peaches. Put peaches into a strainer set over a large bowl. Chop the tomatoes and add to strainer.

3. Chop the onion and put into a small bowl of ice water; cover and refrigerate.

4. Cut the kernels from the corn with a sharp knife. Add to the strainer. Cover and refrigerate.

## STAGE 2 (10 minutes; if doing in two sessions combine with Stage 3)

1. Drain the onion and combine with the other vegetables in one large bowl. Discard the accumulated juices.

2. Add the extra-virgin olive oil and vinegar, toss, and refrigerate.

## STAGE 3 (20 minutes)

1. Remove salad from the refrigerator—you don't want it to be too cold when you eat. Add the bocconcini and salt and pepper to taste, toss, and set aside.

2. Preheat a grill pan or an outdoor grill over medium-high heat. Coat lightly with 1 tablespoon olive oil.

3. While the grill is heating, cut the polenta crosswise into 12 slices and pat dry with a paper towel (this will help achieve those pretty grill marks more quickly).

4. Arrange polenta slices in the grill pan or on the grill, and cook until dark grill marks appear, 6 to 8 minutes, then turn over and cook for 6 to 8 minutes more.

5. While the polenta is grilling, wash and dry the basil, then stack the leaves flat on top of each other. Roll the stack like a cigar, then slice thinly—you'll end up with thin, pretty strips of basil. Add to the salad.

6. Put 3 slices of the polenta on each plate. Top with the salad, and serve.

MAKE BABY FOOD: All that prep makes for perfect finger food! Just cut the cheese into bits before feeding to baby. (If your baby finds tomatoes too acidic, leave them out.) Polenta logs are fantastic for young eaters. Take a slice or two off the grill a few minutes sooner, before the grill marks get really dark, and cut into sticks.

### MAMA SAID
"OMG it was good! Everything was great, easy, no issues. The baby loved the little cut-up bits of everything. He's a huge peach fan now." —Maggie K., mom of two, Pleasantville, NY

# ROASTED VEGETABLE LASAGNA

**Serves 6 to 8**

This is always the most popular dish in my cooking classes. It tastes so decadent and yet is so healthy, and my students are amazed that they're able to prepare something this impressive with a baby on board.

2 medium zucchini, quartered lengthwise and chopped into ¼-inch pieces

1 medium eggplant, skin on, chopped into ½-inch pieces

4 ounces cremini mushrooms, thickly sliced, optional

1 medium red bell pepper, chopped into ½-inch pieces, optional

2 to 3 tablespoons olive oil

Salt and pepper

2 cups ricotta cheese (part-skim or whole milk)

1 egg, beaten

1 teaspoon dried oregano

One 25-ounce jar best-quality prepared pasta sauce

One 8- or 9-ounce box oven-ready lasagna noodles

1 cup frozen chopped spinach, not thawed

3 cups shredded mozzarella cheese (part-skim or whole milk)

## STAGE 1 (35 minutes)

1. Preheat oven to 425°F, and set racks to upper and lower levels. Line or grease two baking sheets.

2. Chop the zucchini and eggplant and the mushrooms and pepper, if using, and spread on the sheets in a single layer. Drizzle with the olive oil and season with salt and pepper.

3. Roast vegetables for 12 minutes. Stir, then rotate baking sheets, and roast for another 12 minutes.

4. Remove from oven and set aside (no need to refrigerate).

## STAGE 2 (15 minutes)

1. Combine the ricotta, egg, and oregano in a medium bowl and set aside.

2. Grease a 9 x 13-inch baking dish. Spread about 1 cup pasta sauce in the bottom of the baking dish. Cover with 4 noodles, overlapping them slightly. They don't need to reach the edges of the pan since they'll expand during baking.

3. Top with half of the ricotta mixture, then half of the roasted vegetables, half of the spinach, and about ¾ cup of sauce. Sprinkle with 1 cup mozzarella.

4. Repeat with 4 more noodles, the remaining ricotta mixture, the remaining vegetables, another ¾ cup of sauce, and another cup of mozzarella.

5. Top with 4 more noodles (you will have a few noodles left over), the remaining sauce, and remaining 1 cup mozzarella. Cover with aluminum foil and refrigerate.

## STAGE 3 (1 hour 15 minutes, 15 minutes active)

**NOTE:** These baking instructions are for Ronzoni brand no-boil noodles. If you're using Barilla or another brand, read the instructions on the box. Each brand calls for slightly different oven temperatures and cooking times.

1. Preheat oven to 350°F. Remove the baking dish from the fridge and let it sit on the counter while the oven heats.

2. Bake, covered, for 30 minutes.

3. Remove the foil and bake an additional 10 to 15 minutes, until the cheese is bubbling and lightly browned. Remove from oven and let sit 5 to 10 minutes before serving.

MAKE BABY FOOD: Serve this cut up as finger food, or puree.

**MAMA SAID**
**"This worked perfectly and was really delicious. I would never have thought to roast mushrooms, but they were great!" —Beth P., mom of one, Los Angeles, CA**

## OTHER USES FOR ROASTED VEGETABLES

Roasted vegetables are just about the best way I know to put naptime to good use. The basic technique remains the same, no matter the variety: Preheat oven to 425°F. Cut vegetables into uniform chunks (but go smaller with hard vegetables, like carrots or potatoes, to keep the cooking times equal), toss with olive oil, salt, and pepper, and roast on a baking sheet for about 25 minutes, stirring things around halfway through. And once that's done, you can use those meltingly sweet morsels in myriad ways:

- **Quesadillas:** Put a tortilla into a dry skillet over medium-high heat. Add shredded Cheddar or Jack cheese, and scatter roasted vegetables on top. Cover with a second tortilla. Cook until the cheese melts and the bottom tortilla begins to brown, then flip and cook the other side. Serve with salsa and sour cream. If you've got large tortillas, leftover rice, and a can of black beans, roll everything into burritos instead.

- **Pasta:** In addition to the lasagna and cauliflower-and-fig pasta recipes in this chapter, it's super-simple to make an impromptu pasta primavera with roasted vegetables. Roast some unpeeled garlic cloves with the veggies, and save some of the pasta cooking water. Once your pasta's drained, return it to the pot over low heat, dump in the roasted vegetables (squeeze the garlic out of the skins), and stir. Add reserved cooking water until it looks saucy. Serve with grated Parmesan cheese. Even easier: Doctor some good-quality jarred sauce with a cup or two of roasted vegetables.

- **Soup:** My Roasted Vegetable Beef Barley soup is well worth the effort, but if you're really pressed for time, transform roasted vegetables into a simple pureed soup. You can use just one type of vegetable, like butternut squash, or a mixture of your favorites. Simmer the roasted vegs for a few minutes in a quart of low-sodium broth—chicken, vegetable, whatever—with a bay leaf tossed in. Remove the bay leaf, then puree the whole thing in a blender or food processor (be careful when pureeing hot liquids). Sprinkle your favorite grated cheese on top, cut up some crusty bread, and dinner's ready.

- **Pizza:** Buy some pizza dough from your favorite pizzeria (they'll sell it to you, just ask!) and roll it out. Transfer to a baking sheet and top with jarred sauce, shredded mozzarella, and roasted vegetables; bake in a hot oven (450° to 500°F) for 10 to 15 minutes.

- **Ravioli:** For this one you'll need wonton wrappers, available in the produce aisle of many supermarkets. Use a fork to mash roasted vegetables with some ricotta cheese. Put a spoonful in the center of a wonton wrapper. Dip your finger in water and run it around the edges of the wrapper, then top with a second wrapper and press to seal out all the air. Simmer the ravioli gently in a little water or chicken broth for about 5 minutes—they're too delicate to boil like regular pasta—and top with your favorite sauce.

- **Panini:** If you've got a panini press (or even a George Foreman grill) you're halfway there. If not, use a grill pan or a skillet. Top one slice of hearty bread with prepared pesto or olive tapenade, roasted vegetables, and mozzarella, provolone, or Fontina cheese. Put another slice of bread on top. If you're using a skillet, place a foil-covered, heavy pan on top of the sandwich, in order to press it evenly. Cook until both slices of bread are crisp and the cheese is melted (flipping halfway through, if using a skillet).

- **Frittata:** Preheat oven to 325°F. Grease a 9 x 13-inch baking dish and set aside. Put 4 egg whites, 3 whole eggs, 2 tablespoons water, 2 tablespoons grated Parmesan, and salt and pepper to taste into a blender and whir for 10 seconds, until foamy. Pour egg mixture into a bowl and add 2 cups roasted vegetables; stir together. Pour into the prepared baking dish and disperse the solids evenly. Bake for 15 minutes. Rotate the dish and bake for another 10 to 15 minutes, until top is firm and lightly golden. Serve warm or at room temperature.

· · · · · · · · · · · · · · · · · · · · · · · · · · · · · · · · · · · · · · · · ·

## MARC MEYER'S LEMONY BROCCOLI AND CHICKPEA PASTA

**Serves 4 to 6**

Marc Meyer is the chef/owner of Cookshop, Five Points, and Hundred Acres, three acclaimed New York City restaurants devoted to fresh, seasonal food. I'm a huge fan, so when I saw this recipe in *Food & Wine* a few years ago, I had to try it. I've made some minor adjustments (less oil, whole-grain pasta), but it's essentially his concoction with Nap-Friendly Cooking techniques applied. And boy, is it good.

2 medium heads broccoli, cut into florets (it's fine to use pre-cut)

5 large garlic cloves, very thinly sliced

One 19-ounce can chickpeas, drained and rinsed

⅓ cup lemon juice (from 2 large lemons)

½ cup plus 2 tablespoons olive oil, divided

Salt and pepper

One 12- to 14.5-ounce box whole-wheat or whole-grain rigatoni or penne

½ teaspoon red pepper flakes

1 cup grated Parmesan cheese

### STAGE 1 (10 minutes)

1. Cut the broccoli, cover, and set aside. No need to refrigerate.

2. Slice the garlic, put in a small bowl, cover, and refrigerate.

### STAGE 2 (20 minutes. If doing in two sessions combine with Stage 3; remove the broccoli from the boiling water with a slotted spoon, then cook the pasta in that same pot)

1. Bring a large pot of salted water to a boil (covered to speed things up). While you wait for it to boil, combine the chickpeas with the lemon juice and ½ cup of the olive oil in a medium bowl. Season with salt and pepper to taste, and set aside (no need to refrigerate).

2. Add the broccoli to the boiling water and cook until just tender, about 4 minutes. Drain in a colander and rinse under cold water until cool. Drain well again, put in a bowl, cover, and refrigerate.

### STAGE 3 (35 minutes)

1. Bring another large pot of salted water to a boil, and cook the pasta according to package directions. Drain while it is still quite al dente.

2. Remove the garlic and broccoli from the refrigerator. Heat the remaining 2 tablespoons olive oil in a large, deep nonstick skillet over medium heat. When it shimmers, add the garlic and red pepper flakes and cook, stirring, until the garlic is golden but not browned, about 2 minutes.

3. Add the broccoli and cook until tender, about 5 minutes. Add the chickpea mixture and cook until heated through, 1 to 2 minutes.

4. Drain the pasta, reserving ¼ cup of the cooking water. Add the pasta and the reserved cooking water to the skillet, and season with salt and pepper to taste. Cook over medium heat, stirring, until the pasta is coated with a light sauce.

5. Remove from heat and stir in half of the Parmesan cheese—the cheese will melt and become part of the sauce. Serve topped with the remaining Parmesan.

MAKE BABY FOOD: If you're on purees, leave several broccoli florets in the pot for a few minutes longer, until they're fully cooked, and puree with some plain pasta, a handful of chickpeas, and some olive oil or cooking water—or if you know your baby likes lemon, go ahead and puree the finished dish. For finger foods, leave out the red pepper flakes. Chop the broccoli and pasta and mash the chickpeas lightly with a fork to prevent choking. If he finds lemon too acidic, reserve some of the cooked broccoli, the plain rinsed chickpeas, and the pasta, chop it all roughly, and toss with olive oil.

**MAMA SAID**
"This recipe is a staple around here, ever since it appeared on your blog. We've found that the leftovers are great cold. I try to plan ahead, and grate a little more Parmesan and drizzle a little more lemon juice over it before it goes into the fridge, and then it's ready to go. Our two-year-old inhales the pasta, tastes the broccoli, and won't touch the chickpeas. She used to eat them, but has gone decidedly anti-bean." —Michelle P., mom of two, Kirkland, WA

• • • • • • • • • • • • • • • • • • • • • • • • • • • • • • • • • • • •

# PASTA WITH ROASTED CAULIFLOWER, FIGS, AND MINT

**Serves 4**

This recipe has ingredients that might leave you scratching your head: Cauliflower, figs, anchovy paste, and mint, all in one dish? Trust me, if you set aside your skepticism, you'll be rewarded with a meal filled with sweetness, heat, and *umami* (a fancy word for "savoryness"), a satisfying, almost-vegetarian main course that's perfect for a chilly night. Leave out the anchovy paste for a truly vegetarian version.

1 medium head cauliflower, cored and separated into small florets

A good handful of fresh mint, finely chopped

1 tablespoon finely chopped fresh rosemary

3 tablespoons olive oil, divided

Salt and pepper

10 small dried figs, chopped (I like Mission figs, but any will do)

2 tablespoons pine nuts, toasted

3 large garlic cloves, minced

½ teaspoon anchovy paste

½ teaspoon red pepper flakes

One 12- to 14.5-ounce box whole-wheat or whole-grain pasta of your choice

## STAGE 1 (45 minutes, 15 minutes active)

1. Preheat oven to 425°F. Line or grease a baking sheet.

2. Cut the cauliflower and chop the mint and rosemary separately. Put the mint in a small bowl and refrigerate, covered.

3. Toss the cauliflower in a large bowl with 1 tablespoon olive oil, the rosemary, and salt and pepper to taste. Spread on the prepared baking sheet in a single layer, and roast for 20 minutes. Stir, then roast an additional 15 minutes. Remove from oven and cover loosely; no need to refrigerate.

4. While cauliflower is roasting, chop the figs and put in a small bowl. Add ½ cup boiling water, cover the bowl, and set aside. Mince the garlic and refrigerate in a small covered bowl.

**STAGE 2 (10 minutes. If doing in two sessions combine with Stage 3.)**

1. Toast the pine nuts in a dry, large nonstick skillet over medium heat, shaking the pan frequently, until golden brown. Watch closely; they go from brown to burned in a heartbeat. Remove from pan and set aside; no need to refrigerate.

2. Add the remaining 2 tablespoons olive oil to the skillet. When it shimmers, add the minced garlic and cook, stirring, until fragrant, about 30 seconds. Add the anchovy paste and break it up with the back of a spoon. It will dissolve into the garlic and oil. Stir in the red pepper flakes.

3. Pluck the figs from the bowl and add to the skillet, along with a tablespoon or two of the soaking water (reserve remaining soaking liquid). Cook until liquid in pan has almost evaporated.

4. Combine fig and cauliflower mixtures and set aside (no need to refrigerate). Reserve remaining fig soaking water, separately.

**STAGE 3 (25 minutes)**

1. Bring a large pot of salted water to a boil and cook the pasta according to package directions.

2. Once the pasta goes into the water, put the cauliflower and figs in a skillet large enough to eventually hold the pasta too. Add most of the mint (reserve about 1 tablespoon) and cook over medium-low heat. Add a splash of the reserved fig soaking water if it looks dry. Remove sauce from heat if the pasta's not ready yet— this shouldn't look super-saucy, but you don't want it to be dry, either.

3. Before draining the pasta, reserve ½ cup of the cooking water. When the pasta is cooked to your liking, drain (it's OK if it's still fairly wet) and add to the skillet.

*If your skillet isn't big enough to hold everything, finish preparing the dish in the pasta-cooking pot instead.*

4. Stir everything together and cook over low heat, adding more of the fig soaking water and/or pasta cooking water as needed, until a light sauce forms.

5. Serve with the toasted pine nuts and reserved mint sprinkled over each bowl.

MAKE BABY FOOD: Leave out the red pepper flakes until you remove baby's portion, and if there are food allergies in your family skip the pine nuts, too. If you're on purees, you've got choices: Reserve some of the cauliflower and puree it with some of the plumped-up figs, plain pasta, and a splash of the fig water, or puree the entire dish. For finger foods, the entire dish can be safely served to a baby—just chop the pine nuts to avoid a choking hazard.

**MAMA SAID**

"This was a great pasta dish. I love the earthiness and the unusual pairing of fresh mint and sweet fig with the anchovy paste. I really liked how healthy this pasta is while also having flavors that offer a special treat. This did take time, and was a little complicated, but we had a lot of leftovers to eat throughout the week, so I didn't mind spending extra time to prepare it. Delicious!" —Heather M., mom of two, Los Gatos, CA

. . . . . . . . . . . . . . . . . . . . . . . . . . . . . . . . . . . . . . . . . .

# INDIAN-SPICED BLACK LENTIL STEW

**Serves 6**

Black lentils are sometimes labeled "Beluga" lentils, because they look a lot like caviar. They hold their shape beautifully and don't seem to get mushy, ever. You'll find them in most large supermarkets, specialty stores, and health-food stores.

1 small onion, finely chopped

2 garlic cloves, minced

1 small sweet potato, peeled and chopped

1 large or 2 small carrots, peeled and chopped

2 celery ribs, chopped

2 tablespoons olive oil

1 tablespoon garam masala

1 tablespoon ground cumin

1½ teaspoons ground ginger

¼ teaspoon cayenne

1½ cups black lentils

6 cups low-sodium chicken or vegetable broth

Salt

Cooked couscous or brown rice, for serving

**STAGE 1 (15 minutes)**

1. Prepare all of the vegetables.

2. Put the onion and garlic into a bowl, cover, and refrigerate.

3. Combine the remaining vegetables into another bowl, and measure spices into a third. Cover both (no need to refrigerate).

## STAGE 2 (10 minutes)

1. Heat the oil over medium-low heat in a large, heavy pot or Dutch oven. When it shimmers, add the onion and garlic and cook, stirring frequently, until onion is nearly translucent, about 5 minutes.

2. Add the sweet potato, carrot, and celery, and cook until the vegetables begin to soften, 4 to 5 minutes.

3. Sprinkle the spices over all, stir, and cook for another 30 seconds. Cover and remove from heat (no need to refrigerate).

## STAGE 3 (30 to 40 minutes, 10 minutes active)

1. Sort through the lentils and remove any debris. Rinse the lentils.

2. Return pot to a medium-low flame, and when it's warmed up add the lentils.

3. Pour in the broth and bring to a boil. Lower heat and simmer, covered until the lentils are cooked through but still have a hint of bite, 20 to 30 minutes. Add salt to taste about 5 minutes before the end of the cooking time.

4. Serve over couscous or brown rice.

**NOTE:** This will thicken as it sits, so you may need to add a little more water or broth when reheating.

MAKE BABY FOOD: This one's ready go to as-is; either pureed or as finger food. The cayenne doesn't add much heat, but if you're concerned it's fine to leave it out.

**MAMA SAID**
"I made this recipe with my three-month-old watching me from his bouncy chair in the kitchen and I narrated everything I was doing to keep him interested. My preschooler helped me cook. I figured that, like most stews, it would be better the next day and wow, it sure was! Reheated the next day the flavors melded together and the spices really came out."
—Amber D., mom of two, Woodland Hills, CA

. . . . . . . . . . . . . . . . . . . . . . . . . . . . . . . . . . . . . . . . . . . . .

# CRISPY QUINOA CAKES WITH ROASTED RATATOUILLE

**Serves 4**

Quinoa is terrific for everyone, but it's fantastic for nursing moms—it has all nine essential amino acids so it's a "complete" protein, it's high in iron, and nutritionally it's considered a whole grain. Personally, I don't like the taste of plain quinoa all that much, but when I mix it with Parmesan and pan-fry little patties until they're golden and crunchy, it takes a concerted effort not to eat the whole batch.

**NOTE:** The uncooked patties are quite delicate, so take care when sliding them into the pan and again when turning.

2 tablespoons chopped flat-leaf parsley

1 medium eggplant, skin on, chopped into ½-inch pieces

2 small zucchini, chopped into ½-inch pieces

1 large red bell pepper, chopped into ½-inch pieces

3 plum tomatoes, chopped into ½-inch pieces

1 medium onion, chopped

8 garlic cloves, unpeeled

4 to 6 tablespoons olive oil, divided

Salt and pepper

1 cup quinoa

1 large egg plus 1 egg white, lightly beaten

1 cup grated Parmesan cheese

½ cup low-sodium chicken or vegetable broth

2 tablespoons tomato paste

6 to 8 basil leaves, chopped

## STAGE 1 (40 minutes)

1.  Preheat oven to 425°F. Grease or line two baking sheets.

2.  Chop the parsley, put into a small bowl, cover, and refrigerate.

3.  Prepare the eggplant, zucchini, pepper, tomatoes, and onion and put into a large bowl, along with the garlic. Toss with 2 tablespoons olive oil and salt and pepper to taste, then divide between the baking sheets.

4.  Roast for 15 minutes, then stir the vegetables, and roast for another 15 minutes. Remove from oven, put into a bowl, and cover immediately. (You want a little bit of condensation, which will help keep things juicy later.) Once vegetables have cooled slightly, refrigerate.

## STAGE 2 (35 minutes)

1. In a small saucepan, bring 1¼ cups lightly salted water to a boil.

2. While water is heating, rinse the quinoa well in a fine strainer or sieve.

*If your quinoa package says that it's pre-rinsed, skip this step.*

3. When the water boils, add the quinoa, stir, cover, and reduce heat to low. Cook for 15 minutes, or until almost all the water has been absorbed, then remove from heat. Let sit, covered, 5 minutes.

4. Transfer quinoa to a medium bowl and cool, stirring occasionally, 10 minutes. While it's cooling, put a sheet of wax paper on top of a medium cutting board or tray and set aside.

5. Add the chopped parsley, egg and egg white, and Parmesan to the quinoa, and stir to combine.

6. Coat a ⅓-cup dry measuring cup with cooking spray. Pack solidly with the quinoa mixture, but under-fill just slightly, and unmold onto the wax paper. Repeat with the remaining mixture, leaving a bit of space between each; you should get 8 scoops. Using a spatula, press down gently on the scoops to form 3-inch patties. Cover loosely with plastic wrap and refrigerate.

## STAGE 3 (20 minutes)

1. Heat 2 tablespoons olive oil in a large nonstick skillet over medium heat until hot but not smoking.

2. While it's heating, chop the basil and set aside.

3. With a spatula, gently add the patties. All 8 should fit without crowding—if they don't, cook them in 2 batches. Cook until the bottoms of the patties form solid, golden-brown crusts, 8 to 10 minutes (patties are quite delicate, so don't attempt to turn too soon). You may need to add remaining 2 tablespoons oil.

4. Turn carefully, using two spatulas, and cook until the other side is lightly browned. Transfer to a paper-towel lined plate. If they break in transit don't sweat it—they'll still taste delicious!

5. While the patties are cooking, squeeze the garlic cloves out of their skins and transfer the roasted vegetables to a large saucepan and cook over medium-low heat. Add the

chicken broth, tomato paste, and basil and cook, stirring occasionally, until heated through and lightly thickened. Taste, and adjust seasoning with salt and pepper.

6. Put two patties on each plate, and top with ratatouille.

MAKE BABY FOOD: Texturally, the ratatouille's ideal for babies—you can puree or serve as-is. And quinoa is wonderful for little ones. Either set some aside before you add the egg, cheese, and parsley, and puree along with the ratatouille, or serve a cake as finger food.

**MAMA SAID**
"Awesome! I got 10 patties out of the quinoa mixture, just FYI. My husband and I loved the dish, and my three-and-a-half-year-old daughter ate the quinoa patties dipped in ketchup (which is how she eats most things these days)." —Karen M., mom of two, Barbados

# CHAPTER 3
# QUICK SUPPERS

For me, the hardest part of Harry's infancy was the exhaustion, the bone-melting, please-somebody-carry-*me* exhaustion. First there were the hormones, the physical changes in my body, and, at age 40, my status as an "elderly" mom (yup, that's the medical term). Toss in the fact that you pretty much can't put down a newborn (as a lactation consultant once said to me, "Babies don't *want* to be held. They *need* to be held."), and I felt like Grandma Moses. Or Betty White. Or, you know, a really old lady.

This feeling only intensified when Stephen, my husband, went back to work when Harry was a week old. I'd spend all day with The Boy, mostly just trying to figure out what to *do* with a newborn—which, let's face it, isn't exactly the most interesting phase of childhood. In the beginning, at least, I didn't do a whole lot. I carried him around the apartment, narrating as I went ("And this is your changing table, and here's your mobile . . ."). I bundled him into a sling or his stroller and walked him around the neighborhood. I moved him from his musical swing to his vibrating bouncy seat to his play mat, each of which might buy me as much as ten whole minutes with both arms free. I nursed him, or tried to. I watched him sleep and marveled that this little creature was mine, my son, the thing I'd most wanted for so long.

And then we'd hit the late afternoon, the witching hour. Starting around 5 o'clock, Harry would fuss, squirm, squawk. Even being held didn't please him. It was hell. I see you nodding—you know what I'm talking about. Just about the time when I should've been thinking about making dinner, my sweet pea would transform into a bad seed. That's when I'd start watching the clock, wondering when Stephen would call to say he was on his way, getting irrationally angry with him for not having called yet. That's when I'd fantasize about giving Harry back.

Most nights, by the time Stephen walked through the door the witching hour was over. Lucky him. But I was so wiped out it was all I could do to hand over our now-calm infant and slump into the kitchen. Only then would I troll through the cabinets and pore over the crisper drawers in search of something to make. It had to be easy—I was too tired for anything requiring actual effort. And it had to be tasty—exhausted as I was, my appreciation for good food hadn't left me. If dinner didn't have a bajillion calories, even better.

The recipes in this chapter all satisfy those requirements, deliciously.

What's that? Your baby's already past the witching hour newborn stage? Well, Harry outgrew that phase a few years ago, and I still use these quick recipes regularly. One of them, Hail Mary Pasta, was created in the time it took for Stephen and toddler Harry to walk home from the playground. Turns out, you can never have too many oops-I-forgot-to-plan-dinner options.

**AND DON'T FORGET . . .**

There are quick-cooking recipes in several other chapters in this book:

- Quick Pasta e Fagioli (page 22)

- Quinoa Salad with Chickpeas, Dried Fruit, and Almonds (page 28)

- Tuna and White Bean Salad (page 30)

- Cheater's Chana Masala (page 34)

- Angel Hair Pasta with Garlic and Lemon-Parmesan Breadcrumbs (page 40)

- Spaghetti alla Puttanesca (page 42)

- A Greekish Orzo-Tomato Salad (page 63): Do all the steps consecutively, and you're eating in well under an hour.

- Whole-Grain Pasta with Greens and Beans (page 303)

- Soba Noodle Salad with Tahini-Lime Dressing (page 306)

- Plus just about any recipe in Chapter 7, which is aimed at moms who work outside the home, and Chapter 8, which is aimed at partners and others who can't cook.

## CRIB NOTES

- While I won't play Rachael Ray and promise you a 30-minute meal, in many cases these dishes are ready in about that long. If it takes much longer, like the Butterflied Roast Chicken on page 124 (which is still ready in under an hour), it only requires a few minutes of actual work; the rest is unattended cooking time.

- One way to shave a few minutes off your prep time: Buy pre-cut, fresh vegetables. Most supermarkets carry at least some ready-to-cook options now and many have salad bars; when you're too knackered for knives, that can be a lifesaver. Same thing goes for olives: Buy them already pitted.

- Along those lines, you'll see quite a few recipes in this chapter that call for grape or cherry tomatoes. That's because they're small enough to need very little prep. Many times all you'll have to do is rinse. And, unlike their full-sized cousins, they're tasty year-round.

- Salad is your friend. Think about it: It's pretty hard to make a salad that takes more than half an hour. And if you add a bit of protein, whether it's leftover chicken, canned beans, or hard-boiled eggs cubes of cheese, it can be a meal unto itself. If you're really lucky, you'll have some leftover pasta or couscous to toss in, which will bulk up a salad. (Grandpa's Kitchen Sink Tuna Salad, on page 109, is a great jumping-off point.)

- Keep eggs on hand, and you'll always have the foundation of a quick, healthy meal. Omelets, scrambled eggs, frittatas—whatever the method, eggs cook fast.

- Fish is another reliably fast option. You'll see several recipes in this chapter that call for tilapia. In the Northeast, where I live, American-farmed tilapia is one of the few widely available white-fleshed fish that is sustainable. You can substitute any white-fleshed fish—check the Monterey Bay Aquarium's Seafood Watch site (www.montereybayaquarium.org/cr/seafoodwatch.aspx) for details on what's best to buy where you live.

# CAST-IRON MAC AND CHEESE

**Serves 3 to 4**

**Cooking time: 30 minutes (15 minutes active)**

Mac and cheese can be a time-consuming proposition. My version is on the table in just about 30 minutes total.

The spark for this recipe came from my friend Taryn, who casually combines ingredients without using a particular formula. She goes by feel, adding handfuls of cheese and spoonfuls of flour until the mixture *feels* right. Then she stirs in the cooked macaroni, pours everything into a casserole dish, and runs it under the broiler for a few minutes. The blast of heat creates an instant crust—no need for breadcrumbs.

I've modified Taryn's technique to make things even easier. I prepare the cheese sauce in a large cast-iron skillet, which can safely go under the broiler. It saves on cleanup since there's no casserole dish, and the pan itself makes the dish more nutritious. That's right, cooking in cast iron will actually impart iron to food. Women and toddlers need plenty of that mineral, so it makes this quickie method downright indispensable, as far as I'm concerned.

Since this recipe moves so quickly, make sure you've got everything measured and lined up on the counter before you start.

One 12- to 14.5-ounce box whole-wheat or whole-grain pasta (I like rotini or radiatore, but elbows are nice too)

1 tablespoon butter

1½ cups milk (I use 1 percent)

1 teaspoon dry mustard

½ teaspoon paprika

½ teaspoon salt

2 to 2½ cups (8 to 10 ounces) grated cheese(s) of your choice, divided (the more you use, the cheesier the dish)

4 to 5 tablespoons all-purpose flour

1. Preheat broiler. Bring a large pot of salted water to a boil (covered to speed things up). Heat a large cast-iron skillet (8 to 10 inches across, and 2 inches or more deep) over low heat.

2. When the water boils, add the pasta and cook according to the package directions. Set a timer, since you'll be distracted by the next steps.

*Use a thick potholder with that skillet! Cast iron gets very, very hot. After burning my hand one too many times, I learned to pull a small dishtowel through the hole in the skillet's handle. It serves as a good visual reminder—just be sure it's kept well away from the flame. One of my mom-testers offered another bit of advice: Always use two (potholdered) hands when picking up a cast-iron pan. Otherwise, you might casually try to grab it with your free, bare, hand. Ow.*

3. While the pasta cooks, make the cheese sauce: Put the butter into the now very-hot skillet. It should melt, foam, and begin to brown almost immediately. Pour in the milk, then add the mustard, paprika, and salt, and whisk together.

4. Set aside ½ cup of the grated cheese for topping the final dish. Begin to add the rest of the cheese to the skillet, one handful at a time, whisking between each addition. When it has all melted, sift the flour over the skillet, one tablespoon at a time, whisking after each spoonful. Stop adding the flour when the sauce is almost as thick as housepaint.

*Easiest way to sift small amounts of flour: Use a regular old strainer.*

5. Continue to cook the sauce, whisking constantly, until pasta is cooked. Drain the pasta well and add to the skillet, then remove from the heat.

6. Stir pasta and cheese sauce together until fully combined, then sprinkle the top with the reserved grated cheese. Broil until top is browned and bubbly, 4 to 6 minutes. Cool for a few minutes before serving.

· · · · · · · · · · · · · · · · · · · · · · · · · · · · · · · · · · · · · · · · · · · · · · · · · ·

## VARIATIONS

- Go southwestern by adding a strained 10-ounce can of diced tomatoes and green chiles (such as Ro-Tel) or a generous cup of your favorite salsa, drained. Use Cheddar and Jack cheeses in the sauce.

- Smoke it up by frying 2 diced strips of bacon in the skillet before adding the milk. Skip the butter completely.

- Add 8 ounces frozen vegetables (your choice) to the pasta pot about 5 minutes before pasta is done. Since the water will take a little time to come back up to a boil, increase the cooking time by a minute or two.

- Don't laugh, but a couple of diced hot dogs, cooked in the butter then removed until you stir it back in with the cooked pasta, makes for a surprisingly delicious twist. Use organic, kosher, or even tofu pups.

- Make it secretly healthy by stirring a 10-ounce package of frozen butternut squash puree, defrosted, into the cheese sauce just before adding the pasta.

· · · · · · · · · · · · · · · · · · · · · · · · · · · · · · · · · · · · · · · · · · · · · · · · · ·

MAKE BABY FOOD: I wouldn't give a new eater the crusty bits, but the gooey underneath parts? Yum.

**MAMA SAID**
"Mmmmmmm. I make mac and cheese all the time, but I love your sauce method—totally new for me, and super easy with great results! I used a combo of freshly shredded sharp Cheddar, Swiss, and Parmesan, with a little more Parm and some pre-shredded 'Mexican' Cheddar mix on the top. I loved that the whole thing was done in the time it took to cook the pasta (as did the kids dancing around my feet begging for macaroni and cheese)."
—Sarah B., mom of three, Canterbury, CT

. . . . . . . . . . . . . . . . . . . . . . . . . . . . . . . . . . . . . . . . . . . .

# ZESTY BLACK BEAN, CORN, AND TOMATO SALAD

**Serves 4 to 6**

**Cooking time: 25 minutes (10 minutes active)**

To be perfectly honest, I'm amazed every time I make this salad. So much flavor for so little work! It's great served with baked tortilla chips, crumbled on top of each serving.

**NOTE:** If you've got time, make your own baked tortilla chips following the instructions in the recipe for Chipotle Tortilla Soup on page 21.

### SALAD

3 large ears corn, shucked, or 2½ cups frozen
   corn kernels, defrosted

Two 15-ounce cans black beans, rinsed and
   drained

1 pint grape or cherry tomatoes, halved
   (leave tiny ones whole)

One-quarter medium red onion, minced

1 garlic clove, minced

A large handful of minced flat-leaf parsley
   (about 2 tablespoons)

*This should probably have cilantro in it, but I hate the stuff and it's my recipe, so . . . nope. Of course, when you're making it, go right ahead and use an equivalent amount of cilantro if you like.*

### DRESSING

3 tablespoons fresh lime juice

1 tablespoon rice wine vinegar or other mild
   vinegar

2 tablespoons olive oil

1 chipotle in adobo, minced (scrape out the
   seeds if you want a milder result), plus
   2 teaspoons adobo sauce

Salt

1. If corn is very fresh, cut raw kernels off and add to a large salad bowl. If not, microwave or steam corn for 3 to 5 minutes until crisp-tender. Cool before cutting.

2. Add the beans, tomatoes, onion, garlic, and parsley to the bowl.

3. Put the dressing ingredients in a small air-tight container and shake to combine well (or whisk vigorously in a bowl), and pour over the salad. Stir to combine, and let sit for at least 15 minutes and up to an hour to let the flavors meld.

> MAKE BABY FOOD: Unless your baby's already enjoyed spicy food, the chipotle in the dressing might be a little much. But black beans and corn are wonderful finger foods, so just reserve a little of each before mixing if you want to avoid the spice.

**MAMA SAID**
"Soooo good! Even my husband, who will not touch a bean, had seconds and thirds of this. The dressing is just delicious!" —Kristy P., mom of one, Utica, NY

. . . . . . . . . . . . . . . . . . . . . . . . . . . . . . . . . . . . . . . . . . . . . . . . . . . . . . . . .

### FIVE WAYS TO TURN A CAN OF BEANS INTO DINNER

(Unless you're using unsalted beans, rinse and drain them first.)

1. **Quick Bean Burritos:** Toss warmed red kidney, pinto, or black beans with your favorite salsa. Roll up in a tortilla with lettuce, tomato, shredded carrots, shredded cheese, and chopped avocado. Serve with more salsa and sour cream.

2. **Pasta with White Beans:** Cook the pasta of your choice. While it's boiling, quickly sauté a clove or two of minced garlic for about 30 seconds. Add the drained white beans and chopped sage, rosemary, or thyme leaves and cook until heated through. If you've got baby spinach or arugula around, add a few handfuls of that too. Drain the pasta, reserving 1 cup of cooking water, and combine pasta with the bean mixture. Add as much cooking water as you need to reach a saucy consistency.

3. **Bean and Grain Salad:** Combine a drained can of beans—any kind—with leftover cooked grains like brown rice, bulgur, barley, or quinoa. Add some chopped carrots, cucumber, or any other vegetable. Toss in some chopped fresh herbs if you've got 'em, and the oil and vinegar combo you like best.

4. **Gallo Pinto:** This Latin-American rice and beans dish is as simple as it gets. Sauté chopped onion, garlic, and red bell pepper in olive oil until the onion is translucent and the pepper softens, 5 to 10 minutes. Add equal amounts of cooked white rice and canned black beans, together with enough of the beans' liquid (use unsalted, so you won't have

to rinse) to moisten everything. Toss in some chopped cilantro if there's any on hand. Serve with hot sauce.

5. **Chickpea Salad with Lemon and Parmesan:** This one's courtesy of food blogger Molly Wizenberg, a.k.a. Orangette, and it couldn't be easier. Mix one can of rinsed and drained chickpeas with a squirt of lemon juice, a drizzle of best-quality olive oil, and a handful of grated Parmigiano-Reggiano. Steam some broccoli alongside, and dinner's ready.

• • • • • • • • • • • • • • • • • • • • • • • • • • • • • • • • • • • •

# MONICA'S MONDAY NIGHT POTATOES

**Serves 4**

**Cooking time: 30 minutes (25 minutes active)**

I am lucky enough to be friends with Monica Bhide, author of the wonderful cookbook *Modern Spice: Inspired Indian Flavors for the Contemporary Kitchen.* She is one of the most generous writers I know, always willing to offer advice or assistance. Case in point: this recipe. When I sought her input on my Cheater's Chana Masala recipe (page 34), she sent me her mom's version. It was a bit too complicated for us time-pressed folk, but I asked if she had something simpler that I might use in the cookbook. Monday Night Potatoes was her response.

I realize a pile of potatoes might seem too basic to be terribly interesting, but Monica's way with spices turns spuds into something special. I did wonder about how to serve it, so I went back to her. Monica said, "Believe it or not, I usually serve this on toast. Indians have made an art out of carbs on carbs! My husband likes his toast buttered and this piled on. The kids like it plain. I add some minced cilantro to mine. The key is that the potatoes should be diced small so that the toast can hold them, and things don't fall off."

If Monica's explanation didn't convince you to try this straight up, serve it with a sauce made of plain yogurt, a minced garlic clove, a little curry powder, and some lemon juice.

| | |
|---|---|
| 2 tablespoons vegetable oil | ½ teaspoon red chile powder |
| 1 teaspoon cumin seeds | Salt |
| 4 medium potatoes, peeled and cut into small cubes | 1 large bunch cilantro leaves, finely chopped |
| ½ teaspoon turmeric powder | Water as needed |

1. Heat the vegetable oil in a medium skillet over medium heat. Add the cumin seeds. When they begin to sizzle, add the potatoes and cook until potatoes begin to brown, 5 to 8 minutes.

2. Add the turmeric, red chile powder, and salt to the skillet and cook, stirring continuously, 1 minute. Add the cilantro and cook another minute.

3. Add about ½ cup of water, reduce heat to low, and cook, covered, until the potatoes are tender, 5 to 10 more minutes.

MAKE BABY FOOD: If your baby's OK with a little spice he should enjoy these, either pureed or as-is.

**MAMA SAID**
"I love how few ingredients the recipe required. Also I was really surprised by how quick the recipe was. I was easily able to make it *and* clean up while both boys slept at the same time, which never lasts more than 45 minutes. I like the idea of serving a yogurt dipping sauce with the potatoes. I just mixed yogurt and lemon juice for my older son and he started by only eating the sauce, and finally tasted the potatoes, which he liked too. It could be a great side dish to make a simple dinner of chicken and salad seem a little more elaborate and interesting." —Abigail A., mom of two, New York, NY

# ROASTED CHERRY TOMATOES WITH COUSCOUS

**Serves 4**

**Cooking time: 30 minutes (10 minutes active)**

I'll never forget the first time I tasted a roasted cherry tomato. I was at my friend Will's country house (which is almost as impressive as it sounds; he's got serious style) and we were dining al fresco. The most memorable part of the meal was the simplest: He put a couple of pints of cherry tomatoes into a baking dish along with olive oil, garlic, and basil, then slid the whole thing into a hot oven until the tomatoes burst. They were a brilliant red, goopy, and unbelievably luscious.

I've taken Will's inspiration in a few directions, as you'll see with this recipe and the one that follows, Hail Mary Pasta. This recipe is the lighter of the two, perfect for a summer evening—or any evening, really, when you want something simple, tasty, but not at all heavy.

2 pints cherry tomatoes, stemmed

3 garlic cloves, thinly sliced

A handful of basil leaves, thinly sliced
*The quickest way to do this is to make what's called a chiffonade: Stack up the leaves and roll them into a tight little cigar, then slice thinly. Unroll and you'll have perfect ribbons.*

2 tablespoons olive oil

Salt and pepper

1½ cups couscous, preferably whole wheat

¼ cup pine nuts, toasted

4 ounces goat cheese, crumbled

**Preheat oven to 450°F.**

1. Coat a large baking dish with cooking spray and add the tomatoes, garlic, basil, and olive oil. Toss with salt and pepper to taste. Roast until most of the tomatoes have burst, 12 to 15 minutes.

2. Meanwhile, prepare the couscous according to package directions.

**NOTE:** Most couscous packages call for an equal amount of water and couscous, though sometimes whole wheat requires a little more water. Bring the water to a boil with a little salt, add the couscous, and turn it off to sit, covered, for 5 minutes.

3.  Just before serving, gently combine the tomatoes, couscous, and pine nuts. You don't want to stir too vigorously or the tomatoes will turn to mush. If you like, add a little more of the fresh basil.

4.  Top with the crumbled goat cheese.

> MAKE BABY FOOD: The texture of the cooked tomatoes is certainly soft enough—just pay attention to the skins, as sometimes they're a little tough. Couscous: yes! Goat cheese: certainly! Pine nuts: no, if nut allergies run in your family.

**MAMA SAID**

"Great! Super easy. I loved that it didn't require me to cut very much up. I could pretty much make the whole thing while holding my baby on my hip, which was awesome! It also tasted great—it was warm and refreshing, light yet comforting at the same time. My husband and I both really enjoyed it." —Bethany S., mom of one, Prague, Czech Republic

• • • • • • • • • • • • • • • • • • • • • • • • • • • • • • • • • • • • • • • • •

# HAIL MARY PASTA

**Serves 4 to 6**

**Cooking time: 30 minutes (15 minutes active)**

This was born out of desperation, when I realized that Stephen and Harry were on their way home from the playground and would be expecting dinner, pronto. As long as you cut it into small, quick-cooking pieces, you can substitute almost any vegetable for the zucchini—whatever's in the fridge, threatening to spoil—but don't skip the tomatoes. The sweet juices they release are the base of the sauce.

2 pints grape or cherry tomatoes

2 medium zucchini, quartered lengthwise and
   thinly sliced

3 garlic cloves, thinly sliced

2 tablespoons olive oil

Salt and pepper

One 12- to 14.5-ounce box whole-wheat or
   whole-grain pasta

Grated Parmesan cheese, for serving

**Preheat oven to 500°F.**

1.  Bring a large pot of salted water to a boil (covered to speed things up).

2.  Combine tomatoes, zucchini, garlic, and olive oil in a rectangular baking dish. Season with salt and pepper and stir. Put the dish in the oven before the water boils, if you can manage it. Roast, giving the dish a nearly shake every 5 minutes, until most of the tomatoes have burst, 12 to 15 minutes.

3.  Meanwhile, when the water boils, add the pasta and cook according to package directions, reserving ½ cup of the cooking water.

4.  If you're lucky, the tomatoes will burst before the pasta's done. If not, drain the pasta and put the colander over the pasta pot, then put the pot's lid on top of the pasta to keep it warm.

5.  When the tomatoes have burst, pour a few tablespoons of the reserved cooking water into the baking dish and stir it around, to get all the good stuff off the bottom and sides. Pour the pasta back into the pot, dump in the sauce, and stir. If it seems too dry, add the rest of the reserved cooking water.

6.  Serve topped with the grated Parmesan cheese. Hail Mary.

MAKE BABY FOOD: This one's all good—either pureed or as finger food; the only concern for finger food would be if the tomato skins are too tough for a wee'un. Depending on which pasta you use, you may want to give it a quick chop to prevent the possibility of choking.

**MAMA SAID**
"Oh my goodness, we loved this pasta. The sauce was really nice, not too heavy, not too oily, but tasty and refreshing. My husband is picky, doesn't like vegetables or pasta salads so I was worried that he might not like this. Turns out that he loved it. So, easy, delicious, and healthy." —Monica W., mom of one, St. Louis, MO

· · · · · · · · · · · · · · · · · · · · · · · · · · · · · · · · · · · · · · · · · · · · · · · · · · · · · · · ·

# TWELVE-MINUTE PASTA SALAD

**Serves 6**

**Cooking time: 25 minutes (12 minutes active)**

OK, OK. It's not *ready* in 12 minutes. But it only takes 12 minutes of actual effort, so I'm calling it Twelve-Minute Pasta Salad. It's reminiscent of A Greekish Orzo-Tomato Salad on page 63, only with less cooking and a very different combination of flavors. While that one's heavily Mediterranean, this salad feels like a light and breezy American summer.

**NOTE:** If you're making this ahead of time, add just enough dressing to moisten the pasta, and hold the rest until you're ready to eat. Pasta salad has a tendency to absorb all available liquid, which would leave you with limp, soggy, and yet oddly dry pasta.

3 large ears corn, shucked, or 2½ cups frozen corn kernels, defrosted

1 pint grape or cherry tomatoes, halved (*it's especially good with Sun Gold, those supersweet, orange-yellow cherry tomatoes*)

Your choice of protein: edamame, leftover cooked chicken, tuna, beans, cheese (*bocconcini, those little balls of fresh mozzarella, are fun here*)

6 to 8 large basil leaves, thinly sliced

One 12- to 14.5-ounce box medium-size whole-wheat or whole-grain pasta

¼ cup flavorful extra-virgin olive oil

3 tablespoons sherry vinegar or fruit-infused vinegar

Salt and pepper

1. Bring a large pot of salted water to a boil (covered to speed things up).

2. If corn is very fresh, cut raw kernels off and add to a large salad bowl. If not, microwave or steam corn for 3 to 5 minutes until crisp-tender. Cool before cutting.

3. Add the tomatoes, protein, and basil to the salad bowl.

4. When the water boils, cook pasta according to package directions. Drain in a colander and rinse under cold water (skip this step if you'd like to serve salad warm). Add pasta to the bowl with the oil and vinegar, and season with salt and pepper to taste. Toss and serve.

> MAKE BABY FOOD: Pasta salad makes for some fine finger food. If your baby's OK with the acidity in raw tomatoes, there's nothing here she can't have, as long as everything's chopped into small pieces. NOTE: Never give a little one whole grape or cherry tomatoes—they're a choking hazard.

**MAMA SAID**
**"This was delicious and a big hit with all the eaters around here! I used Barilla Plus penne, frozen corn, teeny grape tomatoes (like the size of my fingernail), and chunks of Cheddar cheese. Super fast and easy to make—did it while the baby was lying on the floor, which doesn't usually buy me much time, what with the big girls and dog trampling over him. Definitely going into the summer rotation!" —Sarah B., mom of three, Canterbury, CT**

· · · · · · · · · · · · · · · · · · · · · · · · · · · · · · · · · · · · ·

# GRANDPA'S KITCHEN SINK TUNA SALAD

**Serves 4**
**Cooking time: 15 minutes**

Most of my happy memories of my grandfather revolve around food. He, not my grandmother, was the cook in the household, and he was prone to improvisation. His most memorable dish was tuna salad.

It was never the same twice. Besides tuna, I'm not sure it had any set ingredients. But it was ambrosial, mysterious, and unpredictable, and I loved it. Grandpa would go into the cupboards and pull canned vegetables and condiments and spices and toss them all in. Sometimes corn niblets, sometimes quartered baby white potatoes, sometimes Veg-all, a canned combo of squishy peas, beans, potatoes, celery, carrots, lima beans, and corn. Caraway seeds. Carrots. Green onion. Pickle relish. Occasionally lettuce. Maybe some mustard. Very little mayo, if he used any at all—I'm pretty sure it was mostly held together by the juices of the various ingredients. To be clear: this is eat-with-a-fork tuna salad, a Jewish Yankee's Salade Niçoise. This does not get slathered on white bread. It gets eaten out of a bowl, with napkin placed firmly in lap.

Grandpa's version is a little, let's say, strange. When I make it, I usually include the following ingredients. Please consider this a jumping-off point for your own tunariffic flights of fancy.

- - - - - - - - - - - - - - - - - - - - - - - - - - - - - - - - - - - - - - - - - - - - - - - - - - - -

### A NOTE ABOUT MERCURY IN FISH

As long as you use *light* tuna, you don't need to stress about mercury—the EPA and FDA recommend that women and young children eat up to 12 ounces of lower-mercury fish (like canned light tuna) each week. Albacore ("white") tuna is higher in mercury, so the limit is 6 ounces weekly.

- - - - - - - - - - - - - - - - - - - - - - - - - - - - - - - - - - - - - - - - - - - - - - - - - - - -

Two 6-ounce cans light tuna in olive oil, drained

A variety of lettuce leaves, torn (I particularly like the combination of Lolla Rossa, red Boston, and romaine)

2 medium carrots, halved lengthwise and chopped

1 cucumber, peeled if it's waxed, halved lengthwise, seeded, and chopped

1 scallion (white and light green parts), chopped

1 to 2 cups cooked couscous, rice, or small pasta

12 to 15 olives, pitted and roughly chopped

6 Peppadew peppers, quartered, or 1 large roasted red pepper, chopped

½ teaspoon caraway seeds

Juice of 1 lemon (about 3 tablespoons)

2 teaspoons Dijon mustard

¼ cup flavorful extra-virgin olive oil

Salt and pepper

1. Combine everything but the last four ingredients in a large bowl.

2. Put the lemon juice, mustard, olive oil, and salt and pepper to taste into a small air-tight container and shake to combine well (or whisk vigorously in a small bowl). Pour over the salad, toss, and serve.

MAKE BABY FOOD: Since this recipe's ingredients are so variable, you'll have to determine what's appropriate for your baby.

**MAMA SAID**

"The tuna salad I grew up with was very WASPy stuff—tuna, mayo, pickle relish, and occasionally, if we were getting exotic, some chopped celery. This was really different, in a good way. I love a recipe that can absorb bits and bobs of leftover good things from the fridge. I added capers because I love tuna with capers and I had an almost-empty jar to use up. I think slivered almonds or dried currants might be interesting additions too." —Beth P., mom of one, Los Angeles, CA

· · · · · · · · · · · · · · · · · · · · · · · · · · · · · · · · · · · · · ·

# FISH NIÇOISE

**Serves 2**

**Cooking time: 35 minutes (25 minutes active)**

I love the Mediterranean flavors of this dish. If you have a skillet large enough to hold everything the recipe doubles well, though it may take a few minutes longer for the sauce to reduce.

Two 6-ounce tilapia fillets (or any other white-fleshed fish)

Salt and pepper

1 tablespoon olive oil

1 fennel bulb, stalks trimmed and discarded, halved vertically, cored, and sliced as thinly as possible
*If you want to get fancy, reserve some of the fennel fronds and use them to garnish the final dish.*

1 garlic clove, minced

½ cup dry white wine or vermouth

One 14.5-ounce can diced tomatoes, with juice

¼ cup chopped, pitted Niçoise or other brine-cured black olives
*Save time by buying pitted olives.*

2 tablespoons capers, rinsed and drained

2 tablespoons thinly sliced basil leaves
*The quickest way to do this is to make a chiffonade: Stack up the leaves and roll them into a tight little cigar, then slice thinly. Unroll and you'll have perfect ribbons.*

Lemon wedges, for serving

1. Season both sides of the fish with salt and pepper and set aside.

2. Heat the olive oil in a large, nonstick skillet (that can be covered) over medium heat. When it shimmers, add the fennel, season lightly with salt and pepper, and cook until fennel starts to brown, 8 to 10 minutes.

3. Add the garlic and cook until fragrant, about 30 seconds. Add the wine and raise heat to medium-high. Simmer until wine reduces slightly, about 2 minutes.

4.  Add the tomatoes along with their juice. Simmer until the sauce thickens and the fennel is soft, 6 to 8 minutes.

5.  Reduce heat to medium-low. Stir in the olives and capers. Add the fish, nestling it into the sauce. Cover skillet and simmer until fish is opaque all the way through, 8 to 10 minutes.

*Fish overcooks quickly, so watch carefully. For fillets thinner than one inch, check at the 7-minute mark. If the fish is opaque, it's done.*

6.  Gently stir basil into the sauce, and serve with lemon wedges.

> MAKE BABY FOOD: This is fine for babies, either pureed or cut up—the only thing to give you pause is the alcohol. Much of it cooks off, but since the cooking time is relatively short there will still be some remaining in the sauce. For the record, fennel, olives, and capers were among Harry's favorite foods when he was about eight months old.

**MAMA SAID**
"Super easy and super delicious. I had never chopped fennel or cooked with Niçoise olives or capers before, even though I've eaten all of those things plenty of times, so it was a big success for me. And cooking fish, well I *never* do that right, except I did this time, and it was so easy!" —Lee P., mom of two, Pittsburgh, PA

- - - - - - - - - - - - - - - - - - - - - - - - - - - - - - - - - - - - - - - - - - - - - - - - - - -

### MAKE IT FASTER

An even quicker version of this dish is Spicy Sauteed Fish with Olives and Grape Tomatoes, which is ready in under 20 minutes: Salt and pepper the fish, then cook in about two tablespoons of olive oil for 3 minutes on each side. Transfer to a platter and keep warm. Add ¼ cup chopped fresh basil, ½ teaspoon red pepper flakes, 1 pint grape tomatoes, halved, ¼ cup chopped, pitted Niçoise or Kalamata olives, 3 garlic cloves, minced, and the grated zest and juice of ½ lemon to the pan and cook until the tomatoes are soft and juicy, about 3 minutes. Season the sauce with salt and pepper, then spoon over the fish and serve with rice to catch all those delicious juices.

- - - - - - - - - - - - - - - - - - - - - - - - - - - - - - - - - - - - - - - - - - - - - - - - - - -

# BAKED FISH WITH ARTICHOKES AND OLIVES

**Serves 4**

**Cooking time: 30 minutes (20 minutes active)**

If this were, say, the 1950s, I'd probably write something like, "This is perfect for those times when hubby calls to say he's bringing his boss home for dinner—and they'll be there in half an hour!" But since we're in a whole different century, I'll say that it's perfect for nights when you come home from work exhausted, but you've invited the neighbors over and you need something quick and elegant to serve them.

Four 6-ounce tilapia fillets (or any other white-fleshed fish)

Salt and pepper

1 tablespoon olive oil

3 garlic cloves, thinly sliced

1 medium shallot, finely chopped

Two 9-ounce packages frozen artichoke hearts, defrosted

¾ cup dry white wine or vermouth

1 tablespoon finely chopped rosemary

⅔ cup chopped, pitted Kalamata or other brine-cured black olives

Lemon wedges and cooked rice, for serving
*Start cooking a bag of Success rice when you turn on the oven, and it'll be ready with time to spare.*

**Preheat oven to 425°F.**

1.  Grease a baking dish large enough to hold the fish in 1 layer, and lay the fish inside it. Season with salt and pepper.

2.  Heat the oil in a medium nonstick skillet over medium heat. When it shimmers, add the garlic and shallot and cook, stirring frequently, until softened, 2 to 3 minutes.

3.  Add the artichoke hearts, season with salt and pepper to taste, and cook just until heated through, 2 to 3 minutes.

4.  Add the wine and raise the heat to medium-high. Let it bubble away until wine evaporates slightly, 5 to 8 minutes, then stir in the rosemary and olives.

5.  Pour artichoke and olive sauce over the fish. Bake fish for about 15 minutes. To test for doneness, stick a fork in the thickest part of the fish and pull slightly. If the center of the fish is opaque all the way through, it's ready.

6.  Serve the fish immediately with the lemon wedges and rice.

MAKE BABY FOOD: There is alcohol in this dish; most of it will have cooked off, but it's your call whether to serve the sauce to your baby. The fish, yes. The olives, yes. The artichokes, not so much—they can be difficult for little eaters to chew. If you're on purees, though, by all means include some in the food processor.

**MAMA SAID**

"This smelled soooo good! It was definitely quick and impressive. I put everything through the food processor, which made it go even faster—garlic and shallots, then olives. My eldest said it 'smelled like hot dogs,' which is pretty much her highest praise." —Anita J., mom of two, San Ramon, CA

## HONEY-SOY ROASTED SALMON

**Serves 4**

**Cooking time: 35 minutes (5 minutes active)**

You've got to love a marinade with only three ingredients. I serve this with rice and something green and steamed—think broccoli, bok choy, snow or sugar snap peas, or spinach. If you enjoy a saucy fish (sounds like a British come-on, doesn't it?), double the marinade ingredients.

⅓ cup honey

¼ cup reduced-sodium soy sauce

1 teaspoon Sriracha sauce or other Asian chili sauce, or to taste

Four 6-ounce salmon fillets, skinned
*Ask the fishmonger to skin the fish for you. Or, if you like the skin, leave it on!*

Cooked rice and a green vegetable, for serving

**Preheat oven to 450°F.**

1. Whisk together the honey, soy sauce, and Sriracha in a shallow bowl. Add the salmon, turning to coat, and marinate for 20 minutes at room temperature, and up to 1 day refrigerated.

2. Grease a baking dish large enough to hold the fish in 1 layer. Remove salmon from the marinade and arrange in the dish (skin-side down, if you've left it on). Reserve marinade.

3. Roast fish just until it's opaque all the way through, 12 to 14 minutes.

4. While the fish is roasting, pour the reserved marinade into a small saucepan and bring to a boil. Cook until thickened, 4 or 5 minutes. (Watch carefully or you'll wind up with something akin to tar.)

5. Serve the fish with the rice and a green vegetable, and pass the sauce separately.

> MAKE BABY FOOD: Salmon, with all that omega-3 goodness, is great for babies. However, due to botulism fears, honey is a no-no for the under-one set. Set aside a small piece of salmon before marinating and bake that separately for your baby.

**MAMA SAID**
"Delicious! I *loved* the honey flavor, and everyone else agreed. One trick I learned with a similar recipe: I buy double the amount of salmon, combine half with a batch of marinade and put it straight into the freezer, and then make the other half. A couple weeks later, the second half marinates while it thaws, and voilà, that second batch is even faster (if possible) than the first." —Ariella M., mom of two, Brookline, NH

· · · · · · · · · · · · · · · · · · · · · · · · · · · · · · · · · · · · · · · · · · · · · ·

# SWEET AND SOUR CHICKEN

**Serves 4 to 6**
**Cooking time: 35 minutes**

If you're expecting deep-fried chunks of chicken in a gelatinous sauce, think again. This is a quick stir-fry that's reminiscent of the Chinese restaurant classic, but lighter and healthier. As with most stir-fries, the most time-consuming part here is the prep; once you've got your ingredients chopped, measured, and lined up next to the stove in order of use, you'll be at the dinner table in less than 15 minutes.

**NOTE:** Since the garlic, ginger, and bell peppers all go into the pan together, it's fine to combine them in one prep bowl. Saves on cleanup later! And if you don't have any pre-cooked rice in the house (or the time to make some from scratch), pick up a container of rice at any Asian takeout restaurant.

1 egg white

3 teaspoons cornstarch, divided

1 pound boneless, skinless chicken breasts, cut into bite-size pieces

One 8-ounce can pineapple chunks in juice, drained and juice reserved
*The recipe will work with fresh pineapple, but the taste will be sharper and more astringent. In this instance, I prefer canned.*

1 tablespoon dark brown sugar
*Make this easier for next time by quadrupling the sauce ingredients. Store the excess in a sealed container in the fridge and it'll stay good for weeks. It's math, I know; sorry—use a generous half-cup of sauce each time.*

2 tablespoons reduced-sodium soy sauce

2 tablespoons rice wine vinegar (cider or balsamic work too)

1 tablespoon dry sherry

2 to 3 tablespoons vegetable oil

2 garlic cloves, minced

1½ teaspoons grated ginger
*Keep a knob of ginger in the freezer, tightly wrapped, and you'll always have some on-hand. Frozen ginger grates more easily too.*

2 bell peppers, any color, chopped into 1-inch pieces

½ cup unsalted cashews

Cooked brown or white rice and sliced scallions (optional), for serving

**NOTE:** I set aside the tenders when I'm preparing a chicken cutlet dish like Sauteed Chicken in Mushroom Sauce (page 118), cut them up, and put them in a small resealable freezer bag that's labeled "for stir-fry." Defrost in a pan of cold water for 30 minutes, and it's good to go. You can also buy the tenders separately, and they'll only need a few cuts to be bite-sized.

1. Combine the egg white and 2 teaspoons of the cornstarch in a bowl large enough to hold the chicken. Add the chicken, stir to coat, and set aside while you prepare the other ingredients.

2. Heat 2 tablespoons oil in a large nonstick skillet over medium-high heat. When the oil is hot but not smoking, transfer the chicken with a slotted spoon and arrange in a single layer (leaving excess egg white mixture in the bowl). You may need to do this in two batches; if so, the second batch may require that additional tablespoon of oil. Cook chicken until lightly browned on each side, about 3 minutes per side. Use a clean slotted spoon to transfer chicken to a clean bowl.

3. While chicken is still cooking, combine ¼ cup of the reserved pineapple juice (discard any remainder) with the brown sugar, soy sauce, vinegar, and sherry in a small bowl, and set aside. Combine the remaining teaspoon of cornstarch with 1 teaspoon water in another small bowl, and set aside.

4.  There should still be a light coating of oil in the pan; if not, add a teaspoon more. Add the garlic, ginger, and bell peppers and cook, stirring frequently, until softened but not browned, 3 to 5 minutes.

5.  Stir in the pineapple chunks, cashews, and pineapple juice mixture and raise heat to medium-high. Boil until slightly thickened, 1 to 2 minutes, then reduce heat to medium and return chicken to the pan. Stir, and if the sauce seems thin, add the cornstarch-water mixture. (If the sauce already looks good to you, just omit it.) Cook until slightly thickened, 1 to 2 minutes.

6.  Serve over rice and top with the scallions, if using.

> MAKE BABY FOOD: There is a teeny-tiny bit of alcohol in this dish from the sherry, but since it's only a tablespoon to begin with, after cooking it's pretty much vapors. Other than that this is fine for babies, either pureed or as finger food—just chop the cashews finely. If there are food allergies in your family, don't feed to baby until your pediatrician says it's OK, or skip the nuts entirely.

**MAMA SAID**
"My family loved the sweet and sour chicken recipe! It really was a quick dinner. I couldn't find any 8-ounce cans of pineapple, so I got a can twice as large and used half of it. It worked out well because the kids loved the pineapple and ate the remainder before I had finished cooking dinner. I used my rice cooker to make rice in the same amount of time it took to cook the meal. There were lots of leftovers, and it tasted great for lunch the next day." —Laura P., mom of two, Colorado Springs, CO

# SAUTEED CHICKEN IN MUSHROOM SAUCE

**Serves 4**

**Cooking time: 40 minutes**

All cooks should have a dish like this in their repertoire: It's simple, it's quick, and the results are impressive enough for company. I like to serve it with rice or couscous (Israeli couscous is especially nice) to soak up the sauce.

**NOTE**: Sherry gives the sauce a wonderful nuance, but if you don't have any use white wine or dry vermouth instead. It won't be quite the same, but it will still be lick-the-plate good.

3 tablespoons all-purpose flour

½ teaspoon sweet or smoked paprika

Salt and pepper

4 boneless, skinless chicken breasts (about 6 ounces each)

2 to 3 tablespoons olive oil

1 pound cremini or white button mushrooms, sliced

*Save time by buying pre-sliced. It's not my first choice, but if it means you cook instead of ordering in, I'm all for it!*

2 garlic cloves, minced, or 1 medium shallot, minced

1 teaspoon fresh thyme leaves, or ½ teaspoon dried thyme

½ cup low-sodium chicken broth

½ cup dry sherry

2 teaspoons honey

2 teaspoons sherry vinegar or red wine vinegar

1 tablespoon butter, optional

1. Combine the flour, paprika, ½ teaspoon salt, and ¼ teaspoon pepper in a gallon-sized resealable bag and set aside.

2. Place each chicken breast between two pieces of plastic wrap and using a meat mallet or the bottom of a heavy saucepan gently pound to an even ½-inch thickness. Add chicken to the resealable bag, seal, and shake to coat all the chicken evenly. (Even easier: ask your butcher to flatten the breasts for you.)

3. Heat 2 tablespoons olive oil in a large nonstick skillet over medium-high heat. When it shimmers, add the chicken (as you pull each breast from the bag, tap lightly to remove any excess flour). You may need to do this in two batches, in which case you'll use that additional tablespoon of the oil for the second round.

4. Cook chicken until it is golden brown and cooked through, about 3 minutes per side. Stick a fork into the meat, and if the juices run clear, it's done. Transfer chicken to a

plate and keep warm. (I usually just stick it in the oven. Even turned off, it'll do the trick.)

5.  Add the mushrooms, garlic, and thyme to the skillet. Season with salt and pepper to taste, and cook, undisturbed, until the mushrooms begin to release their liquid, about 1 minute, then stir. If it seems like your garlic is going to burn, reduce the heat to medium. Cook, stirring occasionally, until mushrooms are lightly browned and most of the liquid has evaporated.

6.  Add the broth, sherry, honey, and vinegar to the skillet, and raise heat to high. Scrape the skillet (use only wooden or plastic spoons on nonstick pans) to make sure all the crusty bits are absorbed into the sauce. Bring to a boil and cook until the sauce is slightly reduced, to a consistency you like, 5 to 8 minutes.

7.  Reduce heat to low. For a richer sauce, stir in the optional butter. Return the cooked chicken to the pan, along with any accumulated juices. Spoon the sauce over the top to coat each piece, remove from the heat, and serve.

MAKE BABY FOOD: There's honey in here, as well as alcohol. Most of the alcohol will evaporate off, but there will still be some remaining. To solve both problems, you can substitute white grape juice or apple juice for the sherry, and leave out the honey.

**MAMA SAID**
"The chicken dish was absolutely delicious; I really enjoyed the sauce. I didn't have any sherry so used white wine and wine vinegar and it was still tasty with those. (As we're big garlic fans I used both garlic and shallot, which was also tasty.) Honestly, this was good enough to go into our old favorites/standby list." —K.L.Z., mom of one, Cambridgeshire, UK

- - - - - - - - - - - - - - - - - - - - - - - - - - - - - - - - -

# PASTA WITH CHICKEN, ASPARAGUS, AND MUSHROOMS

**Serves 4 to 6**

**Cooking time: 35 minutes**

This is one of those magical "in the time it takes to boil pasta . . ." dishes—as long as you choose a pasta that takes a little while to cook. Super-fast angel hair won't fly here, so go for something with some bite to it like penne or farfalle. Here's how it works:

- Put a pot of water on the stove.
- Prepare the other ingredients while waiting for the water to boil.
- Start cooking the sauce as soon as the pasta hits the water.

Just be sure to have all the sauce ingredients ready before you add the pasta to the water. Once you start cooking, you won't have time to stop!

If your pasta *is* ready before the sauce, drain it and place the filled colander on the pasta-cooking pot. Top it with the pot's lid to keep it hot until the sauce is ready.

1½ pounds boneless, skinless chicken breasts, cut into strips

1 medium onion, halved and thinly sliced

3 garlic cloves, minced

8 ounces cremini or white button mushrooms, sliced
*It's fine to use a package of pre-sliced mushrooms here.*

1 pound asparagus, tough ends snapped off, chopped into 1-inch pieces

8 sun-dried tomato halves, thinly sliced
*If your tomatoes are packed in oil, you'll have no problem slicing them. If not, sometimes*
*they can be a little tough. If that's the case, soak them in hot water for 10 minutes while you're waiting for the pasta water to boil, then drain and slice.*

One 12- to 14.5-ounce box whole-wheat or whole-grain pasta

2 tablespoons olive oil

Salt and pepper

½ tablespoon fresh thyme leaves or ½ teaspoon dried thyme

Juice of 1 lemon (about 3 tablespoons)

Grated Parmesan cheese, for serving

1. Before you start chopping anything, bring a large pot of salted water to a boil (covered to speed things up). Now prepare the chicken and vegetables.

2. When the water boils, add the pasta and cook according to package directions.

3. Heat the oil in a nonstick skillet large enough to hold all the ingredients over medium-high heat. When it shimmers, add the chicken strips without crowding the pan (you may need to do this in two batches, adding a little more oil for the second batch). Season with salt and pepper and add the thyme. Cook, stirring occasionally, until lightly browned and fully cooked, 6 to 8 minutes. Transfer to a clean bowl and set aside.

4. Add the onions to the skillet and cook, stirring occasionally, until softened and translucent, about 3 minutes.

5. Add the garlic and cook until fragrant, about 30 seconds. Add the mushrooms, asparagus, and sun-dried tomatoes. Scoop out about ½ cup of the cooking water from the pasta pot and pour that in too. Season with more salt and pepper.

6. Cook, scraping up the brown bits and stirring every so often, until vegetables are crisp-tender. Return the chicken to the pan and cook, tossing, until warmed through, about 2 minutes.

7. By now the pasta should be done. Drain it and add it to the skillet, along with the lemon juice. Cook, stirring, until the pasta has absorbed some of the liquid and what remains looks saucy.

8. Serve with Parmesan cheese.

MAKE BABY FOOD: If you're on purees, whir the entire dish, including the pasta. The only thing here that might not work for finger food is the sun-dried tomatoes, which can be tough (you be the judge), but they're easy enough to pick out.

**MAMA SAID**
"It was delicious and so easy! I love that this is pretty much a one-pot meal (except for the pot you boil the noodles in)—very little to clean up afterward. My toddler loved it too. Also, it made lots of leftovers, which is a huge bonus in my book!" —Robin M., mom of one, Chicago, IL

• • • • • • • • • • • • • • • • • • • • • • • • • • • • • • •

# BUTTERFLIED ROAST CHICKEN WITH MAPLE-MUSTARD SAUCE

**Serves 4**

**Cooking time: 45 to 60 minutes, depending on the size of the chicken (15 minutes active)**

Roast chicken was my nemesis for years; I tried dozens of techniques and it was always under- or overcooked. But I finally found a foolproof method: Butterfly it first. This simply means to cut out the backbone and flatten the chicken so it (sorta) looks like a butterfly. It takes about two minutes, and it cuts the cooking time substantially. This is a roast chicken you can make on a busy weeknight. I like to serve it with brown rice and steamed green beans.

The oven's high heat makes for quite a smoky kitchen, so turn on the exhaust fan and open some windows before you start.

## FOR THE CHICKEN

2 tablespoons olive oil, plus more for the pan

2 garlic cloves, peeled

Salt and pepper

1 whole chicken (3 to 4 pounds)

## FOR THE MAPLE-MUSTARD SAUCE

1 cup low-sodium chicken broth

2 tablespoons Dijon mustard

1 tablespoon pure maple syrup

1 tablespoon butter, softened

**Preheat oven to 500°F.**

1. Drizzle a generous tablespoon of olive oil into a large oven-safe skillet or roasting pan, spread it around, then set the pan aside.

2. Roughly chop the garlic, then sprinkle ½ teaspoon salt all over it. Holding the flat side of your knife almost parallel to the cutting board with the sharp edge angled down and away from you, repeatedly drag the knife across the mixture to mash the salt into the garlic. You'll wind up with a paste. Mix in as much of the pepper as you like and set the whole thing aside. (If you've got some fresh herbs, feel free to mince them and mix in here.)

3. Place the chicken, breast side-down, on a cutting board, drumsticks pointing at you. Using kitchen shears, cut along one side of the backbone (about half an inch from the center of the back)—go all the way up the chicken, until you've completely freed one side. Now cut all the way up the other side of the backbone. When you're done, you'll be holding the backbone and looking at an inside-out chicken. If you like to make chicken stock (for example, the Overnight Chicken Broth on page 141), save the backbone for later use. If not, discard. Remove and discard any visible gobs of fat from the chicken. (If you want to make this even easier, ask the butcher to butterfly the chicken for you.)

4. Turn the chicken right-side up and push down with the heels of your hands on the meaty part of the breast—you'll hear bones cracking and feel the chicken flattening out. Work your fingers between the skin and the meat to loosen it as much as you can without tearing, then spread the reserved garlic paste underneath the skin, all over the breasts, thighs, and drumsticks (don't sweat it if you can't get it into the drumsticks, just do your best). Rub 2 tablespoons olive oil and more salt and pepper all over the outside of the chicken.

5. Next, using a very sharp knife cut a half-inch slit in the excess skin at the rear end of each breast (the side where the cavity used to be), and tuck the drumstick through the hole. (Be careful not to cut too close to the edge of the skin, or the drumstick might tear through during roasting.)

6. Put chicken, skin side up, into the prepared skillet or roasting pan.

7. Roast about 30 minutes for a 3- to 3½-pound chicken, or about 45 minutes for a 4-pound chicken. The chicken is done when a meat thermometer inserted into the thickest part of the thigh reads 165°F. Let the chicken rest for 10 minutes before carving.

**While it's resting, make the sauce.**

1. Using a soupspoon or a turkey baster, remove as much of the fat as possible from the pan. Heat the skillet or roasting pan on the stove, over medium-high heat. (A roasting pan will likely need two burners.)

2. Add the chicken broth, increase heat to high, and bring to a boil, stirring to release the browned bits. Cook until reduced by half, about 5 minutes, then remove from heat.

3. Whisk in the mustard and maple syrup, then stir in the butter. Taste, and season with salt and pepper if needed. Serve with the chicken.

MAKE BABY FOOD: Roast chicken, especially the dark meat, makes babies happy. Puree, or serve cut into small pieces.

**MAMA SAID**

"Cool! Chicken origami! I have shared your frustration with making the perfect roast chicken and as a consequence I rarely make it. But this came out wonderfully! I was a little intimidated by the butterflying but forged ahead, and it wasn't difficult at all. I loved the maple-mustard sauce. So simple and really satisfying." —Beth P., mom of one, Los Angeles, CA

# WHADDYA GOT FRIED RICE

**Serves 2 to 4, depending on what you pull out of the fridge**

**Cooking time: 30 minutes**

If you've been reading along, you've heard my spiel about how authenticity doesn't matter much to time-pressed cooks—moms or otherwise. This recipe is a perfect example. When I make fried rice, I pull out every vegetable I can find in our fridge. That might mean leftover cooked broccoli, half a zucchini, a couple of carrots, even artichokes. It's endlessly versatile, since you really can use just about any scraps of vegetables and protein you've got handy. This is my master recipe. As long as you add hard vegetables, soft vegetables, and cooked ingredients at their specific times, you can substitute just about anything you like. I've also been known to stop at the local Chinese takeout and buy cooked rice—for a buck or two, it makes this feast even easier. When you get home, spread the rice out on a plate and refrigerate it. You want the rice to be cold, or it may turn mushy.

Another one of my spiels is about mise-en-place, and the need to have all your ingredients prepped and ready to go before you start cooking. It's especially crucial here, since you won't have time to stop and chop once you turn on the burner. Line your ingredients up next to the stove, in order of use. If you're a mom whose kid still naps, this is an excellent candidate for the technique explained in Chapter 2, "Nap-Friendly Cooking." Devote 20 minutes of naptime to prepping the vegetables and leftover protein of your choice. Stow it all in the fridge in individual containers. This will be your mise-en-place come cooking time.

2 tablespoons vegetable oil

1 medium onion, chopped

2 garlic cloves, minced

2 carrots, chopped into ¼-inch pieces
(also good: celery, cauliflower,
broccoli)

3 tablespoons reduced-sodium soy sauce,
divided

½ a medium zucchini, chopped into ¼-inch
pieces (also good: red bell pepper,
mushrooms)

2 cooked boneless chicken breasts, chopped
(also good: steak, tofu, shrimp)
*I especially like to make this with leftover
Polynesian Flank Steak, from page 126.*

A handful of frozen peas

2 to 3 cups leftover brown or white rice

3 to 4 teaspoons toasted sesame oil

1. Heat vegetable oil in a very large nonstick skillet over medium heat. When it shimmers, add the onion and cook, stirring occasionally, until translucent, 3 to 5 minutes.

2. Add the garlic and cook until fragrant, about 30 seconds, then add the carrots or whatever hard vegetables you're using. Cook for 1 more minute, then stir in about 1 tablespoon of soy sauce. Raise heat to medium-high and cook, covered, 2 to 3 minutes. (You're actually steaming the hard vegetables, which will help them cook faster.)

3. Add the zucchini or other soft vegetables, adding another tablespoon of soy sauce or water if it looks like it's going to burn, then cover and cook until zucchini is softened and maybe even a little brown, about 2 minutes. Add whatever already-cooked ingredients you're using, including the protein, rice, and peas—they can all go in at once. Cook until everything is heated through.

4. Season with the remaining tablespoon of soy sauce and drizzle with sesame oil. Stir and taste, adjusting soy sauce and sesame oil until you like the way it tastes.

MAKE BABY FOOD: This will depend entirely on what you have put into it. At the very least, your baby should be able to eat the rice, peas, and some of the softer vegetables.

**MAMA SAID**
"The fried rice was an easy, quick, and perfect family dinner—for my toddler, who happily fed herself everything except the zucchini, for my husband, who doused his in Sriracha, and for me— most of the way through the first trimester with #2, I'm ravenous by the time dinnertime rolls around, and this really hit the spot. We made it with Quorn instead of chicken and added a little pineapple to the basic line-up (my daughter's request), and it was fantastic." —Susan B., mom of one, with a baby on the way, Portland, OR

· · · · · · · · · · · · · · · · · · · · · · · · · · · · · · · · · · · · · · ·

# POLYNESIAN FLANK STEAK

**Serves 6 to 8**

**Cooking time: 40 minutes (10 minutes active)**

I'm not sure if this could be any easier—or tastier. Serve the steak with rice, to catch the sauce, and steamed broccoli.

**NOTE:** Flank steak is prone to toughness; cutting across the grain helps make it more tender. Position the flank steak so the visible lines running the length of the meat are parallel to your body, then cut across.

½ cup pineapple juice
*If you like, use the juice from a can of pineapple rings, then grill or broil the rings alongside the steak.*

½ cup reduced-sodium soy sauce

3- to 4-pound flank steak

1.  Combine the pineapple juice and soy sauce in a large resealable bag or bowl.

2.  Using a sharp knife, score the steak lightly across the grain, several times on each side, and place the steak in the bag with the pineapple juice and soy sauce. Refrigerate at least 30 minutes and up to 8 hours.

3.  Preheat the broiler, a stovetop grill pan (over high heat), or charcoal or gas grill. Remove steak from marinade (reserving marinade) and cook steak for 3 to 4 minutes on each side for medium-rare.

4.  While steak is cooking, bring the remaining marinade to a boil in a small saucepan. Lower heat and simmer vigorously, until reduced, 5 to 8 minutes. Remove from heat.

5.  Transfer steak to a cutting board, cover loosely with foil, and let steak rest 10 minutes before cutting it (I'm not kidding, this really makes a difference).

6.  Thinly slice steak on an angle across the grain. Serve with the reserved sauce.

MAKE BABY FOOD: Flank steak can be chewy so I wouldn't expect a baby to actually *eat* this, but if you give her a strip to gnaw she'll get the juices and flavors. Or you can puree with a bit of broth or water (don't use the sauce, which will be too salty for an infant).

**MAMA SAID**
"Wow, this was a winner at our house. My meat-averse toddler had three helpings! So easy to prepare too. Took the steak out to thaw one morning, mixed it up the next, used a rice cooker for mindless rice making, microwaved a fresh veg. None of it took me away from the kiddos for much time at all so everyone was happy." —Heather B., mom of two, Westmont, IL

. . . . . . . . . . . . . . . . . . . . . . . . . . . . . . . . . . . . . . . . . . . . .

# AMERICAN "CHOP SUEY"

**Serves 4 to 6**

**Cooking time: 40 minutes (15 minutes active)**

There's nothing remotely Chinese about this dish. Ground meat, macaroni, onions, bell peppers, tomato sauce, Worcestershire. . . . It's more like homemade Hamburger Helper, about as Asian as a Twinkie. But one thing it is, is delicious. Filling, comforting, satisfying— and for me, a reminder of my childhood. My mom made this for us regularly when I was growing up, and back then I never questioned its origins. It was just supper. Not a supper anybody I knew had ever eaten, but when you're a kid who stops to think about that?

So imagine my surprise when, with Stephen on our honeymoon, I saw it on the menu at Moody's Diner in Waldoboro, Maine. Turns out it's a New England dish, which makes sense since my mom is originally from Newton, Mass. It's one of those cultural mish-mash recipes from the early 20th century, when the great influx of immigrants was shaking things up in myriad ways.

2 tablespoons olive oil, divided

1½ pounds ground meat (growing up it was plain ol' beef, but now I use either extra-lean ground beef or a combo of ground turkey breast and "regular" ground turkey)

½ pound (about 2 cups) whole-wheat or whole-grain elbow macaroni (uncooked)

1 small onion, finely chopped

1 medium red bell pepper, chopped, or 2 celery ribs, chopped (or a combination)

Two 8-ounce cans tomato sauce

1 cup water

1½ tablespoons Worcestershire sauce

Salt and pepper

1.  Heat 1 tablespoon olive oil in a large, heavy skillet over medium heat (if you're using ground beef, you probably won't need the oil). Cook the meat, breaking it up with the back of a spoon, until browned, 3 to 5 minutes, and remove to a bowl. If using beef, discard any accumulated fat.

2. Wipe out the pan, and add a little more oil. When it shimmers, add the uncooked macaroni, onion, pepper, and/or celery and cook until vegetables are softened, 3 to 5 minutes.

3. Return the browned meat to the pan and add the tomato sauce, water, and Worcestershire sauce. Season with salt and pepper to taste. Bring to a boil, then lower the heat and simmer, covered, until the macaroni is cooked through and the pan looks saucy but not wet, 20 to 25 minutes.

MAKE BABY FOOD: The consistency of this dish should make your baby very happy. It also purees nicely.

**MAMA SAID**

**"This was delicious and quick. I'm definitely adding it to our regular repertoire. I'd made it before but had cooked the pasta separately; this was easier and vastly tastier. And baby loved it, perfect for self-feeding and a balanced meal in one dish. I sprinkled a few cubes of Cheddar cheese on before serving, mmmm." —Martha W., mom of one, St. Louis, MO**

. . . . . . . . . . . . . . . . . . . . . . . . . . . . . . . . . . . . . . . . . . .

# TANGY MINI-MEATLOAVES WITH LOW-FAT MASHED POTATOES AND PAN-ROASTED CARROTS

**Serves 6**

**Cooking time: 50 minutes (35 minutes active)**

Who doesn't love a good meatloaf? Problem is, they're hardly quick—most recipes call for 45 minutes to an hour just for baking. Not exactly what I'm looking for after a long day of working and wrangling Harry.

Mini-meatloaves to the rescue! Smaller portions cook much faster, so once you've got your mixture you're only 20 minutes away from eating. This version uses reconstituted dried mushrooms, which add a nice, meaty moistness, and a glaze of barbecue sauce mixed with mustard. If you're not a fan of that flavor combo, adapt your usual recipe to my mini method. The best part of minis: the leftovers are ideal for freezing.

The potatoes and carrots are optional, but I thought you might like to have a full meal laid out, no thinking required. You're welcome.

## FOR THE MEATLOAVES

½ ounce dried mushrooms (about ½ cup like
    porcini)

1 small onion, peeled and quartered

1½ pounds extra-lean ground beef

1 egg

¾ cup dry breadcrumbs

¼ cup plus 2 tablespoons barbecue sauce,
    divided

*If you're buying jarred barbecue sauce, read
labels carefully. Buy one whose ingredients you
recognize, without high-fructose corn syrup.*

Salt and pepper

1 tablespoon Dijon mustard

**Preheat oven to 425°F**

1.  In a small bowl, cover the dried mushrooms with about 1 cup boiling water. Grease or
    line a baking sheet with nonstick spray and set aside for at least 15 minutes.

**NOTE:** You can add the boiling water to the mushrooms at any point during the day,
even before you leave for work in the morning. No need to wait until dinnertime's
looming!

2.  Pluck mushrooms from the bowl (don't include their soaking water, as it might have
    gritty sediment at the bottom) and transfer to a food processor. Add the onion and
    process until a slightly chunky paste forms (you'll have to scrape down the sides of
    the bowl once or twice).

3.  Transfer mixture to a large bowl and add the ground beef, egg, breadcrumbs, ¼ cup
    barbecue sauce, and salt and pepper to taste.

4.  Mix, gently, with clean hands until combined. Don't be obsessive about it, or the final
    result will be unpleasantly dense.

5.  Divide the mixture into 6 roughly equal portions, each about the size of a softball.
    Arrange on the prepared baking sheet and, using your hands, form each ball into a
    loaf shape, 3 to 4 inches long and 1 to 2 inches high.

6.  Combine the mustard and the remaining barbecue sauce in a small bowl. Spread a
    generous teaspoon of this mixture on each meatloaf.

7.  Bake until a meat thermometer inserted into the center of a mini-loaf reads 160°F,
    20 to 22 minutes.

## FOR THE LOW-FAT MASHED POTATOES

6 large or 12 small Yukon gold potatoes,
  peeled and chopped
1¾ to 2 cups low-sodium chicken broth
1 tablespoon butter

¼ cup to ½ cup milk, warmed (I prefer
  1 percent, and warm it in the microwave for
  30 to 45 seconds)
Salt and pepper

1. As soon as the meatloaves go into the oven, combine the potatoes and broth in a large saucepan. The broth should just cover the potatoes—if it doesn't, add enough water to do so. Bring to a boil over high heat, then reduce the heat to medium-low, and simmer, covered, until a fork pierces the potatoes easily, 10 to 15 minutes.

2. Leaving the potatoes in the pan, carefully drain off most of the liquid into a glass measuring cup and reserve—you'll need some of it in the next step. Add the butter to the potatoes and start mashing.

3. Add some of the broth back to the potatoes, a bit at a time, until the mashed potatoes no longer look dry. At this point, start adding the milk to the potatoes, again a bit at a time, until the potatoes are as creamy as you like them.

4. Taste, and season with salt and pepper.

## FOR THE PAN-ROASTED CARROTS

1 tablespoon olive oil
1 tablespoon butter
6 large or 10 medium carrots, sliced into
  ¼-inch pieces

Salt and pepper

1. Once the potatoes are simmering, heat the olive oil and butter in a large nonstick skillet over medium heat. When the butter stops sizzling, add the carrots and salt and pepper to taste, stir, and cook, covered, until the carrots are tender, 10 to 15 minutes.

2. Uncover, then stir and cook for 3 to 5 minutes more, until all the liquid has evaporated and the carrots are browned.

MAKE BABY FOOD: Your baby can enjoy everything in this meal, either pureed or as finger food.

**MAMA SAID**

"This recipe was great as far as ease and timing. I used the 20 minutes (or so) while the mushrooms were sitting in the water to unload and reload my dishwasher and start peeling potatoes. I loved that the onions and mushrooms were pureed—it was great for my picky husband who hates chunks of veggies. The potatoes were wonderful! As for the carrots, I don't know if I had my temperature too high or what because I burnt these. But even a little burnt they were still delicious—and more importantly—easy. My husband even took a couple from my plate—and he does not eat vegetables. I was amazed and thrilled." —Monica W., mom of one, St. Louis, MO

# CHAPTER 4

# MOM'S NEW BEST FRIEND: THE SLOW COOKER

For years, I scorned the slow cooker. Sure, my mom had been using hers since the '70s, making cholent, an old-world Jewish dish of beans, potatoes, and beef traditionally served on Shabbat, and "Italian" meatballs and sauce, but it always struck me as a way to make dinner with minimal effort, rather than a way to make a meal that actually tasted good. Plus I was a bit of a food snob. During the economic boom of the 1990s, I had a series of jobs running the advertising departments of several book publishers. As the person controlling the ad spending, I was wined and dined at New York's top restaurants. My palate developed, and so did my efforts at home cooking. I took classes at the city's leading culinary school. I baked artisanal bread! I made recipes with fancy French names! A squat, unassuming machine like a slow cooker did not belong on my kitchen counter next to the top-of-the-line chef's knives, convection toaster oven, and KitchenAid stand mixer.

Uh, yeah. Tell that to a new mom who's been living on Clif bars and egg sandwiches (and by that I mean me, circa September 2006). I began to rethink the slow cooker. On AltDotLife.com, the message board I turned to for been-there, done-that parenting advice, slow cookers were something of a religion. Dozens of recipes were posted, and several cookbooks received enthusiastic endorsements. What the heck, I figured. Slow cooking was better than *no* cooking.

About three weeks after Harry was born, my parents stopped by, a ginormous box in my dad's arms. It wasn't another toy for Harry, but a new gadget for me: a fancy-shmancy, stainless steel, programmable slow cooker. And did I mention it was huge? It held six quarts, the second-largest size available. By this point I knew that a slow cooker could find a place in my kitchen, but I was still a little skeptical. Sure, I thought, I could use this new gadget to prepare the old-fashioned meals of my childhood, but would this device deliver the kind of satisfaction I got from standing over the stove? More importantly, would we actually want to eat the food that came out of it?

The first recipe I tried, for ratatouille, erased any doubts about the machine's helpfulness. The ratatouille was juicy and robust, by far the best I'd ever made. A slow cooker's lid seals tightly, so no steam escapes during cooking and all the flavors intensify. And the best part: I'd put it together during Harry's morning nap, added an ingredient or two a few hours later, and just let it happily bubble away all day. You'll find the recipe on page 143.

I was sold, but soon I realized I didn't even need that fancy-shmancy machine. In fact, I found it more trouble than it was worth; in addition to being too big, it ran hot, which led to more than a few overcooked meals. So I bought myself a smaller, simpler machine for less than twenty dollars. That machine still—nearly four years later—gets used weekly. Thanks, Mom.

. . . . . . . . . . . . . . . . . . . . . . . . . . . . . . . . . . . . . . . . . . . . . . . . . . . . . . . .

### SLOW COOKER SAFETY

- Never put frozen food into the slow cooker. I know it's tempting, especially if you're going to be out all day and you'd like to stretch a relatively short cooking time. But it takes too long for the food's temperature to rise from frozen to the safe zone above 140°F—you'd create a perfect breeding ground for bacteria.

- The WARM setting will keep food warm, safely, for up to four hours. Don't push it.

- The slow cooker is *not* a vessel for reheating cold leftovers. The food will be in an unsafe temperature range for too long.

- Unless it's labeled otherwise, the ceramic insert is not intended for use on a stove, either gas or electric. And it's not meant for storing leftovers in the fridge or freezer, either. Quick changes in temperature can crack the insert.

- Following that logic, let the insert come to room temperature before washing. (You can pour in hot water to keep things from getting too crusty, but never add cold water.)

- On the other hand, it *is* safe to put all your ingredients into the insert the night before and refrigerate the entire thing. The slow heating of the machine won't crack the insert. If the insert is coming straight from the fridge, and you're cooking for more than four hours, the overall time won't change. Under four hours, though, you should anticipate things taking up to 30 minutes longer.

- If you come home to find that the power has gone out, don't risk it: Throw everything away. If you're lucky enough to be home when it blows, transfer the food to an appropriate pot and finish cooking on the stove or in the oven.

## BASIC TIPS FOR THE SLOW COOKER

- Resist the urge to open the lid and peek inside. Part of the slow cooker's magic relies on a water seal that builds up around the rim. Breaking that seal lowers the internal temperature. Because the cooker is intended to heat slowly, it can take up to 30 minutes to come back up to temperature.

- That said, you'll see a handful of recipes that call for adding ingredients several hours into the process. In those cases, go right ahead—there's no other choice.

- If, at the end of cooking time, the food isn't cooked to your satisfaction, replace the lid, turn the cooker to HIGH, and check it no fewer than 30 minutes later. (Remember, it can take that long just to heat back up.)

- Vegetables, especially hard ones like carrots and potatoes, cook slower than protein in a slow cooker. Put them nearest the heat source, which is on the bottom and around the sides of the machine.

## CRIB NOTES

- All of these recipes were prepared in my Rival 4-quart oval slow cooker, which has no timer and three settings: LOW, HIGH, and WARM. You really don't need a fancy machine for slow cooking.

- If your machine is smaller than four quarts, you may have to trim back, proportionately, on some of the recipes to make everything fit. Slow cookers perform best between one-half and two-thirds full; never fill a slow cooker more than one inch from the rim.

- Not ready to buy a slow cooker? Most of the recipes in this chapter work in a Dutch oven with a tight-fitting lid, inside a regular oven set very low. Specific instructions are included at the end of each recipe. Please note that using your oven requires you to be home while it's on—according to an expert at the National Fire Protection Association, it's perfectly safe to have the oven on for long stretches, including overnight, but you shouldn't leave the house.

- Whenever possible, these recipes simply call for putting ingredients into a slow cooker and turning it on. None of them call for browning meat, and only a handful ask you to add things to the machine in stages.

- If you're planning to cook on LOW and you'll be around the home, start on HIGH for the first hour of cooking, then switch to LOW. (Set a timer!) It brings the temperature up to a safe level faster.

- Slow cookers vary in their cooking temperatures. Some run much hotter than others, which means your food will be done sooner. You may find that the HIGH setting is just too high, in which case you should stick to LOW. As you use the machine, you'll get to know its idiosyncrasies and adjust times accordingly.

- If you're new to the slow cooker and would like an entire cookbook devoted to the device, I highly recommend *Not Your Mother's Slow Cooker Cookbook* by Beth Hensperger and Julie Kaufman. It's the book that got me started, and I still use it regularly—in fact, it inspired a handful of recipes in this chapter.

• • • • • • • • • • • • • • • • • • • • • • • • • • • • • • • • • • • •

# OVERNIGHT STEEL-CUT OATMEAL

**Serves 2 to 3**

**Cooking time: 8 to 10 hours on LOW (5 minutes active)**

If you're not familiar with steel-cut oats, they're quite different from their quick-cooking or rolled cousins. Quick-cooking oats are whole oats that have been cut into pieces then flattened and flaked, which makes them cook, well, quickly. Rolled oats are left whole but still flattened and flaked; their larger size gives them a hint of chewiness, but they still cook relatively fast. And steel-cut oats have been cut a few times, but that's it. No further processing. This means they're super-chewy (my favorite texture, by the way) and quite filling. But, oy, do they take a long time to cook. Thirty minutes of simmering is *not* my ideal way to start the day. Enter the slow cooker. Before bed you measure water and oats, and set up a nifty little water bath. Lights out, and in the morning: perfection.

Overnight Steel-Cut Oatmeal saved my sanity when Harry was tiny, for a few reasons. First, the pre-bed setup takes less than five minutes, and thanks to that gentle water bath, the timing is remarkably flexible. I've set this up as early as 9 o'clock at night and as late as midnight, and it's creamy every time. Second, it's an absolute pleasure to wake up and find breakfast waiting for me. Third, thanks to the variability of toppings, oatmeal never gets boring. And the fourth and perhaps most important reason (for me, at least, thanks to my breastfeeding problems), oatmeal is a wonderful galactagogue—it helps increase breastmilk supply. (For more recipes using galactagogues, see Chapter 9.)

**NOTE:** I make this in a 4-quart slow cooker, and the largest container I've found that will work within it is a 4-cup measure. If your slow cooker is larger, by all means use a larger bowl and increase proportionately the amounts of water and oatmeal. You'll be able to serve more people or have leftovers, which reheat nicely with a little milk stirred in.

3 cups cold water
1 cup steel-cut oats
Pinch of salt

1. Combine all ingredients in a glass 4-cup measure (or a similar heat-safe bowl that can hold at least 4 cups). Put the measuring cup inside your slow cooker's insert.

2. Carefully add more cold water in the space between the cup and the wall of the insert (you're making a water bath). You want the water level to come up just slightly higher than the level inside the cup; this will keep things creamy, not crusty.

3. Cover and turn the cooker to LOW.

4. Head to bed and when you wake up in the morning, the oatmeal will be ready to serve.

**MAKE IT IN THE OVEN:** I'm not exactly sure of the science behind it, but when you make this in the oven, inside a Dutch oven, the proportion of water to oats must be adjusted to avoid a texture akin to wallpaper paste. Use 4 cups of water for each cup of oatmeal. It will no longer fit in a 4-cup glass measure, but any kind of deep baking dish will work. Bake in a 200°F oven for 8 to 10 hours. Note that it's safe to leave the oven on overnight, but please don't leave your home while it's on.

MAKE BABY FOOD: While oatmeal is often among baby's first foods, it shouldn't be this hearty variety—the type you buy specifically for baby is finely ground and quite thin. Pureed with extra milk, though, this recipe is perfect.

MAMA SAID
"I am never eating quick oats again! Crockpot oatmeal is so creamy and delicious! Instead of using a 4-cup measure (which we didn't have), I used two 1-cup glass measures (each with 1 cup water plus ⅓ cup oats) so we had 2 servings when we woke up. I ate mine with blueberries and milk." —Kristy P., mom of one, Utica, NY

· · · · · · · · · · · · · · · · · · · · · · · · · · · · · · · · · · · · · · · ·

# ITALIAN WEDDING SOUP

**Serves 6 to 8**

**Cooking time: 8 to 10 hours on LOW, 4 to 5 hours on HIGH (30 to 40 minutes active)**

This is a slow cooker recipe for days when you're in and out of your home, because it requires some attention midway through. But oh, is it worth it! And it makes quite a bit, so you'll get several meals out of it. It freezes well too.

3 large carrots, chopped

1 medium head escarole (about ¾ pound), roughly chopped (kale or spinach work well too)

8 cups low-sodium chicken broth

1 Parmesan rind, approximately 2 inches long, optional

1 pound ground turkey breast

⅓ cup dry breadcrumbs

⅓ cup grated Parmesan cheese

1 egg

1 large garlic clove, minced

A large handful of flat-leaf parsley or mint, minced

Pepper

½ cup small pasta, such as ditalini or acini de pepe

Salt and pepper

Grated Parmesan cheese, for serving

1.  Combine the carrots, escarole, broth, and Parmesan rind, if using, in the slow cooker. Cook on LOW for 4 to 5 hours or HIGH for 2 to 3 hours.

2.  When you have the time (about 20 minutes), make the meatballs. Combine the turkey, breadcrumbs, grated Parmesan, egg, garlic, parsley, and pepper to taste in a medium bowl. Mix gently, as ground turkey breast gets tough with too much handling. Shape mixture into mini-meatballs, about ½ tablespoon each. Arrange meatballs on a plate or cookie sheet, mixture should yield 30 to 35 balls. If you make them in advance, cover and refrigerate.

**NOTE:** The Parmesan is plenty salty—don't add any salt to the meatball mixture.

3.  After the soup has cooked for about 4 hours on LOW or 2 hours on HIGH, add the meatballs. Cook for another 3 to 3½ hours on LOW or 1½ to 2 hours on HIGH.

4.  Add the pasta and cook for another 30 minutes (LOW or HIGH), or until the pasta is tender. Taste, and season with salt and pepper.

5.  Serve with the grated Parmesan cheese.

**MAKE IT IN THE OVEN:** Put the carrots, escarole, broth, Parmesan rind, if using, *and meatballs* in a Dutch oven, and cook at 200°F for 6 to 8 hours. Proceed with the recipe from step 4. Do not leave your home with the oven on.

MAKE BABY FOOD: If you're on purees, go ahead and whir together the whole thing. For finger food, babies love meatballs, and the carrots will have the perfect texture. Plus there are little bits of pasta! Make sure the escarole is finely chopped, or it may be too stringy.

**MAMA SAID**
**"We all really liked this one, 14-month-old included. The turkey meatballs were really, really tasty (and we don't do ground turkey that often as I am normally not a fan) and my toddler** *loved* **them. I plan to make a batch just of the meatballs to freeze and thaw for future meals for her." —Dana N., mom of one, Lexington, KY**

. . . . . . . . . . . . . . . . . . . . . . . . . . . . . . . . . . . . . . . . . . . . . .

# MOROCCAN RED LENTIL STEW

**Serves 6 to 8**
**Cooking time: 6 to 8 hours on LOW, 3 to 5 hours on HIGH (15 to 20 minutes active)**

I adapted this dish from one in *Art of the Slow Cooker* by Andrew Schloss. His version is a soup and requires some stovetop pre-cooking. I've kept Schloss' seductive flavors, but transformed the recipe into something heartier (and simpler—just toss in the ingredients and go).

2 large onions, chopped small

2 garlic cloves, minced

1 medium carrot, chopped small

2 teaspoons ground coriander

1 teaspoon ground cumin

1 teaspoon ground turmeric

½ teaspoon paprika

½ teaspoon ground ginger

¼ teaspoon cinnamon

Pinch of cayenne

Salt and pepper

6 cups low-sodium chicken or vegetable broth

1 cup water

One 28-ounce can crushed tomatoes, with juice

1 pound (about 2¼ cups) dried red lentils, sorted and rinsed

2 medium lemons, 1 juiced, 1 cut into wedges

3 tablespoons chopped fresh flat-leaf parsley

1 tablespoon chopped fresh cilantro

Cooked brown rice, for serving

1. Combine the onions, garlic, carrot, spices, salt and pepper to taste, broth, water, tomatoes with juice, and lentils in the slow cooker. Cover and cook on LOW for 6 to 8 hours or HIGH for 3 to 4 hours, until the lentils are almost dissolved.

2. Add the lemon juice, parsley, and cilantro and stir to combine.

3. Serve over brown rice with the lemon wedges.

**MAKE IT IN THE OVEN:** Combine the ingredients up through the lentils in a Dutch oven and bake at 200°F or lower for 6 to 8 hours. Follow remaining instructions. Do not leave home while the oven is on.

MAKE BABY FOOD: The texture is pretty wonderful for babies, or you could use an immersion blender to make it perfectly smooth. Leave out the cayenne if your baby's not used to heat, then add a splash of hot sauce to your own bowl to make up for it.

MAMA SAID

"The Moroccan Red Lentil Stew was a huge hit. My husband claimed it's the best dinner I've made in recent memory—so I didn't tell him how easy and inexpensive it was." —Sarah L., mom of one, Mill Valley, CA

"Wow, delicious! Big thumbs up. Disclosure: I forgot to start early enough, so instead of using the slow-cooker method I made it as a stovetop stew, which took about an hour. Of course I can't compare it to the taste and texture of a slow-cooker or oven-cooked version, but the lentils were totally broken down after about 45 minutes at a low simmer. The only thing I changed because of the different cooking method was to sauté the onions and garlic with the spices first (in about a tablespoon of olive oil)." —Jody B., mom of two, Boston, MA

# OVERNIGHT CHICKEN BROTH, PLUS CHICKEN NOODLE SOUP

**Makes 2 to 3 quarts**

**Cooking time: 8 to 12 hours (20 minutes active)**

Whenever I have a pile of chicken bones left after a meal—from a whole chicken I made myself, from a rotisserie bird, even from a bunch of chicken parts—I turn it into chicken broth. Using already-cooked bones seems to result in a deeper flavor, and the economy of the whole thing just tickles me. I also like waking up in the morning to fragrant, ready-to-go chicken broth; it gives me time to refrigerate it and skim the fat before transforming it into dinner.

This recipe works best in a large slow cooker. It's one of the few things I make in that 6-quart pot my folks got me when Harry was born. If you've only got a small one you can still make the broth, but you won't be able to fit as much into the pot so your yield will be lower.

Freeze whatever broth you don't use immediately, and it'll stay good for four to six months. I like to fill a large resealable freezer bag and lay it flat on a cutting board inside the freezer. Once it's solid, remove the cutting board and you'll be left with a space-saving, stackable flat of broth.

## FOR THE BROTH

Carcass from a 3- to 5-pound chicken, raw
   or cooked, with bones and scraps of meat
   (discard skin)

2 or 3 large carrots, chopped into big pieces

2 or 3 celery ribs, chopped into big pieces

1 large parsnip, chopped into big pieces,
   optional

1 large onion, unpeeled, quartered

2 or 3 flat-leaf parsley sprigs

1 tablespoon black peppercorns

Cold water

Salt

1. Combine all of the solid ingredients in the slow cooker.

2. Add as much cold water as will fit, stopping an inch below the rim.

3. Cover and cook on LOW for 8 to 12 hours.

4.  Strain the broth, pressing gently on the solids to extract as much flavor as possible. Discard solids.

5.  Add salt to taste and refrigerate.

## FOR CHICKEN NOODLE SOUP (4 servings)

1 large carrot, chopped small

1 celery rib, chopped small

8 cups chicken broth

8 ounces cooked chicken, chopped

6 ounces egg noodles

Salt and pepper

1.  About 30 minutes before you want to eat, bring a large pot of salted water to a boil (covered to speed things up). Skim off and discard any solidified fat from broth.

2.  Combine carrot, celery, and broth in a large saucepan and bring to a boil, then lower heat and simmer, 10 minutes.

3.  By now your water should be boiling; add noodles and cook according to package directions.

4.  Add the chicken to the soup and simmer until the vegetables are tender, about 5 minutes.

5.  Drain the noodles and add to the soup. Taste and adjust seasoning with salt and pepper.

**MAKE IT IN THE OVEN:** Follow all the instructions for making the broth, only use a Dutch oven instead. Set the oven to 200°F. Do not leave home while the oven is on. To make soup, follow the stovetop directions above.

MAKE BABY FOOD: The soup should make baby happy, right down to the noodles. Puree it, or serve the solids separately from the broth (young eaters sometimes have difficulty eating liquids and solids in the same mouthful).

MAMA SAID:

"I used the bones from the Overnight French Onion Chicken (page 151) to make the stock, which made for a very dark and rich stock. I had never made stock in the slow cooker before and it turned out great. I froze more than half of it and used the rest for a pot of soup, with added carrots, whole-wheat egg noodles, and matzo balls (from a mix). It was a great low-maintenance dinner." —Karissa J., mom of one, Vancouver, BC

# RATATOUILLE

**Serves 4 to 6**

**Cooking time: 4 to 6 hours on LOW, 3 to 4 hours on HIGH (30 minutes active)**

Julia Child's version of this classic French dish calls for pre-cooking each vegetable individually, then layering them and simmering, all with near-constant monitoring. The version you see here is much less complicated. Some of the ingredients do get added later than others—so save it for a day when you know you'll be around—but it's still about a thousand times easier than what you're used to and just as delicious.

1 large eggplant (about 1½ pounds), unpeeled, chopped into 1-inch pieces

1 medium onion, roughly chopped

2 bell peppers, any color, chopped into 1-inch pieces

One 14.5-ounce can diced tomatoes, drained (Muir Glen's fire roasted variety are really nice here)

3 large garlic cloves, minced, divided

⅓ cup olive oil

5 small or 3 large zucchini or summer squash (about 2 pounds), cut into 1-inch rounds

3 tablespoons chopped fresh basil or thyme, divided

Salt and pepper

½ cup orzo or other small pasta, optional

1 tablespoon balsamic vinegar

Goat cheese or ricotta, optional

1. Combine the eggplant, onion, peppers, tomatoes, and half of the garlic in the slow cooker. Add the olive oil and toss to coat. Cover and cook on LOW for 2 to 3 hours, or on HIGH for 1 to 1½ hours.

2. Stir in the zucchini. Cover and continue to cook on LOW for another 2 to 2½ hours, or HIGH for 1½ to 2 hours.

3. During the last hour, add the remaining garlic, 2 tablespoons of the basil or thyme, and salt and pepper to taste. The vegetables will be tender but still hold their shape.

4. If the ratatouille seems too soupy at the end of the cooking time, add ½ cup of orzo and cook for another 15 to 20 minutes on either LOW or HIGH. You'll end up with a one-pot meal!

5. Just before serving, stir in the balsamic vinegar and remaining basil or thyme. Top with the goat cheese or ricotta if using.

*If you like, add some chicken cutlets to the mixture at Step 3, and cook for another 1 to 1½ hours.*

**MAKE IT IN THE OVEN:** Set the oven to 200°F, and use a Dutch oven. Follow the instructions for cooking on LOW. Do not leave home while the oven is on.

MAKE BABY FOOD: The texture of the vegetables is lovely for babies. Cut the individual pieces into little bits, or puree.

**MAMA SAID**
"I made this on a day that my baby was home sick. I liked that the prep was easy—I did it during her nap—and that I could throw stuff in and go do something else. We put it on pasta—the goat cheese definitely made it. I think I would include some chickpeas if we made this again, just for some added protein (we eat mostly vegetarian)." —Jennifer N., mom of two, Philadelphia, PA

- - - - - - - - - - - - - - - - - - - - - - - - - - - - - - - - - - - - - - - - - - - -

# (ANOTHER) VEGETARIAN FRIJOLES NEGROS

**Serves 4 to 6**

**Cooking time: 7 to 9 hours on LOW, 4 to 6 hours on HIGH (20 minutes active)**

This recipe is quite similar to the one on page 36, with two main differences: First, it's made in a slow cooker. Second, I've added more vegetables to the mix, which is completely untraditional but considerably more nutritious. (I'll be honest: It was an attempt to trick my toddler into eating some vegetables for once. And it worked. For a while.) To save time, I chop the onions, peppers, chipotle, carrot, zucchini, and garlic all at once in the food processor. Once they've been in the pot for hours, the vegetables melt down so much that they contribute more texture than individual flavors.

Sofrito is a Latin-American flavor base, usually comprised of tomatoes, onion, garlic, cilantro, and bell peppers. Goya makes a fine version. If you can't find it, salsa works well too—just choose one with similar ingredients.

One 1-pound package black beans, sorted and rinsed

1 large onion, finely chopped

1 red or yellow bell pepper, seeded and finely chopped

1 chipotle in adobo, seeded and minced (leave the seeds if you like things spicy)

2 large carrots, finely chopped, optional

1 medium zucchini, finely chopped, optional

2 garlic cloves, minced

1 teaspoon ground cumin

1 teaspoon dried oregano

1 bay leaf

½ cup prepared sofrito or salsa

6 cups water

2 tablespoons red wine vinegar or cider vinegar

Salt

Cooked brown rice, for serving (I like to use Success boil-in bags)

Chopped avocado, corn tortillas, sour cream, shredded Cheddar or Jack cheese, lime wedges, cilantro, and hot sauce, for serving, optional

1. Put all the ingredients except the vinegar and salt in the slow cooker. Cover and cook on LOW for 7 to 9 hours or HIGH for 4 to 6 hours. Make sure the beans are covered with liquid at all times—if they're not, add some boiling water.

2. Check at 7 hours (LOW) or 3 hours (HIGH) to gauge doneness—the beans should be tender and hold their shape, but not falling apart.

3. Remove the bay leaf and stir in the vinegar and salt to taste. Serve over brown rice, with your choice of toppings.

**MAKE IT IN THE OVEN:** Follow the instructions above, but set the oven to 200°F, and use a Dutch oven. The beans should be done in 5 to 7 hours. Do not leave home while the oven is on.

MAKE BABY FOOD: The texture of these beans is just right to puree or for finger food, and many of the toppings are quite infant-friendly as well. If you're concerned about the spice level, use less of the chipotle (or skip it entirely).

### MAMA SAID

"This dish was really, really good. Both of my daughters adored it served over brown rice with grated Cheddar, sour cream, avocado, and toasted crumbles of corn tortillas. This was pretty easy to cook with the kids—the girls helped me sort the beans, dump everything into the crockpot, and stir it, and the prep was fast enough with the food processor that the baby was happy to watch from his seat on the counter. And then it cooked itself while we were outside enjoying the gorgeous weather—definitely what I look for in a meal!" —Sarah B., mom of three, Canterbury, CT

## ALOO DAL GOBI (INDIAN-STYLE POTATO, SPLIT PEA, AND CAULIFLOWER STEW)

**Serves 4 to 6**

**Cooking time: 8 to 10 hours on LOW, 4 to 6 hours on HIGH (15 minutes active)**

Here's a curry that's entirely inauthentic but still filled with all the flavors we expect from a great Indian meal. I've augmented the traditional green peas with yellow split peas, which provide protein and lend the taste of a separate dish of dal without the extra time (and dirty dishes). Don't be surprised if some of the cauliflower melts into the stew much like the split peas do.

1 cup dried yellow split peas, sorted and rinsed

3 medium potatoes, peeled and chopped into ½-inch pieces

1 small head cauliflower, chopped into florets

2 onions, finely chopped

4 cups low-sodium vegetable or chicken broth

4 garlic cloves, minced

1 tablespoon grated fresh ginger

1 tablespoon curry powder

½ teaspoon salt

¼ teaspoon pepper

1 cup frozen green peas, not thawed

Juice of ½ lemon (about 1½ tablespoons)

A handful of cilantro, chopped

Cooked brown or white rice (basmati is best, but a Success boil-in bag is great too!) and plain yogurt, for serving

1. Combine the split peas and potatoes in the slow cooker and stir.

2. Top with the cauliflower and onions, and gently stir those two together (try not to mix with the potatoes and split peas, but don't fret if they mingle).

3. Combine the broth, garlic, ginger, curry powder, salt, and pepper in a 4-cup measuring cup and stir well. Pour over the vegetables immediately, before the spices have a chance to settle.

4. Cover and cook on LOW for 8 to 10 hours, or HIGH for 4 to 6 hours.

5. When the vegetables are tender, add the frozen peas and cook just long enough to heat them through, 5 to 10 minutes. Stir in the lemon juice and cilantro, then taste and add more salt and pepper if needed.

6. Serve with rice and yogurt.

**MAKE IT IN THE OVEN:** Combine everything through the salt and pepper in a Dutch oven and bake at 200°F for 6 to 8 hours. Follow the remaining instructions. Do not leave home while the oven is on.

MAKE BABY FOOD: The soft, nearly mushy texture of this stew makes it for a perfect baby meal—just use a mild curry powder if you're concerned about heat.

**MAMA SAID**
"This was a very easy recipe; I love just putting things into the crockpot without having to do anything else to them first. The flavor turned out just right, not too spicy for my toddler, but lots of flavor for the grownups." —Carol S., mom of one, Venice, CA

- - - - - - - - - - - - - - - - - - - - - - - - - - - - - - - - - - - - - - - - - - - - -

# BUTTERNUT SQUASH RISOTTO

**Serves 4**

**Cooking time: 2 to 3 hours on HIGH (20 minutes active)**

This recipe came to me via AltDotLife.com, the message board where I spent many, many hours during my pregnancy and fourth trimester. The women on the board saved my butt in more ways than I can count; this miraculous dish is just one example.

When buying butternut squash, look for one with a long, thick neck. Because it has seeds and is weirdly shaped, the bulb is a hassle to deal with, so the less of it, the better. If you're too stressed to deal with peeling and chopping a butternut squash, use the pre-cut kind. It usually comes in pretty big hunks so you'll still have to do a little chopping, but it's a whole lot quicker than starting from scratch.

**NOTE:** There are no instructions for cooking this on low, because unfortunately it doesn't really work. When Harry was wee, I'd toss the ingredients into the slow cooker during his afternoon nap.

## HOW TO CUT A BUTTERNUT SQUASH

Intimidated by the mere thought? Here are three basic steps:

1. Using a large knife, cut crosswise right at the point where the neck (the long part) meets the bulb.
2. Peel both sections with a vegetable peeler—after years of using a kitchen knife, I finally realized that a sharp peeler is much, much easier, even though I do have to go over most areas more than once.
3. Cut the peeled neck into slices, then cubes. Cut the bulb in half and scoop out the seeds, then chop.

2 tablespoons olive oil

3 tablespoons minced shallots, (about 1 medium shallot)

1 cup Arborio rice

½ cup dry white wine or vermouth

3 cups (about 1½ pounds) butternut squash, peeled, seeded, and chopped into ½-inch pieces

3 cups low-sodium chicken or vegetable broth

½ cup frozen peas, not thawed

¼ cup grated Parmesan cheese

2 tablespoons softened butter

Salt and pepper

1. Heat the olive oil in a medium skillet over medium heat. When it shimmers, add the shallots. Cook, stirring occasionally, until softened, 3 to 5 minutes.

2. Add the rice and cook for 1 to 2 minutes, stirring to coat each grain with oil, until the rice makes a clacking sound. Add the wine and cook until almost completely absorbed, 5 to 6 minutes more.

3. Scrape the contents of the skillet into the slow cooker. Add the chopped squash and broth, stir, cover, and cook on HIGH for 2 to 2½ hours.

4. Check at around the 2-hour mark; when it's done the liquid will be mostly—but not completely—absorbed and the rice will be al dente. I usually stir at this point to break up the squash. Even if it seems like the rice has a ways to go, pay close attention after this; slow cooker risotto can go from not-done to overdone surprisingly fast.

5. When the risotto is ready, turn off the slow cooker, add the peas, stir, and cover for 5 minutes. The residual heat will cook the peas.

6. Stir in the Parmesan and butter, then season with salt and pepper to taste.

**MAKE IT IN THE OVEN:** Use a Dutch oven instead of a skillet in Step 1, and add ingredients from there—it's a one-pot meal. Set the oven to 250°F to approximate the HIGH setting on a slow cooker. Do not leave home while the oven is on.

MAKE BABY FOOD: This one's pretty darn perfect, just as it is.

**MAMA SAID**
"I thought it was phenomenally tasty, and my nine-month-old ate and ate and ate (as usual, my three-and-a-half-year-old refused to try it). From my perspective, risotto was one of those time-consuming, indulgent dishes I made in the days before children. I didn't think I would get to make it again until our yet-to-be-conceived third child was in college, so I'm pretty psyched to have a risotto I can make with small children clamoring for attention."
—Ariella M., mom of two, Brookline, NH

# SLIGHTLY-LESS-LAZY ITALIAN CHICKEN

**Serves 4**
**Cooking time: 6 to 8 hours on LOW, 3 to 4 hours on HIGH (15 minutes active)**

When I first heard about "Lazy Italian Chicken" on AltDotLife.com, I was put off. It calls for bottled Italian salad dressing, low-fat, no less, which is not something you'll generally find in my kitchen. Honestly, I cringed the first time I read it. But the recipe is just so insanely easy, and it came so highly recommended that I gave it a shot. And I must admit: This is inarguably one tasty dish.

My version differs slightly from the original recipe, with a tweak in the technique and the addition of fresh spinach to make this a complete meal. (That's why I call it slightly less lazy.) One thing I won't change: using low-fat dressing—regular dressing is too oily for this use.

4 medium potatoes, quartered and cut into chunks
4 garlic cloves, peeled and smashed

1 cup low-fat Italian salad dressing (choose a brand with ingredients you recognize—Newman's Own has a light version I particularly like)

1 teaspoon dried oregano

1 teaspoon dried basil

1 cup grated Parmesan cheese

4 boneless, skinless chicken breasts

One bag (5 ounces or more) baby spinach

1. Coat the slow cooker insert with nonstick spray and add the potatoes and garlic. Sprinkle with half of the Italian dressing, half of the dried herbs, and about one third of the grated Parmesan.

2. Place the chicken over the potatoes and top with the remaining dressing and herbs, along with another third of the Parmesan. Cook on LOW for 6 to 8 hours or on HIGH for 3 to 4 hours.

3. When the potatoes are tender, sprinkle on the remaining Parmesan, then add the spinach (you can stir to submerge the spinach in the sauce, or just let it wilt on top). Cook for 10 to 15 minutes more, just until the spinach is completely wilted.

**MAKE IT IN THE OVEN:** Follow all the instructions, only use a Dutch oven instead. Set the oven to 200°F and cook 4 to 6 hours. Do not leave home while the oven is on.

MAKE BABY FOOD: Cut the chicken into tiny bits, and let baby feed herself a chunk of potato. Chop the spinach well, and it'll be fine too. If you prefer, you could also puree everything together.

**MAMA SAID**

"Instead of a slow cooker, I used a Dutch oven at 200°F, for 4½ hours. The chicken was *perfect*: moist, flavorful, delicious. This made a special, lovely, and easy birthday dinner!"
—Anita J., mom of two, San Ramon, CA

# OVERNIGHT FRENCH ONION CHICKEN

**Serves 4 to 6**

**Cooking time: 14 to 18 hours on LOW (30 minutes active)**

The slow cooker is the easiest way I know to caramelize onions—slice them with a mandoline or a food processor fitted with the slicing blade and toss with olive oil, then let them melt away on LOW for 10 to 12 hours. I like to do that part overnight, hence the name of this dish. You'll wake up to an incredible-smelling kitchen (I warn you: You'll likely want to eat a savory breakfast). Serve this chicken with Gruyère-covered crostini to soak up all the deliciously soupy sauce.

Since this requires several stages—overnight cooking of the onions, keeping the onions warm, and finally cooking the chicken—this is a recipe to make on a day when you'll be in and out. It's not complicated, but you will need to attend to the cooker more than once.

**NOTE:** If you'd like a bunch of caramelized onions for another use, slice up a few more onions (you can fill the slow cooker to an inch shy of the rim), add another tablespoon of oil, and remove a cup or two when you wake up in the morning.

6 large onions, halved and thinly sliced

3 tablespoons olive oil

3 fresh thyme sprigs, or 1½ teaspoons dried thyme, divided

1 cup low-sodium chicken broth

½ cup dry sherry (or cognac, brandy, port, or wine of either color)

Salt and pepper

3½ pounds chicken parts, skinned

12 slices Italian bread (day-old is better, but fresh will work too), about ½-inch thick

4 ounces Gruyère cheese, grated

1. Combine the onions, olive oil, and 2 sprigs of the fresh thyme (or 1 teaspoon dried) in the slow cooker. Cover and cook on LOW for 10 to 12 hours. Once cooked, the onions can be kept safely on the WARM setting for up to 4 hours.

2. About 4 hours before you'd like to eat, add the broth, sherry, and reserved thyme to the onions. Season the chicken with salt and pepper, and add to the slow cooker. Stir gently, so that the chicken is just about covered with the onion mixture.

3. Cover and cook on LOW for 4 to 6 hours.

4.  About 30 minutes before serving, preheat oven to 350°F. Grease or line a baking sheet, arrange the bread slices on it, and bake until bread is lightly toasted, about 10 minutes.

5.  Set oven to broil. Sprinkle the Gruyère over the toasted bread (keep slices close together, so that most of the cheese falls onto the bread). Broil just until the cheese is melted and lightly brown, 3 to 5 minutes.

6.  Serve the chicken and onions with the Gruyère crostini.

**MAKE IT IN THE OVEN:** Follow the instructions as written, only use a Dutch oven instead. Set the oven to 200°F. Do not leave home while the oven is on.

MAKE BABY FOOD: The texture of the onions is perfect for young eaters—you can puree them if you like, or serve as finger food. Most of the alcohol from the sherry will cook off, but if you're wary reserve some of the onions before adding the remaining ingredients. The chicken should be falling-off-the-bone tender, great for pureeing or finger food.

MAMA SAID
"Loved this! I like that the most labor-intensive bit is the night before, which makes it a great workday meal that you can start after baby is in bed. And I loved caramelized onions made in the slow cooker. The next morning I thought they were ruined because they were almost black, but I've never made proper caramelized onions on the stovetop, I guess, because they weren't burnt at all, just really intense and delicious. We made a spinach and cheese omelet for breakfast and stole some of the onions for it. The texture of the chicken was very nice, and the crostini were a perfect accompaniment. Also, we had a ton of liquid and onions left in the slow-cooker, so I froze them and plan to use it as a base for French onion soup."
—Karissa J., mom of one, Vancouver, BC

# "ROAST" CHICKEN

**Serves 4**

**Cooking time: 4 to 6 hours on LOW, 2 to 3 hours on HIGH (10 minutes active)**

I'll be the first to admit it: A whole chicken cooked in the slow cooker is not going to win any beauty contests. The skin will be wan and limp, and the chicken itself will likely fall apart on its way out of the cooker. But the meat will be moist and tender, the amount of work is minimal, and the cleanup is a breeze compared to scrubbing a roasting pan. Chicken cooked this way is also perfect for other uses: Shred or chop the meat and add it to burritos, chicken potpie, chicken salad, you name it.

Oh, and there's pretty much zero chance of undercooking the chicken, which always seems to be an issue for me when I traditionally roast one. If anything, you're more likely to overcook the breasts, so be sure to check it at the four-hour mark—it's done when the drumstick wiggles freely (and I mean really wiggles), and the juices run clear. To be absolutely certain, stick a meat thermometer into the thickest part of the thigh. It should reach 165°F.

3 carrots, sliced into ¼-inch pieces

8 to 10 shallots, peeled

One 3- to 4-pound chicken

1 teaspoon salt

½ teaspoon pepper

Adobo seasoning or other seasoning blend, optional

1. Combine the carrots and shallots in the slow cooker.

2. Rub the chicken with the salt, pepper, and seasoning blend, if using, and arrange it, breast-side up, on top of the vegetables.

3. Cover and cook on LOW for 4 to 6 hours or HIGH for 2 to 3 hours. Remove skin before serving.

   **MAKE IT IN THE OVEN:** Set the oven to 200°F. Follow the instructions as written, but use a Dutch oven and check it after 3 hours. Do not leave home while the oven is on.

MAKE BABY FOOD: Either serve the chicken, carrots, and shallots cut up into little bits, or make a puree using some of the juices that accumulate in the slow cooker.

**MAMA SAID**

"Incredibly easy, and it turned out great! The best part was that we had the plain chicken and carrots the first night, and our three-year-old ate it up with green beans. I liked that it was a simple, clean, healthy meal. We also got two sets of leftovers from it: I heated it up with some bottled curry sauce from Trader Joe's and served it over brown rice. And I added it to a white bean chili for the second set." —Maggie K., mom of two, Pleasantville, NY

# BALSAMIC BEEF STEW

**Serves 4 to 6**

**Cooking time: 6 to 8 hours on LOW, 3 to 4 hours on HIGH (20 minutes active)**

The inspiration for this hearty stew came from *Not Your Mother's Slow Cooker Cookbook*, but I've tweaked it so much over the years it's about eight times removed by now. (One of my mom-testers came up with the idea to add the orange zest!) This makes quite a lot of stew, so you'll need at least a 4-quart slow cooker.

5 small or 3 large potatoes, peeled and
    chopped into 1-inch pieces

4 large carrots, chopped into 1-inch pieces

½ cup all-purpose flour

1 teaspoon paprika

½ teaspoon salt

¼ teaspoon pepper

2 pounds beef stew meat, cut into 1-inch
    pieces (I like chuck for this)

2 large onions, cut into 8 wedges each

One 14.5-ounce can low-sodium beef broth

½ cup full-bodied red wine

¼ cup tomato paste

1 tablespoon reduced-sodium soy sauce

3 tablespoons balsamic vinegar

½ teaspoon sugar

¼ teaspoon ground cloves

1 bay leaf

1 tablespoon grated orange zest

Crusty bread, for serving

1. Coat the slow cooker insert with nonstick spray. Put the potatoes in the bottom of the insert, and top with the carrots.

2. In a large resealable bag, combine the flour, paprika, salt, and pepper. Add the beef and onions and toss, shaking off any excess. Add the beef and onions to the slow cooker.

3. In a 4-cup measuring cup, stir together the broth, wine, tomato paste, soy sauce, balsamic vinegar, sugar, and cloves. Pour the mixture into the cooker. Tuck the bay

leaf into the stew. Cover and cook on LOW for 6 to 8 hours or HIGH for 3 to 4 hours, until the beef is tender enough to cut with a fork.

4.  Discard the bay leaf, stir in the orange zest, and serve with the crusty bread.

**MAKE IT IN THE OVEN:** Follow the instructions as written for LOW, only use a Dutch oven instead. Set the oven to 200°F. Do not leave home while the oven is on.

MAKE BABY FOOD: The beef will be very tender, but even so some babies have issues with meat. If yours balks, try making a chunky puree along with some of the sauce and veggies—Harry *loved* it that way. (Note: there's a bit of wine in this dish, but by the time it's ready nearly all the alcohol will have cooked off.)

**MAMA SAID**
"This was great. I liked how the ingredients were simple but the balsamic vinegar and soy sauce gave the gravy a bit of a kick. I also liked that there was no need for browning the meat beforehand. It took me maybe half an hour to prepare *and* clean up afterward. It was a blustery autumn day here so I popped some dumplings on the top when it was nearly done. My husband is a big meat eater and he said it was the best slow-cooked stew I'd made in ages, and 'you can make this again.' That's the highest compliment from him." —Nicola A., mom of one, Melbourne, Australia

## RED WINE–BRAISED SHORT RIBS OF BEEF

**Serves 4**

**Cooking time: 7 to 9 hours on LOW, 4 to 5 hours on HIGH (15 minutes active; best made a
day ahead)**

The first time I made short ribs in the slow cooker, Stephen and I moaned so loudly the
neighbors probably thought something kinky was going on. The results are that luscious.

When I make this recipe, the meat often slips right off the bone while I'm transferring it
from the slow cooker to a serving dish. If that happens, I shred all the meat together, mix
it with some of the rich sauce, and serve it over wide pasta, like pappardelle. Or check
out the tip below from mom-tester Alana, who served hers with couscous.

**NOTE:** Short ribs are extravagantly fatty. I urge you to make this recipe a day ahead of
time—once refrigerated, a shocking amount of fat will solidify, making it much easier to
remove. Plus, this is one of those recipes whose flavor improves with time.

1 cup red wine (I use an Italian table wine)

⅔ cup ketchup

2 tablespoons dark brown sugar

1 tablespoon Dijon mustard

3 tablespoons reduced-sodium soy sauce

1 rosemary sprig

2 garlic cloves, peeled and smashed

Black pepper

4 pounds beef short ribs

2 medium onions, chopped

8 ounces cremini or white button
   mushrooms, quartered

1. Combine the wine, ketchup, sugar, mustard, soy sauce, rosemary, garlic, and black
   pepper to taste in the slow cooker.

2. Add the ribs, submerging them in the sauce. (If they're not submerged completely
   that's OK—just dunk both sides so they're coated with sauce. Eventually the meat will
   soften enough to slide in.)

3. Scatter the onions and mushrooms over the ribs, cover, and cook until the meat starts
   to separate from the bone, 7 to 9 hours on LOW or 4 to 5 hours on HIGH. If you can,
   check the cooker about an hour early and if possible, push down a bit to submerge
   the tops of the ribs, the onions, and the mushrooms.

4. Refrigerate the solids and sauce separately overnight. Discard the fat that congeals on top before reheating. If you don't have time to refrigerate, I suggest pouring the sauce into a fat separator, which is a measuring cup whose spout is attached at the bottom, so the juices flow out but the fat is left behind.

**MAKE IT IN THE OVEN:** Set the oven to 200°F and use a Dutch oven. Check after 5 hours. Do not leave home while the oven is on.

MAKE BABY FOOD: There's a cup of wine in this dish, but it cooks for so long that nearly all the alcohol will have cooked off—it's your call. The meat becomes so soft and succulent, it's perfectly gummable. Or if you prefer, you could puree it with some of the sauce.

**MAMA SAID**

"It was amazingly good. I have never cooked short ribs before, and the bones just slid right out. For a side dish I made couscous with ½ cup water and ½ cup of the sauce from the ribs with 1 cup plain couscous and it worked really well. I was severely anemic post-delivery, and this would have been an awesome red meat dish to help up my iron levels." —Alana D., mom of one, Providence, RI

# BARBECUED BRISKET

**Serves 6 to 8**

**Cooking time: 6 to 8 hours on LOW, 4 to 5 hours on HIGH (10 minutes active)**

Even the most sleep-deprived parent can toss three ingredients into a slow cooker, right? That's all this recipe calls for, and holy cow is it delicious. It's not at all what you'd get if you lived in Texas, where brisket receives the day-long smoking treatment, but on a weeknight it's darn near life-changing. I serve this with baked beans (either canned or, if I have time, I'll make Rick Bayless's recipe for Hickory House Baked Beans, on Saveur.com) and cornbread.

A nice big brisket will give you enough meat for sandwiches the next day. It also freezes well, submerged in the cooking sauce.

**NOTE:** If you're using store-bought barbecue sauce, which I often do in this recipe, please read the labels carefully. Buy a bottle whose ingredients you can pronounce, ingredients that you would use if you were making it yourself.

1 3- to 4-pound brisket, trimmed of as much fat as possible

1 cup barbecue sauce, either homemade or store-bought

1 cup apple juice

1. Put the brisket into the slow cooker (cut it in half across the grain if it won't lie flat). Pour the barbecue sauce and apple juice on top, making sure some of the liquid winds up underneath the meat: the meat should not be fully submerged.

2. Cook on LOW for 6 to 8 hours, or on HIGH for 4 to 5 hours. It's done when a fork pierces it easily. If you feel any resistance, cook for 30 minutes longer on HIGH.

   **MAKE IT IN THE OVEN:** Set the oven to 200°F, and use a Dutch oven. It should take between 6 and 8 hours, but check after 5 to be safe. Do not leave home while the oven is on.

MAKE BABY FOOD: This is tender enough to cut with a fork, so it's great for finger food. But some babies aren't fond of the texture of meat—if yours is one of them, puree it along with some of the sauce.

**MAMA SAID**

"This is, hands down, the easiest brisket I have *ever* made (and we eat a lot of brisket in this house!). I was planning on eating it tomorrow, but when I went to slice the meat and store it in the fridge, my husband said, 'You're putting that away without letting me taste it?' and so the two of us proceeded to shovel the meat into our mouths at 9:30 at night standing over the kitchen counter. It was romance at its best." —Jesse Z., mom of two, Los Angeles, CA

· · · · · · · · · · · · · · · · · · · · · · · · · · · · · · · · · · · · · · · ·

# ROPA VIEJA

**Serves 6 to 8**

**Cooking time: 8 to 10 hours on LOW, 4 to 5 hours on HIGH (20 minutes active)**

When Stephen and I were first dating, he often took me to Café Con Leche, a Cuban restaurant on New York's Upper West Side. Honestly, the food wasn't the best, but their Ropa Vieja never failed me. *Ropa vieja* is Spanish for "old clothes," and that's what the dish looks like, a pile of rags—but the combination of beefy flank steak, peppers, and tomatoes is incredibly satisfying. My version makes no claims on authenticity, as usual, but the flavors take me right back to my dating days, when I ate plate after plate of the stuff in the name of romance.

**NOTE:** This recipe makes quite a lot, and you'll need a relatively large slow cooker—all the ingredients just fit in my 4-quart. Luckily, the meat freezes well, shredded and mixed with the sauce. Traditionally, Ropa Vieja is more juicy than saucy, so don't be surprised if your sauce looks thin at the end.

1 cup low-sodium chicken broth

¼ cup sherry or red wine vinegar

1 large onion, chopped

3 garlic cloves, minced

2 large bell peppers, any color, thinly sliced

1 bay leaf

One 14.5-ounce can diced tomatoes, with juice
*For a spicier result, substitute one 10-ounce can diced tomatoes and green chiles (such as Ro-Tel).*

1 tablespoon ground cumin

Salt and pepper

3 pounds flank steak, trimmed of fat, cut to fit into slow cooker
*If you can't find flank steak, brisket or skirt steak work well too. You want a cut of beef that will shred when it's fully cooked. In a pinch, try top round. It won't be as shreddable, but the flavor will be right.*

½ cup packed fresh cilantro leaves, finely chopped

Corn tortillas, your favorite salsa, chopped avocado, and lime wedges, for serving

1. Combine the broth, vinegar, onion, garlic, bell peppers, bay leaf, and tomatoes in the slow cooker.

2. Combine the cumin with a little salt and pepper, then rub the mixture on both sides of the steak before adding it to the slow cooker. Submerge the steak as much as possible (spoon some of the vegetables on top of the meat, if necessary).

3. Cover and cook until the meat is so tender you can easily shred it with a fork, 8 to 10 hours on LOW, 4 to 5 hours on HIGH.

4. Transfer meat to a cutting board and let rest for 10 minutes. While meat sits, remove and discard the bay leaf, then stir the cilantro into the sauce. Shred the meat with two forks and return it to the slow cooker, then stir to combine everything. Taste, and season to taste with salt and pepper.

5. Serve in heated corn tortillas with salsa, avocado, and lime wedges.

**MAKE IT IN THE OVEN:** Set the oven to 200°F, and use a Dutch oven. It should take between 8 and 10 hours, but check after 7 if you can. Do not leave home while the oven is on.

MAKE BABY FOOD: This meat is plenty soft, but flank steak has a tendency to be stringy. Either cut it up into little bits, or make a puree using the sauce.

MAMA SAID

"This was absolutely delicious and so easy! A few minutes of prep, toss in the cooker, and leave for the day. The aromas when we got home were out of this world, and dinner was a huge success! I added a can of black beans and some cilantro to brown rice for a quick and easy side dish." —Jane B., mom of one, Pleasanton, CA

# CHAPTER 5

# BIG BATCH BONANZA

You know that famed pregnancy nesting instinct, the one that's supposed to kick in during the latter part of the third trimester, when you suddenly have a burst of energy? When magically, you're able to do everything from setting up the nursery to cooking and freezing enough food to get you through the *fourth* trimester? Well, sometimes the instinct doesn't get a chance to work its magic.

When I hit 35 weeks—primo nesting time—my blood pressure started to soar. It wasn't quite pre-eclampsia-level, but it was enough to invoke a stern lecture from my obstetrician. I was ordered to take it easy, because if my pressure spiked any higher he would induce labor immediately. The nurse scheduled me for regular non-stress tests (which in itself was pretty darn stressful). The doctor was fairly certain Harry would arrive sooner rather than later, and he forbade me from spending much time on my feet. There went my grand plan for stocking our freezer with heat-and-eat meals.

For the next two weeks, I felt like a time bomb. Each visit to the OB yielded scary blood pressure numbers and a trip to the hospital for further testing, and each time I was sent home when my BP returned to normal range. And then my water broke. Harry was born at 37 weeks exactly, squeaking in under the full-term wire, but early nonetheless. We were not ready, not by a long shot. We had begun to shape my home office into something resembling a nursery (there was fresh paint on the walls, and a crib!), but we hadn't bought any bedding yet, the artwork we'd designed his room around was still being framed, and most of Harry's wardrobe was in the hamper waiting to be laundered. Enter my mother-in-law.

The indefatigable Pauline arrived the same day as Harry, prepared to sleep on the sofa until we got our parental sea legs. While I was in the hospital she got the laundry done, helped Stephen hang the artwork in the nursery—he'd finally wrested it away from the framer—*and* she made a vat of Little Gram's Sauce (page 177). Little Gram was Stephen's great-grandmother, who at the time was 103 years old. In fact, the best baby gift we received came with Pauline: a batch of Little Gram's Meatballs (page 179), made by the woman herself. Can you imagine, in between dealing with our days-old baby, we feasted on food prepared by a woman who was born in 1902?

The plan was for Pauline to stay long enough to stock the freezer with fully cooked meals, but an impending hurricane forced her to skedaddle just hours after Harry and I came home from the hospital. Not only did we lose our Been There, Done That newborn expert, we also lost our dinner supplier.

Weeks later, when I finally managed to find some kitchen time again, my motto became, "If I'm going to cook, we're getting multiple meals out of it." Big Batch cooking was more than just a smart idea—it was a necessity. Preparing a large amount of food at once, then freezing the extras in meal-sized portions, took a lot of the uncertainty out of dinnertime for the first few months. Even now, four years later, I still make a big batch of something several times a month, just to keep up my freezer stash. Life with a preschooler can be nearly as crazy as life with a newborn, so having a few meals ready to go keeps my blood pressure from spiking. Again.

### COMBO COOKING

When you're investing the time and effort required for Big Batch cooking, it's a smart idea to make complementary recipes together. Here are a few that can be tackled either at the same time or over a weekend:

- Little Gram's Sauce + Little Gram's Meatballs
- Little Gram's Sauce + Baked Macaroni with Ricotta, Spinach, and Mint or Grilled Eggplant Parmesan
- Korean Beef Stew + Asian Barbecue Sauce
- Vegetarian Tamale Pie + Black Bean, Sweet Potato, and Hominy Chili

## BIG BATCH COMPONENTS

Big Batch cooking isn't only for full recipes—it's also mighty handy for making food that will be incorporated into other recipes. For example, when you're roasting a chicken, it's just as easy to roast a second one alongside it. Pull the cooked meat from one chicken off the bones and freeze it in 6-ounce portions. Now it's ready for burritos or Chicken Pot Pie (page 50). By the same token, when you're roasting a tray of vegetables, prepare a second tray to roast at the same time. Freeze those cooked vegetables in 1-cup portions, and use them in soups, quesadillas, or pasta dishes. Other basics that work in big batches: salad dressing (store in the fridge and use within a week or two), mashed potatoes, cooked rice or pasta, caramelized onions, chicken or vegetable broth, and even browned ground meat.

## BIG BATCH BABY FOOD

Since infants eat relatively little at a time, odds are you're pureeing more than baby can eat before the food goes bad. There's a simple solution to this, and you've already got it in your freezer: ice cube trays. Spoon your leftover purees into the trays (measure as you go, so you'll know exactly how much is in each). Lay plastic wrap on top, allowing it to fall flat against the food. Once the contents are frozen solid, pop the cubes out into an air-tight container, label it, and pull a cube or two out as necessary. Defrost in the fridge or in the microwave—or put a frozen cube into a mesh feeder and let baby gnaw away at it. Terrific for soothing teething gums!

· · · · · · · · · · · · · · · · · · · · · · · · · · · · · · · · · · · · · · · · · · · · · · · · · ·

## TIPS ON FREEZING

- To minimize potential food waste, I freeze most leftovers in meal-sized portions—enough for me, Stephen, and Harry. The only exception is for casseroles, which are easier to freeze as described below.

- I'm a big fan of resealable freezer bags: They're handy for individual items like meatballs; they make it easy to freeze liquids in flat, stackable units; and they're a good way to be sure your packaging is airtight.

- If you'd rather avoid plastics completely, choose carefully when buying glass—regular glass can shatter at freezer temperatures. Look for glass containers that are specifically marked for freezer use, and allow food to cool before freezing.

- I know, you're afraid of freezer burn. It's caused when the freezer's air makes contact with food, drying it out. Freezer-burned food is safe to eat, but it's not particularly appetizing. The solution: Wrap everything tightly, and in multiple layers. The less air gets in, the longer your food will stay good.

- That said, remember that liquid expands slightly as it freezes—this doesn't matter so much for casseroles, but when spooning soup or stew into a freezer bag, leave a little bit of headspace at the top.

- Don't forget to label your freezer items! All foil-wrapped packages look alike, don't they? I use a Sharpie on a resealable freezer bag—they usually have a dedicated labeling space on the outside. Include the date the food was made, as well as the number of servings.

- For casseroles, I use a pair of 8-inch square baking dishes rather than a large rectangular one. The following instructions work for freezing the majority of the casseroles in this chapter (exceptions are noted in the recipes):

  - For an entire baking dish: Let the dish cool for 1 to 1½ hours (put it on a cooling rack to allow air to circulate underneath), then stick the whole thing in the freezer, baking dish and all, loosely covered. When it's frozen, the casserole should pop out of the dish easily—dunk the bottom in warm water if you have any trouble. Wrap the frozen food tightly in plastic wrap, then aluminum foil (don't let foil touch food made with tomatoes, as tomato sauce can eat through it!). If you like, put the whole thing in a resealable bag.

  - For individual servings: Wrap each tightly in plastic wrap, then foil, then store all of them together in a resealable bag.

- For all the other recipes, use the following instructions (with exceptions as noted):

- Let the mixture cool for 30 minutes to 1 hour, then spoon into food storage containers or resealable freezer bags (gallon-sized if you want to feed 4 to 6 at a time, quart-sized for 2 to 3). Put the bags on a flat surface like a baking sheet or cutting board, and slide into the freezer. Once the bags are frozen, remove the board.

### TIPS ON REHEATING

- Some storage containers are made to go from oven to freezer and back again—but that's only if the label says so. Don't go back and forth unless you're certain.

- After freezing in plastic (either in freezer bags or reusable containers), transfer to a microwave-safe bowl before reheating there. Chemicals can leech out from plastic in contact with hot food, and only those that are labeled safe have been tested.

- For the majority of the casseroles in this chapter, the following instructions work for defrosting and reheating (exceptions are noted in the recipes):

  - For an 8-inch baking dish: Preheat oven to 350°F. Take out the frozen casserole as well as the baking dish you used the first time around. Grease the dish. Remove all wrapping from the casserole and put the frozen block of food back into that dish. Cover with aluminum foil and bake for 30 to 40 minutes. Remove the foil and bake for 15 to 30 minutes more, until the food is heated through and bubbling.

  - For individual servings: Preheat oven to 350°F. Grease a baking dish. Remove all wrapping, then put the food into the dish. Cover the dish with aluminum foil, and bake for 30 minutes. Remove the foil and bake 10 to 20 minutes more, until food is heated through and bubbling.

- For all the other recipes, use the following instructions (again, with exceptions as noted in the recipes):

  - If you can plan a day in advance, let it defrost overnight in the fridge. Reheat in a saucepan over low heat, or in the microwave. If you're not a planner, the microwave works just fine. Transfer the food from any plastic or foil wrapping into a microwave-safe container, and use the "defrost" setting (usually that's half-power) in 2- to 3-minute increments. Remove portions as they defrost to avoid overcooking those parts while others are still frozen. Once it's fully defrosted, finish reheating in the microwave.

## CRIB NOTES

- Big Batch cooking calls for devoting a substantial chunk of time to recipes that yield enough food to freeze for several future meals.

- The idea of time-consuming recipes may be daunting, but they're definitely worth the extra effort. Wouldn't you love to just pull a homemade dinner from the freezer one or two nights a week? Each recipe includes freezing, defrosting, and reheating instructions too.

- You don't need special equipment for Big Batch cooking, but some of these recipes require a cooking pot that's impressively large—at least 8 quarts. And it helps to own multiple baking dishes.

- If you're in your third trimester, now's the perfect time to do some Big Batch cooking! These recipes should taste as good as the day they were made for approximately three months, provided they're wrapped, frozen, and defrosted carefully. After that they'll still be safe to eat (stored at 0°F, food stays safe indefinitely), but they may lose some of their flavor. Follow the "first in, first out" rule to make sure nothing hangs around that long.

- If you really like the idea of cooking less frequently but in larger quantities, Google "once a month cooking." You'll find enough information to make you dizzy. There are also cookbooks devoted entirely to this method.

. . . . . . . . . . . . . . . . . . . . . . . . . . . . . . . . . . . . . . .

# BAKED MACARONI WITH RICOTTA, SPINACH, AND MINT

**Serves 8, and doubles well**

**Cooking time: 60 minutes (35 minutes active)**

Did the word "mint" in the recipe's name throw you? Well, surprise, mint is a relative of basil, so it works beautifully in pasta dishes. It adds an unexpected twist and a hit of brightness that I really like. If you want to save a few calories, look for ricotta and mozzarella that are labeled "part-skim."

One 14.5- to 16-ounce box whole-wheat or whole-grain ziti or penne

One 5- to 9-ounce bag baby spinach

1 cup ricotta

⅔ cup grated Parmesan

¼ cup chopped mint leaves

¼ teaspoon pepper

One 24- to 26-ounce jar good-quality pasta sauce, or 3 cups Little Gram's Sauce (page 177)

*When I say "good-quality," I mean a jarred sauce that uses only ingredients you recognize, things you'd use if you were making it yourself. So no high-fructose corn syrup, OK?*

1 cup shredded mozzarella

**Preheat oven to 375°F. Grease two 8-inch square baking dishes or one 9 x 13-inch dish.**

1. Bring a large pot of salted water to a boil (covered to speed things up). Cook the pasta for 2 minutes less than directed on the package.

2. While the pasta is cooking, combine the ricotta, Parmesan, mint, and pepper in a small bowl and set aside.

3. When the timer rings, add the entire bag of spinach to the pot—it will wilt quickly—and cook for 1 minute more. (The pasta should be slightly undercooked.) Drain well, then return pasta and spinach to the pot.

4. Add the entire jar of sauce to the spinach and pasta and stir to combine.

5. If using two 8-inch baking dishes, spread about one quarter of the pasta mixture on the bottom of each prepared dish (use one half of the pasta mixture if using one 9 x 13-inch dish). Spoon all of the ricotta mixture on top of the pasta layer (it will be too stiff to spread). It will remain a separate layer, even after cooking. Top with remaining pasta mixture.

6. Sprinkle the mozzarella on top, and bake until the mozzarella is melted and golden-brown, 20 to 25 minutes.

MAKE BABY FOOD: Everything in here is safe for baby, either pureed or as finger food.

**MAMA SAID**

"I was leery of the mint, as in my world 'mint' is usually followed by 'juleps' or 'chocolate chip ice cream,' but it really worked here. The nuttiness of the whole-grain pasta balanced it nicely, and made the dish filling without being heavy. As a bonus, my 14-month-old twins loved 'helping' me pick the mint out in the garden. Usually I try to cook while they nap, but this recipe was easy enough to throw together with toddlers underfoot." —Tracy A., mom of twins, Portland, OR

# GRILLED EGGPLANT PARMESAN

**Serves 8**

**Cooking time: 60 minutes (30 minutes active)**

Eggplant Parm is one of my favorite Italian-American dishes, but between the breaded-and-fried eggplant (a.k.a. oil sponges) and the mounds of gooey cheese, it isn't exactly helpful when it comes to losing baby weight. This version is about a billion times lighter, thanks to eggplant that's grilled rather than fried. Use part-skim mozzarella if you'd like to save a few more calories.

**NOTE:** Many eggplant recipes call for salting the eggplant before cooking, to draw out the bitterness. When I first started cooking, I did just that, but in all honesty I've never tasted a difference. Once I became a mom, I threw all extra steps out the window. If you feel strongly about this by all means salt your eggplant, but I think you'll be just as happy skipping it.

4 medium eggplants (about 3 pounds), sliced into ¼-inch-thick rounds

1 tablespoon olive oil, plus more for brushing

Salt and pepper

1 cup fresh breadcrumbs, from about a quarter loaf of Italian bread

½ cup grated Parmesan cheese

One 24- to 26-ounce jar good-quality pasta sauce, or 3 cups Little Gram's Sauce (page 177)

8 ounces shredded mozzarella cheese (fresh is really nice here, but the supermarket kind is good too)

8 to 10 basil leaves, torn

*Making fresh breadcrumbs is super-easy: Tear the bread into small, 2-inch pieces and whir it in the food processor, or in batches in the blender with the grater button. If you don't have bread lying around, it's fine to use an equivalent amount of dry breadcrumbs—panko, if you've got it.*

**Preheat oven to 400°F. Grease two 8-inch square baking dishes or one 9 x 13-inch baking dish.**

1. Prepare your outdoor grill, or place a grill pan over medium-low heat. (If you don't have either, you can use the broiler for this too. Check for doneness a few minutes sooner, and don't forget to lower the heat before baking the casseroles.)

2. Brush both sides of the eggplant slices with olive oil and season with salt and pepper. Grill, in batches if necessary, until eggplant is tender and has dark grill marks, about 8 minutes per side.

3. While the eggplant is cooking, combine the breadcrumbs, 1 tablespoon olive oil, and Parmesan in a small bowl.

4. Reserve about 1 cup each of the sauce and mozzarella and set aside. If using two 8-inch baking dishes, spread about ½ cup of the remaining sauce on the bottom of each prepared dish (use 1 cup sauce if using one 9 x 13-inch dish). Alternate layers of grilled eggplant slices, followed by sauce, basil, and mozzarella until the dish is full. You should have 3 layers of eggplant, but don't pull out your hair if it's not perfect. Spread the reserved sauce on top, then top with the reserved mozzarella. Finally, sprinkle the breadcrumbs over everything.

5. Bake until the cheese is browned and the sauce is bubbling, 25 to 30 minutes.

MAKE BABY FOOD: This dish should be fine, either pureed or as finger food—just avoid giving baby pieces of eggplant peel, which can be tough.

**MAMA SAID**
"I liked: (1) Vegetarian but filling; (2) Easy prep and easy clean-up; (3) The eggplant had a great consistency; (4) I could use a lot of ingredients that I already had on hand—I usually have tomato sauce, bread crumbs, and mozzarella in the freezer, I always have Parmesan, and there is basil growing outside; (5) The crunchy top was great!" —Jennifer F., mom of one, Montreal, Canada

# MUSHROOM POT PIE WITH AN HERBED CRUST

**Serves 8**

**Cooking time: 1 hour 40 minutes (60 minutes active)**

Yes, I know, this looks complicated, but please don't be intimidated. Although there are quite a few steps, it's a straightforward process and the flavors are wonderfully rich and hearty. It does take a while, so make sure you (and your baby) are up for it.

**NOTE:** For years we were told never to wash a mushroom—use a brush to clear away the dirt. Bah! Who has time for such things? Go right ahead and wash them, quickly, under cold running water, and dry them off immediately. If you don't let them sit in water, they won't have time to soak any in.

1 sheet frozen puff pastry

2½ pounds assorted mushrooms, caps thickly sliced, stems reserved
*Use a food processor fitted with the slicing blade and this will be done in no time. To clean it easily afterwards, add a drop of dishwashing detergent and fill about ⅓ of the way with warm water. Whir for about 10 seconds, then rinse.*

1 thyme sprig, plus 1 tablespoon chopped fresh thyme leaves

3 garlic cloves, minced, plus 1 garlic clove, peeled and smashed

1½ cups low-sodium vegetable broth or water

⅓ cup dry sherry

2 tablespoons reduced-sodium soy sauce

1 tablespoon balsamic vinegar

2 tablespoons olive oil

2 shallots, finely chopped

3 celery ribs, chopped

2 large carrots, chopped

¼ cup all-purpose flour, plus more for rolling

Salt and pepper
*If you like, stir 2 cups cubed tofu or chopped cooked chicken into the mushroom mixture just before you pour it into the baking dish(es).*

1 egg, beaten lightly with 1 tablespoon water

2 tablespoons finely chopped mixed herbs (I like a combo of thyme, rosemary, and chives)

**Preheat oven to 400°F. Grease two 8-inch square baking dishes or one 9 x 13-inch dish.**

1. Remove the puff pastry from the freezer, and let it soften at room temperature for 30 to 40 minutes.

2. Place the mushroom stems (*not* the sliced caps) into a small saucepan, along with the thyme sprig, smashed garlic clove, broth or water, sherry, soy sauce, and balsamic vinegar. Bring to a boil over high heat, then reduce heat to medium-low and simmer for 15 minutes. Strain broth into a bowl, pressing gently on the solids to extract as much liquid as you can. Set the broth aside, covered to keep warm, and discard the solids.

3. Heat the olive oil in a large nonstick skillet over medium-low heat. When it shimmers, add the minced garlic, shallots, celery, and carrots and cook, stirring occasionally, until the vegetables are softened but not browned, 5 to 8 minutes.

4. Sprinkle the flour over the vegetables and cook, stirring constantly, until flour turns golden, about 1 minute.

5. Add the sliced mushroom caps, chopped thyme, and salt and pepper to taste. Raise heat to medium-high and cook, stirring occasionally, until mushrooms begin to soften, 5 to 8 minutes.

6. Pour in the reserved mushroom broth and bring to a boil, then reduce the heat to medium-low and simmer for 5 minutes. Season with salt and pepper to taste. Pour mixture into the prepared baking dish(es).

7. Roll out puff pastry on a lightly floured work surface until it's large enough to cover the baking dish (roll, then cut in half if you're using 2 square dishes). Carefully lay pastry over mushroom mixture and trim the excess. Brush with the egg wash, then sprinkle with the chopped herbs. Slash the crust a few times with a sharp knife.

8. Bake until crust is puffed and golden brown and filling is bubbling, 25 to 30 minutes. Let rest 10 minutes before serving.

**A NOTE ON FREEZING:** Because puff pastry is quite delicate, I'd recommend baking this in two square dishes and freezing one whole (following the standard instructions), rather than attempting to freeze individual servings.

MAKE BABY FOOD: The recipe calls for alcohol—⅓ cup of sherry—most of which will cook off. If you'd rather not give your baby even a trace, pluck out some mushroom chunks, leaving the sauce behind, and either puree with some broth or serve as finger food with bits of the crust.

**MAMA SAID**

"I loved this, and I am so glad to have another one in the freezer. The mixed mushrooms make it a nice and hearty meatless option. My son really liked this one as well." —Alana D., mom of one, Narragansett, RI

● ● ● ● ● ● ● ● ● ● ● ● ● ● ● ● ● ● ● ● ● ● ● ● ● ● ● ● ● ● ● ● ● ● ● ● ● ● ● ● ● ● ● ● ● ●

# VEGETARIAN TAMALE PIE/ TAMALE PIE FOR MEAT-EATERS

**Serves 6 to 8**

**Cooking time: 1 hour 20 minutes (35 minutes active)**

There are a lot of spices in this recipe but they all go in at once, so when you're setting up your mise-en-place (surely by now I've convinced you to pre-measure everything?) you can put them all in the same small dish.

**NOTE:** If you're not cooking for vegetarians, substitute 1 pound browned, extra-lean ground beef or turkey for the carrots, zucchini, and red kidney beans. Add the meat to the pan after the garlic, in Step 2.

## FOR THE FILLING

1 tablespoon olive oil

1 large onion, chopped

1 bell pepper, any color, chopped

2 carrots, chopped

3 medium garlic cloves, minced

1 medium zucchini, quartered lengthwise and chopped into ¼-inch pieces

One 14.5-ounce can black beans, rinsed and drained

One 14.5-ounce can red kidney beans, rinsed and drained

1 cup frozen corn kernels, not thawed

2 tablespoons chili powder

2 teaspoons ground cumin

2 teaspoons ground coriander

1 teaspoon dried oregano

¼ teaspoon cayenne

Salt and pepper

One 10-ounce can diced tomatoes and green chiles, such as Ro-Tel, with juice

1 cup low-sodium vegetable broth

2 teaspoons brown sugar

1 tablespoon cider or red wine vinegar

## FOR THE CRUST

1½ cups cornmeal

½ cup all-purpose flour

3 teaspoons baking powder

1 teaspoon salt

1 cup buttermilk

*If you don't keep buttermilk on hand, make this quickie substitute while the filling ingredients are simmering: Put 1 tablespoon of lemon juice or white vinegar into a measuring cup. Pour in milk until you've got 1 cup. Set aside for at least 5 minutes. It will look curdled and yucky, but that's just fine.*

2 large eggs

¼ cup vegetable oil

**Preheat oven to 375°F. Grease two 8-inch square baking dishes or one 9 x 13-inch baking dish and set aside.**

1.  Heat the oil in a large nonstick skillet over medium heat. When it shimmers, add the onion and bell pepper. Cook, stirring occasionally, until the onion becomes translucent, 3 to 5 minutes. Add the carrots and cook 2 minutes. Add the garlic and cook until fragrant, about 30 seconds. Add the zucchini and cook until it begins to soften, about 3 minutes.

2.  Stir in the remaining ingredients for the filling and bring to a boil over medium-high heat. Reduce the heat to low and simmer for 10 minutes, then transfer the contents of the skillet into the prepared baking dish(es).

3.  Combine the cornmeal, flour, baking powder, and salt in a medium mixing bowl. In a large mixing bowl, combine the buttermilk, eggs, and vegetable oil. Add the dry ingredients to the wet ones, stirring gently—don't overmix. When it's just combined, spread the batter over the filling.

4.  Bake until the crust is lightly browned and the filling is bubbling around the edges, 35 to 45 minutes. Let rest for 5 to 10 minutes before serving.

    **A NOTE ON FREEZING:** For separate portions, let the dish cool for about 30 minutes and then refrigerate; chilling will help the filling and crust hold together as you transfer it out of the dish. Once it's cold, wrap individual servings tightly in plastic wrap, then foil, then put in a resealable bag.

    **A NOTE ON REHEATING:** This is fairly dense, so an entire casserole takes longer to reheat than most of the other recipes. Bake at 300°F, covered with foil, until the food is heated through and bubbling, 1 to 1½ hours. If you'd like to make the top a little crusty, remove the foil for the last 15 minutes.

MAKE BABY FOOD: If your baby's OK with spices, the filling is mighty fine finger food. Think about it: beans, corn, and nice soft vegetables. Still on purees? Add a little broth or water and whir it in the food processor. If you'd rather not go the spicy route, reserve some of the beans and corn before adding it to the skillet. The crust might be a bit dry for baby, but you know what your tot can handle.

**MAMA SAID**

**"This was delicious! All five of us loved it, it was flavorful enough for my husband and me to enjoy and not too spicy for any of the kids. My seven-month-old may have eaten more than my four-year-old, actually! When I put it in the dish to go in the oven, I was afraid it was going to be too juicy and sloppy, but the sauce reduced even more while baking, and it was just right. The cornbread topping was the perfect complement, and I didn't find it dry at all— even the baby chowed it right down." —Sarah B., mom of three, Canterbury, CT**

# BLACK BEAN, SWEET POTATO, AND HOMINY CHILI

**Serves 8 to 10**

**Cooking time: 1 hour (35 minutes active)**

Hominy is whole kernels of corn from which the hull and germ have been removed— either mechanically or by soaking in a weak lye solution. Some hominy is dried and ground into grits, but this recipe calls for canned, which looks sort of like wet popcorn and has a firm, chewy, almost meaty texture. If you can't find canned hominy, several of my mom-testers made this with an equivalent amount of frozen corn kernels and were quite pleased.

The spice mixture as-is makes for a fairly mild chili. If you like things hot, add ¼ to ½ teaspoon of cayenne. Since all the spices go into the pot at once, measure them into one bowl before you start cooking.

2 tablespoons olive oil

1 large onion, chopped

1 red or yellow bell pepper, chopped

4 garlic cloves, minced

1 large sweet potato, peeled and chopped
   into ½-inch pieces

¼ cup chili powder

1 teaspoon dried thyme

1 teaspoon ground cumin

1 teaspoon dried oregano

1 teaspoon ground coriander

½ teaspoon cinnamon

Salt

1 tablespoon pure maple syrup

One 4-ounce can chopped green chiles,
   drained

One 28-ounce can crushed or diced
   tomatoes, with juice

2 cups low-sodium vegetable broth or water

Two 14.5-ounce cans black beans, rinsed and
   drained

One 15-ounce can hominy, rinsed and drained

Chopped cilantro, chopped avocado,
   shredded Cheddar or Jack cheese, sour
   cream, hot sauce, and tortilla chips, for
   serving

1. Heat the oil in a large, heavy pot over medium heat. When it shimmers, add the onion and pepper and cook, stirring frequently, until peppers are softened and onion is translucent, about 5 minutes. Add the garlic and cook until fragrant, about 30 seconds. Add the sweet potato, spices, and salt to taste and cook, stirring, about 1 minute.

2. Stir in the maple syrup, chiles, tomatoes, and broth, and raise heat to high. Bring to a boil, then lower heat and simmer, covered, until the sweet potato is just tender, about 25 minutes.

3. Stir in the black beans and hominy, and simmer, covered, until sweet potatoes are soft and flavors have melded, about 10 minutes.

4. Serve with the cilantro, avocado, cheese, sour cream, hot sauce, and tortilla chips.

MAKE BABY FOOD: This is another recipe for babies who have already enjoyed a bit of spice, either as finger food or pureed. If you're not on spices yet, reserve some of the black beans, avocado, cheese, and sour cream.

**MAMA SAID**

"This was really, really good. My once-upon-a-vegetarian was elated. It was mildly sweet and oh-so-yummy and filling! I didn't serve it *with* anything (avocado, sour cream, etc.), not sure it needed a thing! I put the spices together the night before, chopped the onion, pepper, and sweet potato while the girls ate breakfast, and was able to juggle the baby while I threw the rest together." —Ariella M., mom of two, Brookline, NH

• • • • • • • • • • • • • • • • • • • • • • • • • • • • • • • • • • • • • • • •

# LITTLE GRAM'S SAUCE

**Makes 5 to 6 quarts**

**Cooking time: About 3 hours (30 minutes active)**

Little Gram was Stephen's great-grandmother, born in Sicily in 1902. She lived to be 105, God bless her, and I was lucky enough to spend some time with her while she was still relatively active—she lived alone until just a year or two before she passed away. I knew Stephen's Catholic family would welcome me, his Jewish girlfriend, when this tiny, devout woman pulled me aside at a family gathering, perhaps the second or third one I'd attended, and said to me in her quiet, husky voice, "Debbie, I don't really know you, but I love you."

Her sauce is unlike any other recipe I've seen. It's beautifully smooth, first of all, since it uses only tomato puree and paste. And it's naturally sweet, thanks to an unusual ingredient: baking soda. According to Little Gram, that baking soda pulls the bitterness from the tomatoes to the top of the pot, where it's easy to skim off. I have no idea where this trick came from, but back in Sicily her father worked for a prince and learned many of the family recipes during his time there. Given that, I like to think of this as a royal sauce. It's certainly fit to serve a king—or a child (in my home there sometimes isn't much of a difference).

3 tablespoons olive oil

1 large onion, finely chopped
*As long as we're discussing Little Gram, here's her tip to avoid weeping while chopping onions: Light a candle, and keep it close by (though not near the baby, obviously). Apparently it burns away the fumes that make your eyes tear!*

12 garlic cloves, minced
*And here's a tip from Little Gram's great-grandson, a.k.a. my husband: A mini-food processor minces a dozen cloves of garlic in the blink of an eye. I'm not saying it's worth buying one just for this recipe, but Stephen certainly did . . . Smash each clove with the flat side of a large knife and the peels should slip right off.*

Two 28-ounce cans tomato puree

Two 18-ounce cans tomato paste

56 ounces water (fill the two empty cans from the tomato puree to measure!)

Pinch or two of baking soda (about ¼ teaspoon)

2 tablespoons dried basil

2 teaspoons salt

½ teaspoon dried oregano

1 pound ground meat, either a combination of beef, veal, and pork or turkey, optional (I leave it out when I know we'll be eating the sauce with meatballs or using it in other meat dishes, like chicken parmesan)

1. Heat the olive oil in a large soup pot over medium-low heat. When it shimmers, add the onion and cook, stirring, until golden, 5 to 8 minutes.

2. Add the garlic and cook until fragrant, about 30 seconds. Add the tomato puree, tomato paste, and water, and raise heat to high. When the sauce comes to a boil, lower the heat to a gentle simmer.

3. Stir in the baking soda, which will cause the sauce to foam gently. Skim off foam with a spoon and discard.

4. Add the remaining ingredients, crumbling the raw ground meat, if using, with your fingers as you add it in bits. Cover and simmer, stirring frequently, 2 to 2½ hours (Little Gram stirred the pot every 10 minutes). Make sure your spoon reaches all the way to the bottom of the pot, to prevent the sauce down there from burning.

5. Serve over pasta, with Little Gram's Meatballs (page 179), or use it in any recipe calling for pasta sauce.

   **NOTE:** The sauce will thicken as it cools. Thin it out with a little water when reheating.

   MAKE BABY FOOD: The smoothness of this sauce is absolutely perfect for little ones.

**MAMA SAID**
"I don't usually make red sauce, because it seems like too much work and time for something I can easily buy, but this was better than the jarred one we usually get, and not too much work. I started it at lunchtime while the kids were all eating, and was able to get it to the leave-and-simmer point by the time they needed hands-on attention, which made it easy to fit into our day. My bigger kids loved the foaming baking soda action! I bagged and froze the extra, and defrosted some in the fridge for homemade pizza and some for your Baked Macaroni with Ricotta, Spinach, and Mint. The texture and flavor were exactly the same after defrosting, so that worked perfectly!" —Sarah B., mom of three, Canterbury, CT

# LITTLE GRAM'S MEATBALLS

**Makes 38 to 40 meatballs**

**Cooking time: 40 minutes (15 minutes active)**

Here they are: The meatballs that Stephen and I feasted upon during Harry's earliest days. I've made two departures from Little Gram's original recipe. First, thanks to the ingenious suggestion of one of my mom-testers, I add the garlic at the same time as the eggs; in Little Gram's version, the garlic is meticulously integrated, bit by bit, after everything else has already been mixed in. And second, the current generation of Stephen's family bakes their meatballs. Little Gram fried them gently in olive oil. If you're not counting calories and you have the time (it requires stovetop monitoring), they really are spectacular cooked that way.

**NOTE:** You're using a mise-en-place, right? If you're not, in this case pre-measuring everything is a necessity—you don't want to be pulling out ingredients with your hands all full of goo. Combine the cheese, breadcrumbs, and salt in a small bowl, and beat the eggs with the garlic, before you touch the meat.

2 pounds combined lean ground beef, veal, and pork
*If you'd like to make a lighter version, substitute lean ground turkey for the pork. The flavor won't be quite the same, but they'll still make you sigh with pleasure.*

6 eggs, lightly beaten
2 garlic cloves, minced

2 cups dry breadcrumbs
2 cups grated Locatelli Romano cheese
*Little Gram insisted on Locatelli, a particular brand of Pecorino cheese, but I don't think she'd mind if you used one that's a bit easier to find.*

1 tablespoon salt

**Preheat oven to 375°F. Line a baking sheet with aluminum foil (to help with cleanup) and place a cooling rack on top. Coat the rack lightly with oil or nonstick spray.**

1. Using your hands, gently combine the ground meat with the eggs and garlic in a large bowl. Then add the breadcrumbs, cheese, and salt. Don't mix too vigorously or squish the mixture through your fingers—this will make the meatballs dense and tough.

2. Start shaping the meat into 2-inch balls. Moisten your hands slightly if the mixture is too sticky. As you roll each one place it on the prepared rack, close but not touching. You should get about 40 meatballs.

3.  Bake the meatballs for 22 to 24 minutes, gently flipping them halfway through. If you wound up with fewer than 35 meatballs, your meatballs are a bit large; they may take longer to cook.

4.  Serve hot with your favorite pasta and sauce (No surprise, I recommend Little Gram's Sauce, on page 177), with additional grated Pecorino on top.

> **A NOTE ON FREEZING:** Let the meatballs cool for 30 minutes to an hour, then put them into a resealable freezer bag, squeeze out all the air, and pop in the freezer.

> **A NOTE ON REHEATING:** Here's the real beauty of this recipe: Just take out however many meatballs you'll need for dinner and plunk them right into the sauce as it heats. Let them simmer for 15 to 20 minutes and you're good to go. If you're in a really big rush, you can also defrost them in the microwave.

MAKE BABY FOOD: Once past purees, babies do great with meatballs. If you like, shape some into batons rather than balls, specifically for your baby. It'll be easier for him to hold and self-feed.

MAMA SAID
"Tonight we dove into Little Gram's Sauce and her meatballs to boot. Both my husband and I felt this was the quintessential 'sketti and meatballs' recipe—like something we would find at our local homey Italian restaurant, only better! I am 38 weeks pregnant with a 22-month-old and we squeezed this in between trips to the playground. My picky toddler hadn't eaten long noodles for weeks but he had two helpings! I look forward to freezing the (considerable) leftovers and enjoying them after the new baby arrives in a couple of weeks."
—Shani A., mom of one, with a baby on the way, San Francisco, CA

# CHIPOTLE SLOPPY JOES

**Serves 6 to 8**

**Cooking time: 35 to 45 minutes (30 minutes active)**

The word "chipotle" probably makes you assume this will be spicy. Well, not quite. It can be, if you use the seeds, but if you include only the flesh of the pepper, the flavor will be quite mild. Basically, it gives the Joes an element of smokiness that I really like.

1 tablespoon olive oil

2 onions, finely chopped
*You can chop all the vegetables together in the food processor. Before you put them in cut them roughly, so that the pieces are about the same size.*

2 garlic cloves, minced

1 red bell pepper, finely chopped

2 celery ribs, finely chopped

2 pounds extra-lean ground beef or lean ground turkey

½ cup water
*When you're setting up your mise-en-place, you can measure all the remaining ingredients together into a 2-cup measuring cup. Makes cleanup easy!*

½ cup ketchup

1 chipotle in adobo, minced (remove the seeds if you'd like a bit less heat), plus 1½ tablespoons adobo sauce

3 tablespoons tomato paste

2 tablespoons brown sugar, or pure maple syrup

3 tablespoons cider vinegar

2 teaspoons paprika

1½ teaspoons dry mustard

2 teaspoons chili powder

1 tablespoon Worcestershire sauce

Salt and pepper

Hamburger buns, for serving (I like whole wheat, which seems to hold up a little better than white)

1. Heat the oil in a large nonstick skillet over medium heat. When it shimmers, add the onions, garlic, pepper, and celery, and cook until softened, 5 to 8 minutes.

2. Add the ground meat, raise heat to medium-high, and cook, breaking up the meat with the back of a spoon, until it's no longer pink, 8 to 10 minutes.

3. Stir in the remaining ingredients and salt and pepper to taste, bring to a boil, then lower heat and simmer for 10 to 15 minutes, until flavors meld.

4. Serve on hamburger buns.

MAKE BABY FOOD: This is for babies who enjoy a bit of spice. It purees nicely.

## THE SLOPPY OH-NOS

Feeding a baby is a messy endeavor, even more so once he begins to feed himself. But there are a few precautions you can take to keep the kitchen, the baby, and you from turning into a full-fledged Jackson Pollock painting:

- First, bibs: We don't own a washing machine (hello, Brooklyn rental!), so cloth was impractical. When I discovered sleeved, waterproof bibs (the brand I used was Bumkins), I thought I'd died and gone to heaven. They cover baby's shirtfront entirely, they're escape-proof, they've got a trough at the bottom to catch dropped food, and they rinse clean and dry fast. Machine washable too, for those of you living the high life.

- If you're in the habit of going directly from dinner to bath, feed baby while he's in nothing but a diaper—and let him play with his food!

- Because we only do laundry once a week, we kept a rather huge stack of soft baby washcloths next to the kitchen sink. At the end of feeding we'd wet one and give Harry a good wipe-down, even his hair.

- I'm not looking to send you on a shopping spree, but another item many parents find helpful is a splat-mat—a waterproof mat placed under the high chair. Unless your baby is a food-flinger, most of the mess will land on the mat. Pick it up, dump the debris in the garbage, wipe it off, and you're ready for the next meal. A shower curtain liner is an inexpensive substitute for the mats marketed to parents.

- My last tip: Trade Felix Unger for Oscar Madison. Expect a mess, especially once your baby begins to self-feed, and accept that you may have to live with a less-than-perfect kitchen—it's all part of the parenting gig. It didn't take long for me to realize that sweeping and mopping after each meal was a major time-suck, especially since it would all be messy again hours later. Food can, and should, be fun for babies, and obsessing over the goop on the ceiling won't make either of you very happy.

**MAMA SAID:**
"*Love* these! So yummy, and they were spicy enough for my husband, but my toddler ate them too. I've never used chipotles before, so it was a real education, and now I'm hooked. We ate them the first night, then froze the rest while we were out of town. They held up beautifully. I froze them in small batches, so I could just pop one container in the fridge in the morning for us to eat that night." —Corrin P., mom of one, Los Angeles, CA

# KOREAN BEEF STEW

**Serves 8**

**Cooking time: 2½ hours (30 to 40 minutes active)**

This dish gets its cue from bulgogi, Korean barbecued beef. I've taken the key ingredients of that dish—soy sauce, sugar, garlic, Asian pear (which actually looks more like a khaki-colored apple, and has natural tenderizing properties)—and applied them to a long-simmering pot of stew. I just love a recipe you can throw together and walk away from. Like many beef stews, this is better the next day.

**NOTE:** As long as your oven is on, make the rice in there too: Put 2 cups white rice, 1 teaspoon salt, and 4 cups boiling water into a casserole dish and cover tightly. When you place the stew in the oven in Step 5, slide the casserole dish of rice in next to it. Check after 20 minutes—if almost all the liquid has been absorbed, just let it sit on the counter, unstirred and covered, while the stew finishes cooking. You'll have enough to freeze along with the stew (packed separately, of course—I like to freeze 2 portions at a time). When you reheat it, add about ½ teaspoon of water to restore the texture.

3 tablespoons all-purpose flour

Freshly ground pepper, to taste

3 pounds beef chuck, excess fat removed, cut into 1-inch cubes

3 tablespoons vegetable oil, divided

3 large carrots, chopped into 1-inch pieces

1 large onion, chopped

6 garlic cloves, thinly sliced

2 teaspoons finely grated ginger
   *Keep fresh ginger, tightly wrapped, in the freezer. It'll stay good indefinitely, and it's much easier to grate.*

1 small Asian pear, grated (no need to peel)

¼ cup light brown sugar

1 cup water

⅓ cup reduced-sodium soy sauce

2 tablespoons mirin
   *Mirin is a sweet Japanese rice wine with a low alcohol content. Look for it in the Asian foods section of your supermarket, or Asian markets. Can't find it? Substitute 2 tablespoons sake, dry sherry, or white wine plus an additional teaspoon of brown sugar, or 2 tablespoons sweet sherry.*

8 ounces white button or cremini mushrooms, quartered

1 tablespoon sesame oil

Cooked white rice, 2 teaspoons toasted sesame seeds, and 2 scallions (green parts only), thinly sliced, for serving

**Preheat oven to 350°F.**

1. Combine the flour and pepper in a gallon-sized resealable bag and add the beef. Seal the bag and toss until all the beef is lightly coated, and shake off excess.

2. Heat 1½ tablespoons oil in a large, oven-safe Dutch oven or heavy pot over medium-high heat. When it shimmers, add half of the beef. Cook, stirring occasionally, until browned, 2 to 3 minutes per side, then transfer to a clean bowl. Repeat with the remaining 1½ tablespoons of oil and beef. You may need to lower the heat a smidge for the second round.

3. Add the carrots and onion to the now-empty pot and reduce heat to medium. Cook, stirring occasionally, until softened, 5 to 8 minutes. (If at any point it seems as if the crusty bits on the bottom of the pot are beginning to burn, add a drizzle of extra oil or water.) Add the garlic and ginger and cook, stirring, 30 seconds.

4. Add the grated pear, brown sugar, water, soy sauce, and mirin, and stir to combine. Scrape the bottom of the pot to loosen all the crusty bits, then return the browned beef to the pot. Raise heat to high and bring to a boil, then remove from heat, cover, and transfer pot to oven.

5. Bake for 1½ hours, then add the mushrooms and return the pot to the oven. (If you're baking white rice, now is the time to put it in the oven.) Cook until the meat is very tender, about 30 minutes more.

6. Stir in the sesame oil and serve over rice, sprinkled with sesame seeds and scallions.

> MAKE BABY FOOD: Puree a bit of the meat, carrots, and mushrooms; add a little water if it's too thick. As finger food, beef can be difficult for babies—many don't like the texture—but this is so tender you may be surprised. And the carrots are a lovely, soft consistency.

**MAMA SAID**
"This was so unbelievably delicious—it's not your mama's beef stew! Easy (even for a woman who is 39 weeks pregnant with a toddler in tow), unique, and super-mega-delicious. It's great to have a new beef stew in our repertoire for foggy San Francisco evenings!"
—Alana D., mom of one, with a baby on the way, San Francisco, CA

# ASIAN BARBECUE SAUCE

**Makes about 1½ quarts**
**Cooking time: 40 minutes (10 minutes active)**

Sweet, spicy, tangy—this barbecue sauce has all the flavors you'd expect, but with an Asian inflection. Which means it's blasphemous to both barbecue experts and Asian food aficionados. I like it best with chicken (marinate 6 to 8 pieces in about 1 cup, then brush onto the chicken during the last 10 to 15 minutes of cooking) or a strong-flavored fish like salmon (skip the marinating part and dunk the fish right before cooking).

There are no freezer instructions for this one, because it'll stay good for weeks in the fridge. This recipe makes enough for at least four meals, maybe more.

One 28-ounce can tomato sauce (make sure it's plain tomatoes, not seasoned; you could also use a box of Pomi "strained" tomatoes)

1½ cups unseasoned rice vinegar

1½ cups mirin
*Mirin is a sweet Japanese rice wine with a low alcohol content. Look for it in the Asian foods section of your supermarket, or Asian markets. If you can't find it, substitute the same amount of sweet sherry or 1½ cups dry sherry, white wine, or sake plus ⅓ cup sugar.*

½ cup reduced-sodium soy sauce

¼ cup fish sauce or Worcestershire sauce (they're not usually interchangeable, but both work here)

¼ cup dry sherry

3 tablespoons dark brown sugar

2 tablespoons grated ginger

1 tablespoon toasted sesame oil

2 teaspoons Chinese five-spice powder
*If you can't find this in your area, just leave it out. The flavor won't be quite as complex, but you'll still get that sweet 'n' tangy zing.*

1 teaspoon red pepper flakes, or to taste

1. Combine all of the ingredients in a large saucepan over medium-high heat.

2. Bring to a boil, then reduce heat to low and simmer, uncovered, 30 minutes.

MAKE BABY FOOD: This is purely a question of seasoning, and whether she's accustomed to spice. There is some alcohol in the recipe, but after simmering for 30 minutes most of it will have cooked off.

**MAMA SAID**

"This was sooooo easy. I could throw all the ingredients in the saucepan in the time it took for my baby to eat his post-nap snack. My husband and I both liked it a lot on chicken breasts; we especially liked how the ginger flavor came through." —Sarah T., mom of one, Calgary, Canada

• • • • • • • • • • • • • • • • • • • • • • • • • • • • • • • • • • • • • • • • • • • • • •

# CHICKEN ADOBO

**Serves 6**

**Cooking time: 1 hour (20 minutes active)**

I first made Chicken Adobo, a soy-sauce-and-vinegar–based Filipino dish that has nothing to do with the canned chipotles in adobo you've seen in other recipes, from a recipe in Mark Bittman's *How to Cook Everything*. And I L-O-V-E-D it. For years I followed his recipe religiously, but then I began to wonder if it couldn't be improved, just a teeny-tiny bit. After digging around online, I discovered that adobo is an incredibly variable recipe—pretty much every Filipino family has their own version. I've taken Bittman's version and added a bit from this recipe, a bit from that. While it won't win any authenticity contests, the end result is just about the most flavorful chicken I've ever eaten. And the leftovers are positively killer in Whaddya Got Fried Rice (page 124).

Serve this with rice to soak up all that fabulous sauce and a salad or some kind of greens, just to keep things balanced.

1 to 2 tablespoons olive oil

6 bone-in chicken breasts or 6 chicken quarters, drumsticks and thighs separated

6 garlic cloves, chopped

1½ cups reduced-sodium soy sauce

1½ cups water

1¼ cups cider vinegar or unseasoned rice vinegar

Two ¼-inch-thick slices fresh ginger, unpeeled, optional

4 bay leaves

1 teaspoon whole black peppercorns

1. Heat 1 tablespoon oil in a large nonstick skillet over medium-high heat. When it shimmers, arrange the chicken in 1 layer, skin side down (you may need to do this in two batches, in which case use that second tablespoon of oil). Brown on all sides, 8 to 10 minutes, and remove from the pan. Drain all but about 1 tablespoon of the remaining fat, and lower the heat to medium-low.

2. Add the garlic and cook, stirring frequently, until lightly golden, 1 to 2 minutes.

3. Add the remaining ingredients to the pan. Scrape the bottom of the pan with a wooden spoon to loosen all the browned bits. Bring mixture to a boil, then reduce heat to medium-low. Return chicken to the pan and simmer, covered, 20 minutes. Uncover and simmer 20 minutes more.

4. By now the chicken should be cooked through and the sauce should be nice and thick. If it's too thin for your taste, remove the chicken and raise the heat to high. Reduce the sauce to your desired thickness. Before serving, discard the ginger slices, if you used them, the bay leaves, and the peppercorns.

**A NOTE ON FREEZING:** Separate the meat from the bones and freeze just the meat and the remaining sauce. (Use those bones to make Overnight Chicken Broth, page 141.)

**A NOTE ON DEFROSTING AND REHEATING:** I hate the taste of chicken that's been microwaved, so I put the frozen chicken in the fridge to defrost a day ahead of time—which requires a little advance planning. Once it's defrosted, simply chop it up and add it to whatever recipe you're following. If you don't share my disdain, by all means defrost in the microwave. Just be careful to remove portions as they defrost, to prevent overcooking.

MAKE BABY FOOD: My only caution here would be about sodium—skip the sauce on baby's portion. If he's still on purees, add a bit of water or chicken broth to the food processor instead of sauce.

**MAMA SAID**
"I gotta say, I was a little reluctant for this big batch cooking—the recipes seemed more involved, as I'm more of a quick-and-easy meal type girl. But I gave it a go with the Chicken Adobo and I think this way of cooking may be a revelation for me. I waited until my girls were in bed and then took my time making the dish that night for the week. I finally understood how cooking could be relaxing—when you didn't have hungry people waiting for the meal right now. So nice to come home after work, do the daycare pick-up, and have dinner ready to go." —Maggie R., mom of two, Pleasantville, NY

# LEMON-YELLOW CHICKEN AND RICE

**Serves 8 to 10**

**Cooking time: 60 minutes (30 minutes active)**

This is a recipe that achieves pretty much all my objectives when it comes to dinner: It's bursting with flavor, thanks to the spices and an abundance of lemon. It's pretty to look at, thanks to the sunny turmeric. And it's a one-pot meal with rice, chicken, and vegetables all cooked together. I love it when I pull a portion out of the freezer and realize that, other than reheating, there is absolutely no work involved in tonight's dinner.

6 boneless, skinless chicken breast halves (about 2½ pounds)

Salt and pepper

3 tablespoons olive oil, divided

1 large onion, finely chopped

3 medium zucchini, halved lengthwise and chopped into ¼-inch-thick pieces
*One of my mom-testers used 2 chopped red peppers instead, which works equally well.*

2 cups long-grain white rice (preferably basmati), rinsed

2 teaspoons ground turmeric

1 teaspoon ground cumin

1 teaspoon ground coriander

¼ teaspoon ground cardamom, optional

2 bay leaves

One 14- to 15-ounce can chickpeas, rinsed and drained

4 cups low-sodium chicken broth

A splash or two of hot sauce, optional

⅓ cup lemon juice (from about 2 lemons), divided, plus 1 lemon, cut into wedges

½ cup frozen peas, thawed, optional

¼ cup chopped cilantro, optional

**Preheat oven to 375°F.**

1. Season the chicken breast with salt and pepper, then cut into 2-inch pieces.

2. Heat 1 tablespoon olive oil in a large Dutch oven or large, oven-safe pot over medium heat. When it shimmers, add half the chicken and cook, stirring occasionally, until the chicken is barely browned, about 3 minutes. Transfer to a bowl and repeat with another tablespoon of oil and the remaining chicken. Transfer chicken to the bowl.

3. Heat the remaining tablespoon oil in the pot. When it shimmers, add the onion. Cook, stirring occasionally, until onion is translucent, about 3 minutes. Add the zucchini and cook, stirring occasionally, until it begins to soften, 3 to 5 minutes more.

4. Add the rice, spices, and chickpeas and stir to combine. Cook for 1 minute, to toast the spices. Pour in the broth, hot sauce, if using, and half of the lemon juice. Return the browned chicken to the pot, and raise heat to high.

5. When the pot boils, remove from heat, cover, and transfer to the oven. Bake for 20 minutes, then remove from the oven and let it sit, covered, for 5 minutes before serving.

6. Remove the bay leaves, then stir in the remaining lemon juice and the peas and cilantro, if using, and serve with the lemon wedges.

**A NOTE ON DEFROSTING AND REHEATING:** If you can plan ahead, transfer from the freezer to the fridge the day before you'd like to eat it, then reheat in a saucepan over low heat, with an additional teaspoon or two of water. If dinner's more of an impromptu thing and you don't share my distaste for microwaved chicken, defrost in the microwave, removing portions as they're defrosted. Reheat in the microwave or in a saucepan, and again, add a teaspoon or two of water to keep it from drying out.

MAKE BABY FOOD: Some babies don't react well to the acidity in lemon juice, but others (ahem, Harry) like to suck on lemon wedges. If your baby is on Team Harry, by all means serve this to her, either pureed with a bit of broth or water, or as finger food.

MAMA SAID
"I loved these flavors! And finishing it in the oven definitely kept the chicken moister than pan sauté versions. This is even better the second day—the flavors have blended more."
—Jane B., mom of one, Pleasanton, CA

- - - - - - - - - - - - - - - - - - - - - - - - - - - - - - - - - -

# CHICKEN TAGINE WITH DRIED FRUIT AND ALMONDS

**Serves 8**

**Cooking time: 1 hour 25 minutes (45 minutes active)**

This flavor-packed recipe is a simplified riff on a recipe I tore out of *Gourmet* years ago. I've reduced the number of ingredients as well as some of the fussier steps, but left the flavor. Major flavor. The sultry spices, the mellow-sweet reconstituted dried fruit, and the bright fresh herbs added at the end make for a sophisticated, company-worthy meal. Think how handy that would be to have in the freezer.

1 teaspoon ground cinnamon

1 tablespoon curry powder

Salt and pepper

3 tablespoons olive oil, divided

8 boneless, skinless chicken breasts or thighs
**The recipe works with either white or dark meat, but do choose one or the other—they have different cooking times.**

1 cup water

1 tablespoon honey

½ cup dried apricots, peaches, nectarines, or plums, halved or quartered
**Don't have any of those dried fruits on hand? I've used dried apples and loved it!**

1 medium red onion, halved and thinly sliced, or 2 shallots, thinly sliced

3 large carrots, halved lengthwise and cut into ¼-inch-thick pieces

4 garlic cloves, minced

1 cup low-sodium chicken broth

⅓ cup sliced almonds

¼ cup chopped fresh mint leaves
**If you don't have fresh mint, cilantro or parsley would work here too.**

Couscous (preferably whole wheat), cooked according to package directions, for serving

1. Combine the cinnamon and curry powder with salt and pepper to taste and 1 tablespoon olive oil in a large bowl. Add the chicken and turn to coat well. Cover and let it sit at room temperature for 20 to 30 minutes.

*This tastes even better with a longer marination, so if you have the time, prepare this several hours ahead or even the night before. If you do, it must be refrigerated.*

2. While the chicken marinates, bring the water, honey, and dried fruit to a boil in a small heavy saucepan, then reduce the heat and simmer, uncovered, until fruit is very tender, about 8 minutes, adding more water as needed. Once the fruit is soft, use a slotted spoon to transfer it to a bowl and simmer the liquid until thickened and deeply colored, 5 to 10 minutes. Return fruit to the pan, and set aside.

3. Heat 1 tablespoon olive oil in a Dutch oven or large, heavy pot over medium-high heat. When it shimmers, add half the chicken and brown it on both sides, about 3 minutes per side, then transfer to a clean plate. Repeat with the remaining tablespoon oil and chicken.

4. Lower heat to medium-low, then add the onion and carrots to the now-empty pan and season lightly with salt. There should be enough fat left in the pan, but if it looks dry add a bit more oil. Cook, stirring frequently, until onion is softened and the carrots are beginning to soften, 3 to 5 minutes. Add the garlic and cook, stirring, until fragrant, about 30 seconds.

5. Add the chicken broth and scrape the bottom of the pot to loosen all the browned bits. Now return the browned chicken to the pot along with any accumulated juices, raise the heat to high, and bring to a boil. Reduce heat to low and simmer, covered, 20 minutes for breasts or 30 minutes for thighs. The chicken is done when it's no longer pink.

6. While the chicken simmers, place a small skillet over medium heat and toast the almonds in the dry pan, shaking the pan occasionally, until lightly browned, 1 to 2 minutes. Keep a close watch—they can go from barely toasted to burned quickly.

7. About 10 minutes before the chicken is done, add the fruit, the reduced cooking liquid, and the mint to the pot.

8. Serve over the prepared couscous, sprinkled with the toasted almonds.

**A NOTE ON DEFROSTING AND REHEATING:** Since they're substantial pieces of chicken, I wouldn't defrost this in the microwave—the outer edges of the chicken will start to reheat and overcook before the middle is defrosted. You'll have to plan a bit, and put the frozen package into the refrigerator 1 or 2 days before you plan to eat. Sorry!

MAKE BABY FOOD: There is a small amount of honey in this recipe; for safety's sake you should leave it out if you'll be feeding the dish to an infant under one year old. The reduced syrup won't be quite as thick, but it won't change the flavor too dramatically. If your baby's OK with spices, he can eat everything else except the almonds, which could be a choking hazard—give these an extra chop for his portion. (Skip the nuts altogether if there are food allergies in your family.) It works well as finger food, and you can also puree the chicken, onions, fruit, and carrots together with a spoonful of sauce.

**MAMA SAID**

"My husband made this dish. While he was cooking it he said, 'This is really fun to make! I think this is going to be really good!' He cooked it right after doing the daycare pick-up, so with a 10-month-old and a three-year-old around. He fed them something else that night and then we ate it ourselves later that night. Yum! Then the whole family had it the next night. Double yum!" —Maggie R., mom of two, Pleasantville, NY

# CHAPTER 6
# ONE-HANDED MEALS

OHT. That stands for One-Handed Typing, and it's an acronym used by new moms on AltDotLife, the message board I've mentioned before. It reflects a fact we all learn quickly, and the hard way: Newborns don't like to be put down. Ever. When Harry was small I'd preface my posts with those three letters, to excuse any typos caused by working with one arm locked into a sweet-smelling, cuddly handcuff.

Using just one hand, I can accomplish all kinds of necessary tasks, such as writing shopping lists, stirring a pot, turning pages, operating the remote, opening doors. . . . What can I say? I'm incredibly talented. So when Harry came along I figured I'd just adapt and do *everything* with one hand. I managed pretty well at first. Mind you, in those early days I wasn't trying to change a fan belt or anything, so don't go thinking

I was Superwoman. I was anything but, especially at mealtimes, when the memory of dual appendages became a cruel joke.

Miraculously, on Harry's second night home, he was asleep in his crib at dinnertime. Stephen and I pulled out real plates and silverware, like normal people, but the anticipation of his cry led us to Hoover our plates clean in about three minutes. So much for the luxury of having both hands free. At other meals we had two choices: Risk waking a sleeping baby—or pissing off a content, awake one—by putting him down, or continue to hold him in one arm and eat with the other. It didn't take us long to decide that the latter was the better choice. As I've since heard countless times, newborns don't *want* to be held; they *need* to be held. OHE (that's One-Handed Eating) was better than not eating at all, so we took turns holding him.

The problem was, I'd neglected to consider how tired my left arm would become from holding a mere six pounds of baby—sure, he was teeny at birth, but he was getting bigger by the minute. And then there was the fact that Stephen would be going back to work soon, so I wouldn't have anyone to trade off with. Fancying myself an earth mother, I came up with what seemed like an obvious solution: instead of carrying Harry, I could *wear* him. I just needed a sling. So on Harry's third day home, Stephen and I tucked him into the stroller and set out for the local kids' store.

Once there, selecting a sling was easy—they sold only one kind, a simple pouch. I had considerably more trouble figuring out how to load Harry into it, but the store's owner helped, and eventually my boy was snuggled safely inside his new cocoon. I wore him home, and all through the next day. It was glorious! I had both hands to work with, and suddenly things that had been tiresome and frustrating were doable.

The trouble developed in the late afternoon. Harry was lethargic and disinterested in nursing. Panicked, I called the pediatrician, then sobbed (thank you, hormones!) while waiting for the return call. I was certain there was something very wrong. I had that mama gut feeling, and mama gut feelings were supposed to be rock-solid. After the doctor called back and I explained the situation, she quickly deduced the problem: Wearing Harry in the sling for an entire day had essentially recreated the womb, and he was in an extremely deep sleep. She suggested I back off on the babywearing a bit.

Here's where I confess one of my (many) new-mom failings: After this episode, I didn't trust my instincts to gauge how much babywearing Harry could handle. So I simply stopped wearing him. I gave up on the idea of freedom—at least until he was a little older—because I was too scared that I might break my own kid. Instead, I adapted. I learned to do *even more* with just one hand, and to ignore the fatigue plaguing the other arm. My friends, this is one of my great regrets. Babywearing is safe, it's good for the baby as well as the parent, and lordy it makes life easier. We did the Björn once he was a little bigger, but Harry soon outgrew it and I'd feel pangs of jealousy every time I saw a friend wearing her kid in a Moby, an Ergo, or a Mei Tai sling. Please don't repeat my mistake!

As for our mealtime challenges: Over Harry's first few weeks, I came up with a list of recipes that were easily eaten with one hand. Now, I love a messy, salsa-topped taco as much as the next person, but they just aren't feasible when there's a baby in your lap; the drip factor is too high. So you'll find no tacos here. Instead, the recipes in this chapter are neat and contained: turnovers, pie-rogies, empanadas, even baked ravioli. Some recipes, like the Chicken (Pot) Handpies, require the investment of a little more time than usual, but one kitchen session makes enough to freeze and enjoy at multiple meals. The best thing about these recipes: Each one is satisfying, nutritious, and delicious enough that you won't miss that other hand. I've grouped the recipes that follow by "container"—the ones that use pizza dough come first, then pie dough, and so on.

. . . . . . . . . . . . . . . . . . . . . . . . . . . . . . . . . . . . . . . . . . . . . . . . . . . . . . .

### YOU CAN EAT THESE WITH ONE HAND TOO

There are dozens of pastas, salads, and stews in the book, none of which require a fork and knife. But these recipes in particular are meant to be eaten with one hand:

Baked Falafel (page 31)
A Really Good Smoothie (page 323)
The Quesadilla Variations (page 264)
Mezze Feast (page 276)
Greek Pita Pockets (page 277)
Grilled Chicken Pesto Heroes (page 279)

. . . . . . . . . . . . . . . . . . . . . . . . . . . . . . . . . . . . . . . . . . . . . . . . . . . . . . .

### SEVEN ONE-HANDED, NO-COOK, NO-FORK LUNCHES (OR LIGHT DINNERS)

- Deli turkey, Peppadew peppers (the small, sweet and spicy red ones; you'll find them in jars or in your supermarket's olive bar), whole grain crackers, and cheddar—go ahead and buy the cubes; this is no time for knife work!

- Whole wheat mini-pitas, stuffed—but not overstuffed—with goat cheese and prepared chutney, and red grapes

- Whole wheat mini-pitas, prepared hummus, baby carrots, and grape tomatoes

- Ricotta drizzled with honey, topped with almonds and berries. Scoop it up with whole-grain crackers, or just use a spoon

- Party-sized rye bread topped with roasted red pepper strips and deli-sliced salami and provolone

- Bocconcini (bite-sized mozzarella balls), black olives (I beg you, don't buy canned—they're artificially cured with lye, which sucks out all the flavor), whole grain crispbread like Wasa, and pears (I like Seckel, those miniature ones)

- Deconstructed egg salad: Hard-boiled eggs (ready-made are just fine), honey mustard for dipping, gherkins, celery sticks (again, buy ready-made), whole-grain roll

### CRIB NOTES

- These are meals to be eaten with one hand. I'm pretty sure nobody's yet invented recipes you can *cook* with one hand.

- Since these are grab-and-go recipes, in many cases you'll want to add a salad or some sort of nibbly food like baby carrots and hummus to make a full meal.

- General tips on using purchased dough: Pizza dough is easiest to work with at room temperature, so leave it on the counter for 30 minutes to an hour before you plan to fill it. Room-temperature pie or empanada dough, on the other hand, will be sticky and squishy. With those types, you only want to soften it just slightly—leave it on the counter until it's loosened up a bit but is still cold.

- Quite a few of the recipes in this chapter work well with my Nap-Friendly Cooking technique. For specifics on how to adapt them, see page 75.

- Any of the recipes using dough will freeze well, once baked. Allow them to cool thoroughly, then wrap tightly and freeze. To reheat, unwrap and place on a baking sheet—no need to thaw. Bake at 350°F for 20 to 40 minutes, depending on the size of the item.

# BROCCOLI AND CHEDDAR PINWHEELS

**Makes 8, and doubles well**

**Cooking time: 1 hour (20 minutes active)**

Among my mom-testers, this was by far the most popular recipe in this chapter. It's easy to assemble, and the secret ingredient—Dijon mustard—gives it a nice zip.

1 pound prepared pizza dough, white or whole wheat

2½ cups finely chopped broccoli, or one 10-ounce package of frozen chopped broccoli, defrosted and finely chopped
*If you don't mind the additional cleanup, you can do the fine-chopping by pulsing in the food processor. It's important that the pieces be quite small, or you'll have trouble in the assembly.*

1 to 2 cups shredded Cheddar cheese, depending on how much you like cheese

1 tablespoon Dijon mustard

Salt and pepper

**Preheat oven to 425°F. Line or grease a baking sheet.**

1. Remove pizza dough from the refrigerator 30 minutes to 1 hour before you plan to use it.

2. Steam the broccoli until just tender, 5 to 6 minutes. Cool slightly, then combine broccoli with the Cheddar, mustard, and salt and pepper to taste.

3. Roll or stretch the dough on a floured work surface into a large rectangle, about 10 x 14 inches. Don't worry if you can't get those exact measurements, but take care not to stretch the dough so thin it rips.

4. Spread the broccoli mixture over about three-quarters of the dough, leaving an uncoated portion at one short side. Begin to roll the dough from the short side covered with the broccoli spread, and keep rolling until you've got a nice, neat log of dough.

5. Using a serrated knife or a pastry scraper, cut the log into 8 equal pinwheels. Carefully lay the pinwheels flat on the prepared baking sheet, and bake until crust is golden brown and the cheese is melted, 15 to 20 minutes.

MAKE BABY FOOD: If your baby's still on purees, reserve a portion of the broccoli-cheese mixture and blend it with a bit of milk or broth. If you're on finger foods, simply cut the pinwheel into itty-bitty pieces.

**MAMA SAID**

"Oh these were so good. And easy to make! They were cheesy, doughy, delicious, and the mustard was a surprise treat. I prepared these by myself while solo-parenting, and had no problems whipping them together. I loved them, couldn't stop eating them, and my toddler loved them too. What a great way to get little ones to eat broccoli if they normally won't!" —Heather M., mom of one, Los Gatos, CA

. . . . . . . . . . . . . . . . . . . . . . . . . . . . . . . . . . . . . . . . . . . . . . . . . . . .

# BAKED VEGETABLE PANZAROTTI

**Makes 4 and doubles well**

**Cooking time: 55 to 65 minutes (20 to 30 minutes active)**

Stephen is from south Jersey. The closest the area gets to its own food specialty is panzarotti, which is basically an entire pizza folded in half, sealed, and deep-fried and is intended to serve one person. OK, just writing that makes my mouth water. But it also makes me a little queasy. Luckily, Stephen's favorite pizza joint—Corrado's in Sicklerville, where he worked as a delivery guy after high school—does a baked version. This is an homage.

1 pound prepared pizza dough, white or whole wheat

½ cup best-quality prepared pasta sauce
   *Little Gram's Sauce (page 177) works well here too.*

1½ to 2 cups chopped vegetables (eggplant, zucchini, peppers, mushrooms, broccoli, onions, olives—whatever you can imagine working on a pizza)

1 cup shredded mozzarella cheese

¼ cup grated Parmesan cheese

Additional sauce, for dipping

**Preheat oven to 400°F. Line or grease a baking sheet.**

1. Remove pizza dough from the refrigerator 30 minutes to 1 hour before you plan to use it.

2. Cut the dough into 4 equal pieces. Place 1 piece on a floured work surface, and loosely cover the rest with plastic wrap. Roll or stretch the dough into an 8-inch circle. Don't worry if you can't get those exact measurements, but take care not to stretch the dough so thin that it rips.

3. Spread about 2 tablespoons sauce slightly off-center on the dough, leaving a 1-inch border. Top with ⅓ to ½ cup chopped vegetables, followed by ½ cup mozzarella, and 1 tablespoon Parmesan.

4. Fold the dough into a half-moon—you may need to stretch it a bit, carefully, to cover the filling—and pinch the edges together firmly. It should feel pretty stuffed, but the vegetables will shrink as they cook. Carefully transfer the panzarotti to the prepared baking sheet and repeat with remaining dough and filling ingredients.

5. Bake until the crusts are golden brown, 25 to 30 minutes. Serve with additional sauce for dipping.

MAKE BABY FOOD: Provided you chop the vegetables small enough for your baby to handle, this will work as finger food—just be careful not to give him any large chunks of stringy cheese. You can also puree the cooked filling with water or a little more sauce.

**MAMA SAID**
"It was easy and delicious! We used what veggies we had around, which was basically carrots and broccoli. I can see myself doing this myself on a Sunday and then taking it out of the freezer later in the week to eat." —Monica W., mom of one, St. Louis, MO

# ROASTED VEGETABLE TURNOVERS

**Makes 8, and doubles well**

**Cooking time: 70 to 80 minutes (30 minutes active)**

These turnovers are similar to the Baked Vegetable Panzarottis on page 198 in that they both use pizza dough, vegetables, and cheese, but the results are completely different. Pre-roasting the vegetables gives them a lovely, melting texture, and the addition of thyme and a mellow, nutty cheese makes these feel downright sophisticated. And they're smaller, so you can almost trick yourself into thinking you're at a cocktail party in a little black dress, rather than home wearing a spit-up-stained T-shirt for the third day in a row.

1 pound prepared pizza dough, white or
    whole wheat
1 medium eggplant, unpeeled, cubed
1 medium zucchini, chopped
6 garlic cloves, unpeeled
1 tablespoon olive oil

1 teaspoon fresh thyme leaves, or ½ teaspoon
    dried thyme
Salt and pepper
2 tablespoons tomato paste
1¼ cups shredded Gruyère, Emmental, or
    Fontina cheese, divided

**Preheat oven to 425°F and set the racks in the upper and lower thirds of oven. Grease or line two baking sheets.**

1. Remove pizza dough from the refrigerator 30 minutes to 1 hour before you plan to use it.

2. Combine the eggplant, zucchini, garlic, olive oil, thyme, and salt and pepper to taste in a large bowl. Spread the mixture onto the baking sheets, and roast vegetables until they are browned and tender, switching placement of the baking sheets halfway through, 20 to 25 minutes.

3. Cool vegetables slightly. Remove and discard garlic skin, then transfer all vegetables to a food processor. Add the tomato paste and pulse 5 to 10 times, until mixture is combined but still chunky. Stir in 1 cup of the cheese.

4. Re-grease or line one of the cleaned baking sheets.

5. Cut the dough into 8 equal pieces. Place 1 piece on a floured work surface and loosely cover the rest with plastic wrap. Roll out or stretch the dough into a 4 x 6-inch

rectangle. Don't worry if you can't get those exact measurements, but take care not to stretch the dough so thin that it rips.

6. Put about 2 tablespoons of the vegetable mixture slightly off-center on the dough, and pull the longer side of the dough over it. Pinch the edges firmly to seal. Carefully transfer the turnover to the prepared baking sheet. Repeat with the remaining dough and vegetable mixture.

7. Sprinkle a bit of the remaining cheese on top of each turnover, then bake until crusts are golden brown, 25 to 30 minutes.

> MAKE BABY FOOD: The filling is just perfect for early eaters—puree it fully if you like, or leave it chunky. For babies who are on finger food, cut the baked turnover into small pieces.

**MAMA SAID**
"We had these for dinner tonight, and they were a hit with me, my husband, and the baby! (I had a feeling, which turned out to be correct, that the preschoolers wouldn't like the filling, so I made a batch for them with just red sauce and cheese—those were popular.) The flavor and texture were just delicious." —Sarah B., mom of three, Canterbury, CT

# CHICKEN CACCIATORE TURNOVERS

**Makes 4, and doubles well**

**Cooking time: 1½ hours minutes (45 minutes active)**

Here's a one-hander that's an ideal candidate for Nap-Friendly Cooking: Chop and measure everything during the morning nap (refrigerate the chicken!), cook the filling during the afternoon nap (again, refrigerate), and assemble and bake just before dinner.

If you like dunking, serve this with a little bowl of prepared pasta sauce.

1 pound prepared pizza dough, white or
   whole wheat

1 tablespoon olive oil

1 boneless, skinless chicken breast, chopped
   into ¼-inch pieces
   *It's easiest to chop chicken when it's slightly
   frozen.*

1 small onion, finely chopped

1 garlic clove, minced

2 ounces cremini or white button mushrooms,
   sliced (3 or 4 good-sized mushrooms)

Salt and pepper

¾ cup crushed tomatoes or diced tomatoes
   and their juices
   *You can also use about 1 cup of Little Gram's
   Sauce (page 177) or good-quality jarred pasta
   sauce, and omit the tomatoes, red wine,
   oregano, and sugar.*

¼ cup red wine

¼ teaspoon dried oregano

Pinch of sugar

1. Remove the pizza dough from the refrigerator 30 minutes to 1 hour before you plan to use it.

2. Heat the olive oil in a large skillet over medium heat. When it shimmers, add the chicken and cook, stirring occasionally, until barely cooked but not browned, about 3 minutes. Transfer chicken to a clean bowl.

3. There should still be oil left in the pan—if it looks too dry, add a bit more, then add the onion. Cook until translucent, 2 to 3 minutes, then add the garlic and cook for 30 seconds more. Add the mushrooms and salt and pepper to taste and cook, stirring occasionally, until mushrooms have released their liquid and liquid has mostly evaporated, about 3 minutes.

4. Return chicken to the skillet, and add the tomatoes, red wine, oregano, and sugar. Simmer, uncovered, until the sauce has thickened nicely, 5 to 10 minutes.

**NOTE:** Tomato sauce has a tendency to spatter; if you'd rather a bit less mess, put a lid on the pot—but only partially, otherwise the sauce won't thicken. Expect it to take a few minutes longer.

5. Transfer mixture to a clean bowl to cool slightly. Preheat oven to 400°F. Grease or line a baking sheet.

6. Cut the dough into 4 equal pieces. Place 1 piece on a floured work surface and loosely cover the rest with plastic wrap. Roll or stretch the dough into an 8-inch circle.

7. Put about ⅓ cup of the filling just slightly off-center on the dough and fold the dough over it to form a half-moon. Pinch edges firmly to seal. Transfer turnover carefully to the baking sheet. Repeat with remaining dough and filling.

6. Bake until the crusts are browned, 25 to 30 minutes.

MAKE BABY FOOD: If your baby's on purees, remove some of the filling and simmer it a little longer, to ensure that the chicken is cooked thoroughly and to allow more of the alcohol to evaporate (there's very little to begin with—just 2 ounces of wine for the whole recipe—but the longer it cooks the less likely it is for even a trace to remain). Cool, then puree, with a splash of water or broth if it's too thick. If she's on finger food, just cut up a cooked turnover and serve.

**MAMA SAID**
**"Big family favorite. My toddler, who usually hates bread, really liked it, eating almost all of it—a first!" —Bethany G., mom of one, St. Paul, MN**

• • • • • • • • • • • • • • • • • • • • • • • • • • • • • • • • • • • •

# SFIHA (MIDDLE EASTERN MEAT PIES)

**Makes 4, and doubles well**

**Cooking time: 1 hour 15 minutes (50 minutes active)**

In Brooklyn, there's an ethnic neighborhood for pretty much any group you can think of. One of the strongest is the Arabic enclave centered around Atlantic Avenue, but you can find terrific Middle Eastern food all over the borough. If you're lucky, in addition to the usual falafel and slowly turning cylinders of shawarma, you'll find an assortment of handpies filled with spiced ground meat or spinach. This recipe is a nod to those tasty pies. It's filled with ground beef, vegetables, and toasted pine nuts and scented with cumin and lime juice. The pizza dough crust isn't exactly authentic, but I can live with it if you can.

1 pound pizza dough, white or whole wheat

6 ounces lean ground beef

1 small onion, finely chopped

1 small red bell pepper, finely chopped

1 medium tomato, seeded and finely chopped
   *Easiest way to seed a tomato? Cut it in half across the equator, then hold each half over the sink and squeeze gently. All the goo should slip right out.*

½ tablespoon ground cumin

Juice of ½ lime (about 1 tablespoon)

Salt and pepper

2 tablespoons pine nuts, toasted

**Preheat oven to 400°F. Grease or line a baking sheet.**

1. Remove pizza dough from the refrigerator 30 minutes to 1 hour before you plan to use it.

2. Cook the meat in a medium skillet over medium heat, breaking up clumps with the back of a spoon, until it's no longer pink, 3 to 5 minutes. If there is a considerable amount of grease, drain all but about 1 tablespoon and discard.

3. Add the onion and pepper and cook, stirring occasionally, until the vegetables begin to soften, 3 to 4 minutes. Add the tomato, cumin, lime juice, and salt and pepper to taste and cook until mixture looks saucy but not wet, 3 to 5 minutes. Taste and adjust the seasoning. Transfer to a bowl to cool, and stir in the pine nuts.

4. Cut the pizza dough into 4 equal pieces. Place 1 piece on a floured work surface and loosely cover the rest with plastic wrap. Roll or stretch the dough into an 8-inch circle.

5. Put about ⅓ cup of the filling slightly off-center on the dough, and fold dough over it to form a half-moon. Pinch the edges together firmly to seal. Transfer the turnover carefully to the baking sheet. Repeat with remaining dough and filling.

6. Pierce the top of each turnover a few times with a fork. Bake until crust is dark golden brown, 20 to 25 minutes. Transfer turnovers to a wire rack to cool for about 10 minutes before serving.

> MAKE BABY FOOD: If there are no food allergy concerns, this is fine for babies, either as finger food (chop the pine nuts before adding) or pureed (add a bit of water or broth if it's too dry). To be allergen-free, leave out the pine nuts.

MAMA SAID
"Delicious! I used the leftover filling for a topping on pita chips, as a type of nacho."
—Alana D., mom of one, Providence, RI

• • • • • • • • • • • • • • • • • • • • • • • • • • • • • • • • • • •

# BUTTERNUT HANDPIES

**Makes 8, and doubles well**
**Cooking time: 1 hour 20 minutes (40 to 50 minutes active)**

I won't lie: peeling and cutting butternut squash is a pain. But it's fine to buy the pre-cut kind and just chop it down further—for this recipe it needs to be fairly small in order to cook all the way through before the pie crust burns. If you *are* using a whole squash, buy a 2½- to 3-pounder, halve it lengthwise, and use the other half for the Crispy Butternut Ravioli on page 224. Unfortunately, frozen isn't a good substitute here, since sometimes the water content is rather high—it'll make things too soggy.

2 unbaked pie crusts either storebought or homemade (not pie shells)
1½ cups chopped butternut squash (¼-inch pieces)
⅓ cup finely chopped leeks (whites and palest greens parts)

½ cup shredded Gruyère or Fontina cheese
Generous pinch of grated nutmeg
Salt and pepper
1 egg, beaten with 1 tablespoon water

**Preheat oven to 350°F, and set the racks in the upper and lower thirds of oven. Grease or line two baking sheets.**

1.  Remove the piecrusts from the refrigerator 20 to 30 minutes before you plan to use them. Combine the squash, leeks, Gruyère, nutmeg, and salt and pepper to taste in a medium bowl.

2.  Roll out 1 pie crust on a lightly floured work surface (but not too much or it will become too delicate). Use a sharp knife or pizza cutter to cut the dough into 4 wedge-shaped pieces.

3.  Put about ¼ cup of filling off-center on 1 piece of dough, then carefully fold dough over to form a triangle. Crimp the edges with a fork and prick the top a few times for steam to escape. Transfer handpie carefully to the prepared baking sheet. Repeat with remaining pie crust and filling.

4.  Brush tops of pies lightly with the egg wash, then bake until golden brown, 30 to 40 minutes. If you're not eating them right away, transfer to a wire rack to cool.

MAKE BABY FOOD: If you're on finger foods, break open a pie and let your baby go to town. For purees, scoop out some of the cooked filling and whir it with a bit of broth or milk.

**MAMA SAID**
"My 10-month-old loved the butternut handpie pieces that we gave him! I did most of it while he was napping or occupied with something else. They were easy to make in stages—a huge benefit. The handpies will make terrific lunches for work while I pump."
—Mary T., mom of one, Ankeny, IA

# POTATO AND MUSHROOM PIE-ROGIES

**Makes 8, and doubles well**

**Cooking time: 1 hour (35 minutes active)**

Imagine the traditional flavors of a pierogi—potato, mushroom, golden-browned onions—but in a hand-held, slightly larger version made with refrigerated pie crust. You're welcome.

2 tablespoons oil

1 medium onion, quartered lengthwise and very thinly sliced

4 ounces regular or light cream cheese (not whipped), at room temperature

1 cup leftover mashed potatoes, at room temperature
*Throw in a few extra potatoes when you make Cottage Pie (page 71). Or buy prepared mashed potatoes, as long as they're made with ingredients you recognize.*

4 ounces cremini or white button mushrooms, roughly chopped

1 teaspoon fresh thyme leaves, optional

Salt and pepper

1 unbaked piecrust, either storebrought or homemade (not pie shells)

1 egg, beaten with 1 tablespoon water

Sour cream, for serving

**Preheat oven to 425°F. Grease or line a baking sheet.**

1.  Heat the oil in a large skillet over medium heat. When it shimmers, add the onion and cook, stirring occasionally, until golden-brown, 8 to 10 minutes.

2.  While the onion cooks, stir together the cream cheese and mashed potatoes in a medium bowl, then set aside.

3.  Add the mushrooms and thyme, if using, to the onion, and season with salt and pepper to taste. Cook, stirring occasionally, until mushrooms are tender and all the liquid they've released has evaporated, 3 to 5 minutes. Transfer to the bowl with the potato mixture and stir to combine. Set aside to cool. Remove the pie crust from the refrigerator so it can soften slightly.

4.  On a lightly floured work surface, roll out the pie crust into a rough rectangle (don't roll it too thin or the pie-rogies will fall apart). Use a sharp knife or pizza cutter to square off the rounded edges, then cut the dough into 8 equal rectangles.

5. Place a heaping tablespoon of filling about an inch from the bottom of 1 piece of dough, then carefully fold the dough over. Crimp the edges together with a fork. Transfer completed pie-rogies to the prepared baking sheet.

*You may have some filling left over—lucky you, it's perfect for baby food! Puree it with a splash of milk if your baby's not on chunky foods yet.*

6. Brush tops of pies lightly with the egg wash, then cut a slit in the top of each to allow steam to escape.

7. Bake until crusts are golden brown, 25 to 30 minutes. Transfer pies to a rack to cool.

> MAKE BABY FOOD: Once it's cooled a bit, this is just fine as finger food. Or, as mentioned above, puree the filling.

**MAMA SAID**
"The Pie-rogies were just delish, and would definitely be perfect for those early nursing/newborn days of one-handedness. They turned out beautifully (literally, like a picture in a cookbook!). The prep and assembly were quick enough to do while the baby was occupied by himself, and my three- and four-year-olds helped to chop the mushrooms, which kept them busy and happy. I didn't have any leftover mashed potatoes, so I threw a few potatoes in the microwave and gave them a quick mash with milk and salt before adding the cream cheese." —Sarah B., mom of three, Canterbury, CT

# CHICKEN (POT) HANDPIES

**Makes 8, and doubles well**

**Cooking time: 1 hour 10 minutes (45 minutes active)**

All the flavors of chicken pot pie, but handheld!

1 medium potato, peeled and chopped into ¼-inch pieces
*Substitute ½ cup thawed frozen corn kernels here, if you prefer. Add with the carrot and celery in Step 2.*

1 tablespoon vegetable oil

1 small onion, finely chopped

1 carrot, quartered lengthwise and chopped

1 celery rib, halved lengthwise and chopped

4 ounces boneless, skinless chicken breast or thighs, chopped
*Got some cooked chicken? Add it with the potatoes in step 3 instead.*

Salt and pepper

1 tablespoon all-purpose flour

½ cup chicken broth

½ teaspoon fresh thyme leaves

2 unbaked pie crusts, either store bought or homemade (not pie shells)

1 egg, beaten with 1 tablespoon water

1.  Simmer the potato in a small pot of salted water until just tender, 8 to 10 minutes, then drain and set aside.

2.  Heat the oil in a large skillet over medium heat. When it shimmers, add the onion and cook, stirring occasionally, until translucent, 2 to 3 minutes. Add the carrot, celery, and raw chicken, season with salt and pepper to taste, and raise the heat to medium-high. Cook until the vegetables are softened and the chicken is just about cooked, 3 to 5 minutes.

3.  Sprinkle the flour over everything, stir, and cook for 1 minute. Add the broth, thyme, and reserved potatoes, and simmer for 2 minutes more. Transfer the mixture to a bowl and refrigerate until cool, 15 to 30 minutes. Remove the pie crusts from the refrigerator so they can soften slightly.

4.  When the filling is cool, preheat oven to 425°F and set the racks in the upper and lower thirds of oven. Grease or line two baking sheets.

5.  On a lightly floured work surface, roll out 1 pie crust into a rough rectangle (don't roll it too thin or the handpies will fall apart). Use a sharp knife or pizza cutter to square off the rounded edges, then cut the dough into 4 equal pieces.

6. Place about ¼ cup of filling slightly off-center on 1 piece of dough, then fold the dough over to form a rectangle. Crimp the edges together with a fork, and prick the top a few times for steam to escape. Carefully transfer pie to the prepared baking sheets. Repeat with remaining pie crust and filling.

7. Brush each pie lightly with the egg wash, then bake until golden brown, 20 to 25 minutes.

MAKE BABY FOOD: These are a slam dunk for little ones—either cut a pie into pieces and let baby feed himself, or cook the filling a minute or two longer (to be certain the chicken is cooked through) and puree some of it with a bit more broth.

**MAMA SAID**
"The taste was great. I really enjoyed all the bits and pieces. I made them the night before and stuck them in the freezer, and my husband reheated them for dinner the next day. And boy, does that work out well. The fact that I could also make a double batch on a Sunday and pull them out during the week is incredibly appealing." —Monica W., mom of one, St. Louis, MO

# MEAT PASTIES

**Makes 8, and doubles well**

**Cooking time: 1½ hours (30 minutes active)**

I'd never heard of a pasty (pronounced PAH-stee) until I worked at a New York City restaurant owned by a lovely woman from Michigan. Turns out these humble little meat pies are a specialty of the state's Upper Peninsula, where miners (immigrants from England, where pasties originated) would take them along for a one-handed, compact lunch. They're plain as can be—no special ingredients and virtually no seasoning—but that simplicity is why I like them so much. Traditionally, pasties are formed into a half-moon shape, but since we're using pre-made pie dough that's a pretty tall order. We're going with rectangles, my friends.

2 unbaked pie crusts, either store bought or homemade (not pie shells)

½ pound beef, trimmed of excess fat, chopped into ¼-inch pieces

*Almost any cut of boneless beef would work here: chuck, bottom round. Several mom-testers even used ground beef.*

1 medium potato, peeled and chopped into ¼-inch pieces

1 carrot, quartered lengthwise and chopped into ¼-inch pieces

½ cup chopped leeks (white and palest green parts)

Salt and pepper

4 teaspoons butter, optional

1 egg, beaten with 1 tablespoon water

**Remove the pie crusts from the refrigerator 15 to 20 minutes before you plan to use them. Preheat oven to 350°F, and set the racks in the upper and lower thirds of the oven. Grease or line two baking sheets.**

1. Combine the beef, potato, carrot, leeks, and salt and pepper to taste in a medium bowl.

2. On a lightly floured work surface, roll out 1 pie crust into a rough rectangle (don't roll it too thin or the pasties will fall apart). Use a sharp knife or pizza cutter to square off the rounded edges, then cut the dough into 4 equal pieces.

3. Place about ⅓ cup of filling slightly off-center on 1 piece of dough. Put ½ teaspoon butter, if using, on the filling, then fold the dough over. Crimp the edges together with a fork, and prick the top a few times for steam to escape. Carefully transfer pasty to the prepared baking sheets. Repeat with remaining pie crust and filling.

4.  Brush tops lightly with the egg wash and bake until golden brown, 50 to 60 minutes. If you're not eating them right away, transfer to a wire rack to cool.

> MAKE BABY FOOD: The texture of the meat inside the baked pies can be a little tough for young eaters. If you like, reserve some of the uncooked filling, mix it with a bit of water or broth, and bake, covered with foil, alongside the pies for 30 to 40 minutes. You can puree this or serve it as finger food.

**MAMA SAID**
"The meat pasties were a great success! I made them with ground beef, as that's what we had on hand. It turned out to be really great for this recipe, because it formed a nice mixture with the chopped vegetables and the result was that the pasties held together very well. I had a clingy-toddler moment right when I was forming them, and so I ended up forming long big rectangles (think a large calzone or small stromboli) kind of frantically and yet they kept their shape even after I cut them. Yay for a forgiving recipe." —Christine G., mom of four, Tokyo, Japan

# CURRIED KALE AND APPLE EMPANADAS

**Makes 10 to 12, and doubles well**

**Cooking time: 1 hour (30 minutes active)**

We're a travel-for-food kind of family. In days gone by (read: when we were care- and child-free), Stephen and I would drive for hours to sample an especially promising hot dog. These days we still jump in the car and go, but it's more likely to be within 30 minutes of home. One of our favorite spots is Empanadas Café in Corona, Queens, where they offer dozens of varieties of the South American turnover. They haven't yet come up with a curried option, but I have a feeling the café's owners would approve of this one.

**NOTE:** If you live in an area that has a South- or Latin-American community, you should have no trouble finding frozen empanada shells. No luck? Substitute prepared pie dough.

1 tablespoon vegetable oil

1 medium onion, finely chopped

2 teaspoons curry powder

Salt and pepper

1 tart apple, peeled, cored, and roughly chopped

4 cups roughly chopped kale (from about 1 large bunch), leaves only, with some water clinging to leaves

½ cup shredded Cheddar cheese
*If you're a cheese fan, you can use up to 1 cup.*

12 frozen empanada shells, thawed
*Depending on the brand, packages are sold in quantities of 10 or 12. If yours has only 10, there will be some filling left over—makes a handy snack.*

1 egg, beaten with 1 tablespoon water

**Preheat oven to 350°F. Grease or line a baking sheet.**

1. Heat the oil in a large skillet over medium heat. When it shimmers, add the onion and cook, stirring occasionally, until translucent, 3 to 5 minutes. Stir in the curry powder and salt and pepper to taste, and cook until fragrant, about 1 minute. Add the apple and cook, stirring occasionally, until it begins to soften, 2 to 3 minutes.

2. Stir in the kale, lower the heat, and simmer, covered, until kale loses some of its toughness, 3 to 4 minutes.

3. Transfer mixture to a bowl. When it's cool, stir in the Cheddar cheese.

4. Remove the thawed shells from the refrigerator 10 to 15 minutes before you plan to use them. The shells should be slightly colder than room temperature, and flexible but not squishy.

5. Before you start assembling the empanadas, line up the bowl of filling, a small bowl with a few tablespoons of water, and another with the egg wash.

6. Remove 4 shells at a time, leaving the rest in the packaging to prevent them from drying out. Lay them flat on a work surface, and put a generous tablespoon of filling on each. Dip a finger into the water and wet the entire diameter of the dough, then fold it in half, stretching gently as you pull the dough over the filling. Press firmly to seal, then crimp with a fork. Transfer empanadas to the prepared baking sheet, and repeat with remaining shells and filling.

7. Brush the egg wash over the empanadas, then bake until deep golden brown, 25 to 35 minutes.

8. Cool the empanadas slightly. If you like, serve with the Apricot-Ginger Dipping Sauce on page 222.

> MAKE BABY FOOD: The filling is a lovely texture for finger food—just make sure the kale is well-chopped. If you're on purees, add a bit of water, apple juice, or broth.

**MAMA SAID**
"This was probably one of our favorite recipes so far. We didn't have kale in the house, so we used Swiss chard (it was in our farm share) and it was fine. They take a while to make, so we froze the extras. We reheated one in the microwave tonight (for 1 minute) and it was just as good as the night before. "Our four-year-old loved helping to make the empanadas. We see this as a fun, family meal to make!" —Alexandra S., mom of two, Baltimore, MD

. . . . . . . . . . . . . . . . . . . . . . . . . . . . . . . . . . . . . . .

# BBQ CHICKEN EMPANADAS

**Makes 10 to 12, and doubles well**

**Cooking time: 50 minutes to 1 hour (25 minutes active)**

Of the three empanada recipes in this chapter, this one is the easiest. The filling comes together in about 10 minutes—the most challenging part of the entire recipe is the assembly.

12 frozen empanada shells, thawed
*Depending on the brand, packages are sold in quantities of 10 or 12. If yours has only 10, there will be some filling left over. Use it to make a quick burrito or quesadilla.*

¾ cup chopped or shredded cooked chicken

¾ cup corn kernels, either fresh (from about 2 ears) or frozen (no need to defrost)

½ cup canned black beans, rinsed and drained

¼ cup shredded Cheddar cheese

¼ cup prepared barbecue sauce, plus more for serving

1 egg, beaten with 1 tablespoon water

**Preheat oven to 350°F. Grease or line a baking sheet. Remove the thawed shells from the refrigerator 10 to 15 minutes before you plan to use them. The shells should be slightly colder than room temperature, and flexible but not squishy.**

1. Combine all of the ingredients except for the empanada shells and egg wash in a medium bowl.

2. Before you start assembling the empanadas, line up the empanada shells, the filling, a small bowl with a few tablespoons of water, and another with the egg wash.

3. Remove 4 shells at a time, leaving the rest in the packaging to prevent them from drying out. Lay them flat on a work surface, and put a generous tablespoon of filling on each. Dip a finger into the water and wet the entire diameter of the dough, then fold it in half, stretching gently as you pull the dough over the filling. Press firmly to seal, then crimp with a fork. Carefully transfer empanadas to the prepared baking sheet. Repeat with the remaining shells and filling.

4. Brush the egg wash over the empanadas, then bake until deep golden brown, 25 to 35 minutes.

5. Cool empanadas slightly. Serve with additional barbecue sauce, for dipping.

> MAKE BABY FOOD: This is another filling that works, either pureed or as finger food. Choose a mild variety of barbecue sauce if your baby isn't used to spicy food.

**MAMA SAID**
"Between the BBQ chicken empanadas, the broccoli Cheddar pinwheels, and the taco empanadas, this was my husband's favorite. Overall the recipe was pretty easy to make—I couldn't find frozen empanada shells so I made do with pie crust. That worked out just fine."
—Monica W., mom of one, St. Louis, MO

## TACO EMPANADAS

**Makes 10 to 12, and doubles well**
**Cooking time: 1 hour 15 minutes (40 minutes active)**

Remember how, in the introduction to this chapter, I said you wouldn't find any tacos? Well, I lied. These beauties encase a ground-meat taco filling in dough, which makes for a much neater eating experience. Your baby's head should get through the meal drip-free.

**NOTE:** Looking for a super-fast method? Make the filling using a package of taco seasoning, prepared according to package directions. Look for one with ingredients you recognize and the lowest sodium count you can find. Start the recipe at Step 4.

1 tablespoon chili powder

1½ teaspoons ground cumin

½ teaspoon paprika

½ teaspoon salt

¼ teaspoon garlic powder

¼ teaspoon onion powder

¼ teaspoon red pepper flakes

¼ teaspoon dried oregano

¾ pound lean ground beef or turkey

1 teaspoon brown sugar

2 teaspoons cider vinegar

12 frozen empanada shells, thawed
*Depending on the brand, packages are sold in quantities of 10 or 12. If yours has only 10, there will be some filling left over. Wrap it in a lettuce leaf and call it the chef's treat.*

1 egg, beaten with 1 tablespoon water

Salsa, for dipping

**Preheat oven to 350°F. Grease or line a baking sheet. Remove the thawed shells from the refrigerator 10 to 15 minutes before you plan to use them. The shells should be slightly colder than room temperature, and flexible but not squishy.**

1. Mix together the spices in a small bowl and set aside.

2. Cook the meat in a large skillet over medium heat, breaking it up with the back of a spoon, until completely browned, about 5 minutes. Stir in the spice mixture and ½ cup water, then lower the heat and simmer, stirring occasionally, until mixture is moist but not liquidy, 10 to 15 minutes.

3. Stir in the brown sugar and vinegar and simmer 2 to 3 minutes more, then transfer the filling to a bowl to cool.

4. Before you start assembling the empanadas, line up the shells, the filling, a small bowl with a few tablespoons of water, and another with the egg wash.

5. Remove 4 shells at a time, leaving the rest in the packaging to prevent them from drying out. Lay them flat on a work surface, and put a generous tablespoon of filling on each. Dip a finger into the water and wet the entire diameter of the dough, then fold it in half, stretching gently as you pull the dough over the filling. Press firmly to seal, then crimp with a fork. Transfer empanadas to the prepared baking sheet. Repeat with remaining shells and filling.

6. Brush the egg wash over the empanadas, then bake until deep golden brown, 25 to 35 minutes.

7. Cool empanadas slightly. Serve with salsa, for dipping.

MAKE BABY FOOD: If your baby likes spice, she should have no trouble eating this. If you're still on purees, add a splash of water or broth.

**MAMA SAID**
"Mm, these were good. We had trouble finding empanada shells so for this recipe we actually used puff pastry, but it worked out just fine. The taste was fantastic, with or without salsa for dipping. Making them was really easy too. I made the meat on Sunday, baked on Thursday, and we had them for dinner on Friday. I can see my husband making these the day of as well. These were really easy to reheat—another lifesaver." —Monica W., mom of one, St. Louis, MO

# GREEK RICE BALLS WITH HERBED YOGURT SAUCE

**Makes 20, and doubles well**

**Cooking time: 45 minutes (20 to 25 minutes active)**

These might not make a meal all by themselves, but add a salad (chopped, for ease of eating) and pita bread, and you've got yourself a feast. Or do as one mom did and stuff the salad and the rice balls into the pita, drizzle on some sauce, and eat the entire thing with one hand, all at once—just be aware that overstuffed pitas are prone to falling apart. Tricky, if baby's in your lap.

**NOTE:** These freeze well. Reheat straight from the freezer, in a 350°F oven for 20 to 30 minutes.

## FOR THE HERBED YOGURT SAUCE

1 cup plain Greek-style yogurt
  *If your store doesn't carry Greek-style yogurt, it's fine to use regular—just expect the consistency of the sauce to be thinner.*

1 large garlic clove, minced

¼ cup finely chopped fresh mint, dill, or parsley, or a combination

Salt and pepper

Lemon juice to taste, optional

## FOR THE RICE BALLS

¾ cup panko breadcrumbs, whole wheat or regular

Salt and pepper

4 cups frozen chopped spinach (use two 10-ounce boxes or one 1-pound bag), thawed, water squeezed out

4 scallions (whites and pale green parts), finely chopped

¼ cup olive oil

1 cup leftover cooked brown rice
  *Frozen or shelf-stable cooked brown rice works well. Why cook if you don't have to?*

2 tablespoons finely chopped fresh mint, dill, or parsley, or a combination

½ cup crumbled feta cheese (use more if you really like feta, but add less salt)

¼ cup chopped black olives

2 tablespoons lemon juice

1 or 2 egg whites

**Preheat oven to 350°F. Grease or line a baking sheet.**

1. Make the sauce: Combine the yogurt, garlic, mint, and salt and pepper to taste in a small bowl. If the sauce needs a bit more tang add lemon juice to taste. Set the sauce aside to let the flavors meld.

*The garlic flavor will become more pronounced the longer this sauce sits, so don't be surprised if, tomorrow, it tastes completely different.*

2. Make the rice balls: Mix the panko with salt and pepper to taste in a medium bowl.

3. Combine the spinach, scallions, olive oil, rice, mint, feta, olives, lemon juice, and 1 egg white in a large bowl. Use your clean hands to mix; it's much easier than a spoon in this case. Roll a tablespoon of the mixture into a compact ball. If it doesn't hold together, mix in the second egg white.

4. Roll each rice ball gently into the bowl of crumbs (work in batches of two or three balls at a time). The balls won't be completely coated, but that's OK. Arrange the rice balls on the baking sheet.

5. Bake until crumbs are nicely browned, 20 to 25 minutes.

6. Serve with the dipping sauce.

> MAKE BABY FOOD: This whole dish is great for babies. If you're on purees, mix the rice balls and yogurt sauce together in the processor.

**MAMA SAID**
"The recipe was easy and fun with a young toddler. My daughter loved tasting small bits of some of the ingredients—the scallions, the mint leaves, and the spinach for instance—and she found it fascinating watching me separate the egg. I think it would have been easy to manage with a younger baby in a sling too. The flavor was lovely. We demolished the lot between us, even with baked potato and various other things." —April M., mom of one, Musselburgh, Scotland

· · · · · · · · · · · · · · · · · · · · · · · · · · · · · · · · · · · · · ·

# SICILIAN SPINACH ENVELOPES

**Makes 8, and doubles well**

**Cooking time: 1 hour (30 minutes active)**

These sweet-and-tangy pies use, of all things, refrigerated crescent roll dough. Are you shocked? Believe it or not, brands exist that don't include trans fats and unrecognizable ingredients. Look in larger health food stores; the Immaculate Baking Company makes a good product, as does Trader Joe's. If you can't find any, use pie dough instead, following the assembly and baking instructions on page 207.

2 tablespoons golden raisins, black raisins, or currants

2 tablespoons olive oil

1 small onion, finely chopped

4 cups frozen chopped spinach (use two 10-ounce boxes or one 1-pound bag), thawed, water squeezed out

2 tablespoons pine nuts, toasted
*Toast pine nuts in a dry skillet over medium heat, shaking frequently, until lightly browned, about 3 to 5 minutes.*

1 cup ricotta cheese

¼ cup grated Parmesan cheese

Pinch of ground nutmeg

Salt and pepper

2 packages (8-count) refrigerated crescent rolls

**Preheat oven to 350°F and set the racks in the upper and lower thirds of the oven. Grease or line two baking sheets.**

1. Put the raisins in a small bowl, cover with hot water, and set aside to plump up.

2. Heat the oil in a small skillet over medium heat. When it shimmers, add the onion and cook, stirring occasionally, until translucent, 3 to 5 minutes. Transfer to a large bowl, and stir in the spinach, pine nuts, ricotta, Parmesan, nutmeg, and salt and pepper to taste. Drain the raisins, discarding liquid, and stir them in.

3. Open 1 package of crescent rolls, and separate the dough into two halves—this should happen naturally, right down the middle—then separate each half into two rectangles. Each package will yield four of these rectangles. Place 1 rectangle on a lightly floured work surface, and pinch together the perforation that runs diagonally across it. Roll the rectangle with a lightly floured rolling pin into a 5- to 6-inch square.

4.  Place ⅓ cup of filling in the center of the dough. Pull opposite corners of the dough up and over, and pinch them together in the center. Do the same with the other corners. They will look like little pouches. It's perfectly fine if there are gaps where filling peeks through—the end result will be quite attractive—but it's important that the gathered dough at the top is sealed. Repeat with remaining dough and filling. Transfer the pouches to the prepared baking sheets.

*If your dough won't stick together in the center, wet it lightly with your fingers and try again.*

5.  Bake until deep golden brown, 18 to 22 minutes. If you won't be eating right away, transfer to a wire rack to cool.

> MAKE BABY FOOD: The filling is perfect for babies—no need to cook, even. Puree or, if you'll be serving as finger food, chop the pine nuts before adding to the mixture, to prevent a choking hazard. (If there are food allergies in your immediate family, leave them out completely.)

**MAMA SAID**
**"The combination of sweet and savory is really interesting here. My Italian husband says that it is very typical of southern Italy. It's the North African influence. And I'm thrilled to hear that there are pre-made doughs available that aren't full of trans fats." —Jane B., mom of one, Pleasanton, CA**

# BAKED EGGPLANT AND CHICKPEA SAMOSAS WITH APRICOT-GINGER DIPPING SAUCE

**Makes 10, and doubles well**
**Cooking time: 1 hour 20 minutes (30 minutes active)**

The very first time I went to an Indian restaurant, among the few dishes I was intrepid enough to try were the deep-fried goodies: bhajias, spicy vegetable fritters; poori, bread that inflates like a balloon in the hot oil; and samosas, curry-scented, oversized dumplings. I was in love from the very first lick of my greasy fingers. At home, though, it's been a long time since I deep-fried anything. Instead, I make baked samosas using eggroll wrappers. Rather than the usual triangular shape, these are formed into a pouch, and a brushing with oil helps the wrappers to crisp up beautifully. Not exactly traditional, but trust me: You won't miss the extra fat.

## FOR THE SAMOSAS

1 tablespoon oil, plus more for brushing

1 small onion, finely chopped

2 teaspoons grated fresh ginger

1 teaspoon ground cumin

1 teaspoon ground coriander

½ teaspoon ground turmeric

¼ teaspoon cayenne

Salt

One 10-ounce can diced tomatoes and green
  chiles (such as Ro-Tel)
  *If you can't find this, use most of a 14.5-ounce
  can of diced tomatoes, along with about half of
  a 4-ounce can of diced green chiles, drained.*

1 medium potato (Yukon gold or russet),
  peeled and chopped

½ pound eggplant, peeled and chopped

One 15- to 16-ounce can chickpeas, drained
  and rinsed

10 eggroll wrappers

## FOR THE DIPPING SAUCE

12 dried apricot halves, chopped

2 tablespoons apple cider vinegar, rice
  vinegar, or lemon juice

2 teaspoons honey

½ teaspoon ground ginger

Pinch of cayenne

Pinch of salt

**Preheat oven to 400°F. Grease or line a baking sheet.**

1. Make the samosas: Heat the oil in a large skillet over medium heat. When it shimmers, add the onion and cook, stirring occasionally, until translucent, 3 to 5 minutes. Add the fresh ginger, cumin, coriander, turmeric, cayenne, and salt to taste and cook for 30 seconds more.

2. Stir in the tomatoes, potato, and eggplant, and simmer, covered, until vegetables are softened but not fully cooked, 10 to 12 minutes. Stir in the chickpeas, remove from heat, and set aside to cool.

3. Working with 1 wrapper at a time and keeping the rest covered, place about ⅓ cup of the filling in the center. Dip a finger into a small bowl of water and moisten the edges of the wrapper, then pull the corners up until they meet in the center. Don't worry about it looking pretty—you're making a little pouch. Press all the edges down to seal. Repeat with remaining wrappers and filling. Carefully transfer the samosas to the baking sheet.

5. Brush samosas lightly with oil. Bake until crisp and deep golden brown, 20 to 25 minutes.

6. Meanwhile, make the sauce: Put the apricots in a small bowl and cover with 1 cup boiling water. Soak the apricots for 15 minutes.

7. Transfer the softened apricots, along with the soaking liquid, to a food processor or blender. Add the remaining sauce ingredients and process until smooth. Add water, a tablespoon at a time, to get your desired consistency.

8. Serve the samosas with the dipping sauce.

> MAKE BABY FOOD: If your baby likes spice, the filling works as either a puree or finger food—just taste it first to be sure you're comfortable with the level of heat. If you like, leave out the chiles entirely and use plain diced tomatoes. The apricot sauce is off-limits due to the honey, which isn't recommended for babies under 1 year old due to the risk of botulism, a deadly food-borne illness.

**MAMA SAID**
"The samosas were a wonderful vegetarian dish that had the kind of flavor and bite I crave. My children really enjoyed it, too—anything that's dippable is a big hit around here."
—Christine G., mom of four, Tokyo, Japan

# CRISPY BUTTERNUT RAVIOLI WITH WALNUT-RICOTTA DIPPING SAUCE

**Makes 16, and doubles well**

**Cooking time: 2½ hours (40 minutes active)**

Don't let that cooking time scare you—while it does take quite a while to get from the first step to dinner, for most of that time you're not actually doing anything. This is a prime candidate for Nap-Friendly Cooking, in fact. And the crunchy, savory dumplings that result are well worth the effort. In fact, as long as you're doing the work, make a double batch and freeze half before baking. Then when you've got a hankering, cook them in simmering salted water, just as you would store-bought ravioli, and serve with top-quality olive oil and grated Parmesan cheese.

**NOTE:** If you'd rather not fuss with raw butternut squash, it's fine to substitute a 12-ounce package of frozen squash puree, thawed, and skip Step 1. If it seems watery, add it to the pan with half of the shallot-rosemary mixture in Step 2 and simmer for a few minutes, until it thickens.

1½ pounds butternut squash, halved vertically
*If you can't find a squash that small, use only half of it here. Save the other half for another use, like the Butternut Handpies on page 205.*

Salt and pepper

1 tablespoon olive oil, plus more for brushing

1 shallot, finely chopped

2 teaspoons fresh rosemary, finely chopped

¼ cup grated Parmesan cheese

Pinch of grated nutmeg

32 wonton wrappers

2 tablespoons chopped walnuts, toasted

½ cup ricotta cheese

Juice from ½ lemon (about 1 tablespoon)

Milk, optional

**Preheat oven to 400°F. Grease or line a baking sheet.**

1. Scoop out the seeds from the squash and discard, then season the squash with salt and pepper and place it, cut side down, on the prepared baking sheet. Bake until completely tender, 45 minutes to 1 hour. Set aside to cool.

2. Heat the olive oil in a small skillet over medium heat. When it shimmers, add the shallot and rosemary and cook, stirring occasionally, until shallots begin to brown,

2 to 3 minutes. Transfer half of the mixture to a medium bowl, and refrigerate the other half to use in the dipping sauce.

3. When the squash is cool enough to handle, scoop out the flesh into the bowl with the shallot and rosemary, and add the Parmesan and nutmeg. Mash with a potato masher or the back of a slotted spoon until the consistency is fairly smooth but still has some texture. Taste, and season with salt and pepper if needed. Set aside to cool for at least 30 minutes—cover and refrigerate if you won't be making the ravioli within 2 hours.

4. When you're ready to assemble everything, preheat oven to 375°F. Grease or line two baking sheets.

5. Remove 2 wrappers (cover the rest with a damp towel). Put 1 to 2 tablespoons of filling in the center of 1 wrapper (the amount will depend on the size of the wrappers). Dip a finger in a small bowl of water and moisten the edges, then cover with the second wrapper. Carefully line up the edges, and press to seal, forcing out as much air as possible. Transfer to a prepared baking sheet. Repeat with remaining wrappers and filling.

6. Brush the raviolis lightly with oil, then bake until ravioli are browned and edges are crisp, 15 to 20 minutes. If you're not serving them right away, cool on a wire rack.

7. While the ravioli are baking, make the dipping sauce: Combine the reserved shallot mixture, walnuts, ricotta, lemon juice, and salt and pepper to taste in a blender or mini-food processor. Blend until the texture pleases you—if it's too thick, add a splash of either milk or olive oil. Transfer to a small bowl, and serve with the ravioli.

> MAKE BABY FOOD: The squash mixture is perfect for babies. The ricotta dipping sauce is too—provided there are no food allergies in your immediate family. If there are allergies, walnuts make the sauce a no-no.

**MAMA SAID**
"Spectacular. I liked the use of wonton wrappers as an easy-to-do container for the parcel of butternut squash delight. My butternut squashes were huge and the scales at the store were wrong, so I ended up with huge quantities of the squash mixture left over. I added a couple of pints of broth, some leftover raw spinach that would have gone to the chickens otherwise, some milk, and a little cornstarch, and made soup. Grated a little Parm on top. Holy cow! It was fabulous." —Rachel M., mom of one, Tucson, AZ

# SUMMER ROLLS WITH GINGERY PEANUT SAUCE

**Makes 8, and doubles well**

**Cooking time: 1 hour (30 to 40 minutes active)**

Summer rolls are my go-to appetizer at Vietnamese and Thai restaurants. They look like eggrolls that haven't been fried yet—perfect if you'd rather not deal with deep-frying. The wrapper is a sheet of rice paper that is, in my opinion, a miraculous thing: Just out of the package it's brittle and delicate, but after a quick dunk in warm water, the paper turns soft and pliable, like a giant, translucent noodle. Rolled like a burrito around raw vegetables, herbs, and rice stick noodles—which you'll find shelved near the rice paper at Asian markets and large grocery stores—it's a perfect light dinner, especially good on a warm evening when you just can't face heating up the kitchen.

The assembly is a little fiddly and requires your full attention, so save this for a weekend, or a time when you won't need to be hands-on with the baby right before dinner.

## FOR THE SUMMER ROLLS

Half of a 3.75-ounce package rice stick
    noodles or rice vermicell

8 ounces cooked chicken, shredded, or
    16 cooked jumbo shrimp, or 8 ounces
    firm tofu, cut into 3-inch sticks

2 teaspoons sesame oil

2 teaspoons rice vinegar

1 teaspoon reduced-sodium soy sauce

1 large carrot, shredded

1 cup shredded Napa cabbage

½ cucumber, peeled and cut into thin
    matchsticks

8 sheets rice paper

¼ cup mint leaves

¼ cup basil or cilantro leaves

## FOR THE SAUCE

½ cup creamy natural peanut butter

2 tablespoons reduced-sodium soy sauce

1 tablespoon dark brown sugar

Juice of ½ lime (about 1½ teapoons)

1½ teaspoons rice vinegar

½ to 1 teaspoon grated fresh ginger, to taste

¼ teaspoon red pepper flakes, or to taste

¼ cup hot water

1. Soak the noodles in a bowl of hot water until soft, 30 minutes to 1 hour, then rinse and drain well.

2. While noodles are soaking, make the sauce: Combine the peanut butter, soy sauce, brown sugar, lime juice, vinegar, ginger, and red pepper flakes in a food processor or blender and puree. With the motor running, drizzle the hot water into the mixture, blending until you reach a consistency you like (I like mine about as thick as heavy cream). You may not use all the water.

3. When the noodles are ready, make the summer rolls: Combine the chicken, shrimp, or tofu, sesame oil, rice vinegar, and soy sauce in a small bowl. In another bowl combine the carrot, cabbage, and cucumber.

4. Line up your ingredients, each in its own bowl, in this order: herbs, chicken, shrimp, or tofu, drained noodles, vegetables. Place the rice papers next to a large bowl of warm water.

5. Working with 1 at a time, dip a sheet of rice paper into the warm water for 30 to 40 seconds, until it becomes pliable. Lay it flat on a work surface. Place a few leaves of each herb on the bottom half of the rice paper, leaving about an inch border, cover with some chicken or tofu and a small handful of noodles, then top with a small handful of vegetables.

6. Fold the bottom of the rice paper over the filling, then fold in the sides. Now roll tightly, like you're making a burrito. Transfer the roll to a plate and cover with a damp towel. Repeat with the remaining ingredients.

7. Serve with the prepared sauce. Tightly cover any rolls that won't be eaten right away, or they'll dry out and crack open.

   **NOTE:** If you have leftover sauce, transfer it to an air-tight container and refrigerate; it'll stay good for about a week.

MAKE BABY FOOD: Each individual item in the filling would work well as finger food (chop the noodles into small pieces), or you can puree some of the chicken, noodles, and vegetables with a splash each of rice vinegar and sesame oil.

**MAMA SAID**
**"I have never worked with rice wrappers before, but it was really easy to assemble these! The filling is a great mix of textures. I had a bit of chicken and a bit of noodles and veggies left over—I combined them all with the sauce and it was a great cold noodle salad the next day." —Alana D., mom of one, Narragansett, RI**

# CHAPTER 7

# LUNCHTIME PUMPING AND LAST-MINUTE DINNERS:
## *A Chapter for WOHMs*

Motherhood comes with a lot of acronyms.

Heck, just trying to become a mom has a boatload, if you spend any time at all on message boards: When you're TTC (trying to conceive), you endure half the month in the 2WW (two-week wait), counting down to your chance to POAS (pee on a stick) with that HPT (home pregnancy test), all in pursuit of a sometimes elusive prize, the BFP (big fat positive).

And once you get that BFP, the pregnancy acronyms kick in: EDD (estimated due date), MS (morning sickness, which I was lucky enough to escape, mostly), US (ultrasound, proof that there is, in fact, a baby in there), NST (non-stress test, which I found stressful the minute my OB—obstetrician—suggested I needed one), until eventually you wind up in L&D (labor and delivery).

Get through all that and you've got a new list to learn: BF and FF (breastfeeding and formula-feeding), AP (attachment parenting, whose advocates often practice BW—babywearing—and never let their babies CIO—cry it out), and OHT (one handed typing), which you encountered in the last chapter.

But perhaps the most important acronyms to a mom, and especially a new mom, concern her identity as a parent. I'm a WAHM (work-at-home mom), while most of my friends are either SAHMs (stay-at-home moms) or WOHMs (work-outside-the-home moms).

I kvetch a lot about being a WAHM; I like to say I've got the worst of both worlds, in that I can never completely leave behind either my work or my child. When Harry was very young I hated it—I went back to work at 10 weeks, writing a diary of my first week at home with him for *American Baby* (ah, the irony), and it was pretty hellish. I was so jealous of my friends with "real" jobs, who got three luxurious months of maternity leave and then, I assumed, were spending their lunch hours shopping or at the gym. (Imagine—60 whole minutes to themselves!) And I was equally jealous of the moms whose only job was being a mom; those lucky SAHMs were being pulled in just one direction—toward the baby—while it felt like I was being torn limb from limb.

But you know what? I'm pretty sure that every mom believes every other mom has things just a tiny bit better than she does. Let's call it The Diaper Is Always Cleaner Effect. And in retrospect, I know I've got it pretty good. Since going back to work at 10 weeks, I've spent a lot of time with Harry, but I've also sequestered myself in my home office for a substantial part of each day, a little oasis of child-free peace. When I'm trying out recipes, Harry's in and out of the kitchen, and now that he's older he likes to help, so I get to interact with him even while I'm working. In contrast, my SAHM friends often have no break at all, since paying for childcare with only one salary is challenging. And WOHMs, especially new ones, have a whole other set of problems. If you're living that life, you probably wake to baby's cries (again) at first light, spend time with junior, struggle to get dressed and out the door, work work work (and maybe pump pump pump), commute home, and if you're lucky spend 20 minutes of delicious, non-nursing time with the baby before he goes to sleep. You see the problem here, right? No time to make dinner, never mind a healthy lunch to bring to work the next day.

Well, WOHMs, this chapter is for you: You'll find super-fast, and super-easy, recipes for dinners that are thrown together but sure don't taste that way, as well as tips on everything from how to make the most of your commute to ways to pump while still getting your job done. And because I haven't had to face all the struggles I know you're facing right now, I turned to experts for help: my crew of mom-testers. In that group of more than 100 new moms, a sizable proportion work outside the home. Each woman has figured out her own tricks for getting through the day, and has been kind enough to share that priceless information with you. In fact, WOHMs contributed all the recipes in this chapter—they're tried and tested by women who are dealing with all the same kinds of challenges as you.

These recipes are so terrific, I think they deserve an acronym all their own: YICFM-FWWHDAFTJ. What, you can't figure that one out? It's so obvious: Yes, I can feed my family well, while holding down a full-time job.*

- - - - - - - - - - - - - - - - - - - - - - - - - - - - - - - - - - - - - - - - - - - - - - - - - - - - - - - - - - -

## OTHER RECIPES TO CONSIDER

This isn't the only place you'll find recipes that will work for the WOHM. In addition to the chapters on Quick Suppers, The Slow Cooker, Big Batch Cooking, and Un-Recipes, there are several in Chapter 1, "The New Mom's Pantry":

- Quick Pasta e Fagioli (page 22)

- Quinoa Salad with Chickpeas, Dried Fruit, and Almonds (page 28)

- Tuna and White Bean Salad (page 30)

- Cheater's Chana Masala (page 34)

- Angel Hair Pasta with Garlic and Lemon-Parmesan Breadcrumbs (page 40)

- Spaghetti alla Puttanesca (page 42)

- - - - - - - - - - - - - - - - - - - - - - - - - - - - - - - - - - - - - - - - - - - - - - - - - - - - - - - - - - -

---

* Really, the recipes are useful for all of us. Don't skip them just because you're operating under a different acronym!

## CRIB NOTES

- On days when you get home and have absolutely no idea what to make, preheat the oven and put a big pot of water on to boil while you figure things out. I know, I know, it's not energy-efficient if you wind up not using it, but it'll give you a 15- to 20-minute head start once you decide what to make. And here's a tip from my amazingly helpful editor, Amy: If you've got an electric kettle, it's a safe and easy way to get water boiling quickly.

- Don't be afraid of processed foods as a category! They're the key to many an oh-my-god-it's-5:30-already dinner. I keep things like frozen potstickers, jarred simmer sauces, and boil-in-bag brown rice on hand at all times. The key is to read labels carefully: Look for a relatively brief ingredients list full of things you recognize.

- Along the same lines, it's perfectly fine to buy pre-prepped raw vegetables. Peeled and cubed butternut squash, sliced mushrooms, and broccoli florets have saved many a dinner.

- Eggs are your friend. You'll see them mentioned several times in this chapter because they cook quickly, they're full of protein, and they're super-flexible.

- Another friend: sandwiches. Who says they're only for lunch?

- If you have older kids, don't play short-order cook: There's no time, and you'll be setting yourself up for a lifetime of hair-pulling. Cook what you cook, make sure it's balanced (try to offer a meat or meat alternative, vegetable, whole grain, and fruit), and let the kids choose from there what they eat. Don't force them to eat everything, and try to resist bribing with dessert.

- If you've got like-minded (and taste-budded) friends or neighbors, set up a dinner co-op: Each family prepares one meal a week, in enough quantity to feed everyone. Round up three other families, and you'll have dinner ready and waiting three nights a week!

# LAUREN'S CARROT SOUP

**Serves 8**

**Cooking time: 45 minutes (30 minutes active)**

When it comes to simple, it's hard to beat a big pot of soup. In this case, Los Angeles mom Lauren A. streamlined a recipe from *Splendid Soups* by James Peterson. The natural sweetness of the carrots, the bit of body from the rice, and the utter simplicity of the whole thing make for a sophisticated-yet-effortless meal. It's got a bit (OK, a lot) more butter than my usual recipes, but for something this simple it helps to have a little richness. If you're wary of using an entire stick, start with half that amount and add more if you need it. Serve the soup with crusty bread, and if you'd like something a little more substantial, crumble in some goat cheese or dollop Greek yogurt on top.

"It makes a nice big pot!", Lauren told me. "It freezes very well, and it makes great baby food if you add more broth to make it thinner, a little less broth to make it thicker, depending on the age of the babe."

8 tablespoons (1 stick) butter

2½ to 3 pounds carrots (about 14 big ones), peeled and thinly sliced
*You can use a food processor or a knife to slice them—and it doesn't need to be perfect.*

1 cup basmati rice

1 teaspoon thyme (dried or fresh)

Pinch of sugar, optional (if the carrots aren't super-fresh and sweet)

8 cups low-sodium chicken or vegetable broth

Salt

1.  Melt the butter in a large stockpot over medium-low heat, then add the carrots, rice, thyme, and sugar, if using, and cook until carrots are slightly softened, 5 to 10 minutes.

2.  Add the broth and bring to a boil over high heat. Reduce heat to low and simmer, covered, until rice is tender, about 15 minutes.

3.  Puree the soup with an immersion blender, or in two batches in a regular blender (be careful when blending hot liquids). An immersion blender won't produce a silky-smooth soup, but we like it that way.

MAKE BABY FOOD: As Lauren says in her note, this is perfect for babies—add a splash of broth or milk if your baby prefers a thinner soup.

## DINNERTIME, AND THE LIVING IS EASY

Because I work from home, it's relatively painless for me to take a break to get dinner started—sometimes using the Nap-Friendly Cooking techniques, sometimes by stopping work mid-afternoon and resuming an hour later. But if you work outside the home, obviously this isn't an option. Luckily, my mom-testers have loads of advice to share on how they cut corners and get things done:

"On a weekend **I'll brown five or six pounds of ground beef—no seasonings, and drained to remove all the excess fat. Then I freeze half- or one-pound portions to use at a later date.** I've also done the same with chicken cutlets—I cube them and pan-sear, then portion into freezer bags for later use. All it takes is a short zap in the microwave and it's ready to use." —Karen K., mom of one, Maplewood, NJ

"My advice: plan and prep ahead of time. **If a few recipes require chopped onions, I'll chop a couple on Sunday and then divide them up into individual containers.** If possible I'll cook on Sunday so during the week we're just reheating. Yeah, it takes up a lot of my weekend family time, but otherwise we might live on sandwiches and canned soup all week. With the same idea, **we try to make it easy on ourselves by repeating a lot of meals.** Monday is usually Mexican food night, Friday is usually fish, Wednesday is typically soup or chili. That means Tuesday and Thursday are usually based around whatever other ingredients we have around the house or new recipes we want to try. **We plan all our meals on Sunday and then put them on the calendar so we don't have to remember what we're having for dinner that day.** Putting them on the calendar also helps when we're stuck: 'Oh, two weeks ago we made X, did you like that? Do you want to have that this week?' " —Monica W., mom of one, St. Louis, MO

"**Soups are great because they can be made in advance and reheated quickly.** My toddler and my husband both love it, and I can make soup that my baby will eat too." —Abigail K., mom of two, New York, NY

"**If it's been a really busy day and I didn't prepare something ahead of time, I resort to Breakfast for Dinner,** which is a favorite around these parts and consists of pancakes from a mix and omelets. I can get that on the table in 10 minutes flat and I always have the ingredients at home. Plus my kids love it and eat every bite." —Jesse Z., mom of two, Los Angeles, CA

"**I put the high chair in the kitchen while I cook. I can feed the baby while I'm cooking, at least enough to tide her over until dinner** if I'm making her main meal too (Cheerios and peas keep her busy and semi-satisfied). A bottom drawer in the kitchen is all kid stuff. Some kitchen utensils, some toys, a lot of whatever she puts there. The preschooler can 'cook' while I do. Cooking-wise: **Frozen veggies go in the pot with pasta and get served with jarred sauce on top.**

I cook rice in big batches and freeze instead of using instant rice. And I'm a big fan of grocery store rotisserie chicken." —Heather B., mom of two, Westmont, IL

"Chicken breasts + jar of salsa + slow cooker + 6 to 8 hours on low = filling for tacos at dinner. And I make cheeseburgers by mixing the meat with pre-shredded low-fat cheese. Totally delicious way to liven up extra-lean beef. These can be mixed and formed ahead of time so they're ready to pop into the oven (or onto the grill). I sprinkle them with a little garlic salt, too. Fab on whole-wheat buns with all the fixings." —Amanda G., mom of two, North Brunswick, NJ

"These are two of our go-to meals: Tofu curry: Simmered with a good-quality jarred sauce and a little coconut milk. Usually with a rinsed can of chickpeas, frozen peas, cauliflower or broccoli, and/or diced potatoes thrown in. Rice in the rice cooker. A great, easy meal that takes 20 to 25 minutes, start to finish. Pan-fried fish (usually sole or tilapia) dredged in cornmeal or panko bread crumbs, with sauteed greens and some kind of starch (smashed potatoes or roasted sweet potato are favorites). The kids *love* fish cooked this way. We make an alternative veg for them, or fruit slices, since neither will eat cooked leafy greens." —Jody B., mom of two, Boston, MA

"Here's my top savior for dinner with a baby: our easy-to-clean brick floors, and my dog who's allowed people food. I never have to sweep after dinner—there's not a crumb left."—Kati L., mom of one, Durham, NC

# HEATHER'S SPANISH TORTILLA

**Serves 4**

**Cooking time: 40 minutes**

Back in my single days, I'd regularly meet friends at a Spanish place near my office for a glass of wine (or three) and tapas, little plates of simple, ridiculously tasty food. It felt so chic to wield my oversized glass of red and nibble olive oil–soaked tidbits. One of my favorites was always the tortilla, an oversized potato omelet served in wedges. Until Heather B., a mom of two in Westmont, IL, shared this recipe with me, I'd never attempted to make it at home. I had no idea how easy it was!

Unlike so many of my own recipes, Heather's is authentic—she learned it from her Spanish host mom while living there on foreign study. Now, as a WOHM, she relies on it because, as she said, "It's a one-dish meal, and I can prep it ahead of time or even cook it ahead of time and it still tastes good. The leftovers are great by themselves, or you can do a Spanish-style sandwich and make a *bocadillo* with a slice on a nice hunk of bread. It's even good cold. You can add to it as well—frozen spinach, bell peppers, broccoli . . ."

A few words of advice from Heather: "Note that a high-quality nonstick pan is a must—a well-seasoned cast-iron pan works best for me. Also, this is not a recipe where you want to be shy about oil."

4 eggs

⅓ cup olive oil, or as needed, divided

2 large potatoes, peeled and chopped into
   ½-inch pieces

1 medium Spanish onion, finely chopped

Salt

1.  Beat the eggs in a large bowl. The frothier you can get them, the better. Set aside.

2.  Heat several generous glugs of the oil, about 3 tablespoons, in a large nonstick skillet over low heat and add the potatoes. Cook until potatoes are soft but not brown, 10 to 15 minutes. Add the onions and cook until onions are translucent, 3 to 5 minutes. Season with salt to taste. Using a slotted spoon, transfer the onion-potato mixture into the bowl with the eggs.

3.  Wipe out the pan, taking care because it will be quite hot. Add 2 tablespoons olive oil and tilt the pan to coat with oil. Pour the egg mixture into the pan. Spread the

mixture with a spatula to distribute the potatoes evenly, then let it cook undisturbed. After about 3 minutes, when the eggs are no longer completely liquid, slide the tortilla onto a large plate.

4. Re-coat the pan with another tablespoon or two of olive oil and heat for about 30 seconds. Flip the tortilla back into the pan to cook on the other side until it is golden brown on the outside and moist at the center.

5. Serve the tortilla hot with crusty bread and a green salad or cold as tapas with thin slices of bread on the side.

> MAKE BABY FOOD: Throw a slice of this in the food processor with a little broth, water, or milk to make a puree, or cut it into chunks for finger food.

· · · · · · · · · · · · · · · · · · · · · · · · · · · · · · · · · · · · · · · ·

## AMY'S THAI OMELET

**Serves 2**
**Cooking time: 20 minutes (all active)**

Amy J. was one of my cooking students—she brought her sweet little boy to my kitchen to learn Parents Need to Eat Too in person. Amy's quite the cultural mish-mash: Her mom is Jewish and her dad is Thai, and she lived in Bolivia for a while too. The recipes she gave me for this chapter reflect that influence. This first one is so quick, and so deliciously different, I suspect you'll find yourself cooking it again and again.

And don't worry if your pantry isn't stocked with Thai ingredients. "If you don't have mushroom soy sauce," Amy said, "use a smaller quantity of regular or reduced-sodium soy sauce thinned with a splash of milk."

2 tablespoons vegetable oil

3 eggs

1 tablespoon mushroom soy sauce

½ cup ground chicken or pork

½ cup chopped tomato

½ cup chopped red onion

Chopped cilantro to taste

Cooked jasmine rice
  *Regular white rice would be just fine too!*

1. Heat the oil in a large skillet over medium heat. While it's warming, beat the eggs with the soy sauce in a large bowl. Add the ground meat, tomato, and red onion to the egg mixture and stir to combine.

2. When the oil shimmers, pour the egg mixture into the skillet and cook without stirring, 3 to 4 minutes. When the underside of the omelet is cooked and the meat is browned, flip the omelet over to cook the other side.

*I find it easiest to slide the omelet out onto a dinner plate, then put the skillet over the plate and carefully flip the whole thing over. Use potholders!*

4. Cook the omelet for 3 to 4 minutes more, until the meat is cooked through.

5. Transfer the omelet to a serving dish, sprinkle with the cilantro, and serve over the rice.

> MAKE BABY FOOD: If you're on purees, add a splash of milk before you blend it in a food processor. Or cut the omelet into strips, and an older baby can feed himself.

. . . . . . . . . . . . . . . . . . . . . . . . . . . . . . . . . . . . . . . . . . . . .

## JUGGLE LIKE A PRO WITHOUT JOINING THE CIRCUS

All moms have to be able to multi-task—it's part of the job description. But the number of (often conflicting) responsibilities WOHMs juggle is enough to make me want to curl up in the fetal position and hope someone else will take over. On days when you feel the same way, read over this wise advice from my mom-testers:

"**Cut yourself a lot of slack and don't think you have to be perfect at anything**—your baby will be fine if you don't sanitize pump parts and bottles after every use! Stick 'em in the fridge and go take a nap." —Heather M., mom of one, Los Gatos, CA

"**It's important to keep in mind that with juggling, sometimes you have to drop one ball in order to catch another.** In order to drop off my son at his first day of pre-school, I might have to miss (or reschedule) an important meeting. In order to attend an important meeting on a different day, I may need to skip pumping one afternoon. There are constantly choices to be made and nothing is ever perfect, as tough as that can be to bear sometimes." —Abigail K., mom of two, New York, NY

"**It's a little thing, but I pack my lunch in the cooler bag for my pumped milk.** It keeps my lunch cold until I need to eat it, then the milk goes in the bag when lunch is over. Cuts one bag out of the mix I lug back and forth, which is great. Also, I leave as much as possible at our sitter's house (change of clothes, diapers, even some food products like those Gerber puffs), which means less to lug back and forth." —Heather B., mom of two, Westmont, IL

"Honestly, most weeks I feel like I'm barely holding it all together. When Friday comes it's a relief, no more worry about pumping, milk supply, and getting it all done. But **planning in advance has helped me so much. If I can prep dinner for the week on Sunday I do it, because if I don't chances are I'll say, 'forget about it!' and pick up some fast food.**" —Monica W., mom of one, St. Louis, MO

"**Accept that you can't do it all. Ask for help. And when you ask for help, be OK with things not getting done exactly how you would have done them.** Also, calendars with reminders are your friends. And since I lose track of paper too easily, if there's anything important that I need to do/remember/keep track of, I just email it to myself using a variety of searchable keywords for easier retrieval later. Connecting with other moms on message boards was also hugely important for me. I didn't have that much time for hanging out with IRL (In Real Life) friends, but I could get instant advice/feedback/support from my moms' board friends. " —Amanda G., mom of two, North Brunswick, NJ

"Some things will go wrong no matter how much you plan for them (you'll get spit up all over you on the day you're running late for an important meeting; you'll burn dinner during a long nursing session—it will just happen). **I try to have a back-up plan for anything that might go wrong: always have an extra set of work clothes ready, have my office and the pediatrician's hotline on speed-dial, frozen dinners in the fridge, etc.** So when something goes wrong, I'm prepared for it. No biggie." —Yelena B., mom of two, Houston, TX

# JODY'S FLEXIBLE GRAIN SALAD

**Serves as many as you need**

**Cooking time: 10 to 30 minutes, depending on how much you have to chop**

OK, so technically this one isn't a recipe-recipe. It's more of a really smart guideline, but since it makes feeding the family so delightfully flexible it's perfect for WOHMs. And it comes from one of my favorite people in the world. Yes, some of the mom-testers are my personal friends! Jody B. and I met online when we were both planning our weddings, and met in person when we were both pregnant with our first babies. Her son was one of Harry's earliest playmates. After leaving Brooklyn for Boston she went on to have a daughter, and is now raising two spectacular and precocious little people.

Jody's an artist, and it shows in her improvisational approach to cooking. "These salads are great to have around in the summer, kid-friendly, and you can make them with almost anything you have lying around," she told me. "Make a ton and it will keep for days. The trick is not to use anything that will turn mushy (like tomatoes) or that will dominate the flavor after a day in the fridge (like garlic)."

2 to 4 cups cooked grain (couscous, quinoa, Israeli couscous, orzo, barley, or bulgur)

Handful of fresh herbs, chopped (mint, basil, cilantro, parsley, chervil)

Your choice of seeds or nuts (walnuts, pine nuts, pistachios, sunflower seeds)

A crunchy green vegetable (cucumber, chopped blanched string beans, scallion, kohlrabi, cooked chopped asparagus, edamame)

Handful of dried fruit (raisins, cranberries, chopped prunes)

Olive oil

*The amount of oil and citrus juice you'll need will depend on how much of everything else you're using. In general, go for a ratio of 2:1, oil to juice.*

Fresh lemon or orange juice

Salt and pepper

Toss all of the ingredients in a giant salad bowl. Season with salt and pepper to taste.

MAKE BABY FOOD: This isn't the baby-friendliest recipe in the book. Nuts, hard, raw vegetables, and dried fruit can all be choking hazards. To be safe, hold out some of the cooked grain and serve it to baby with yogurt and fruit.

# ABIGAIL'S SUPER-SIMPLE CHEESY RICE AND BEANS

**Serves 4**

**Cooking time: 35 minutes (5 minutes active)**

I'm not a big cheese fan, but there's something about the straightforwardness of this recipe that I really love, especially after those days that leave me unable to think, never mind cook. You barely even need to measure! Abigail K. was inspired to create this quick casserole by a recipe on the blog One Hungry Mama. I'm doubly happy to include it here, since that's one of my favorite blogs. It's written by a friend of mine, Stacie Billis, who's raising two little boys not far from me in Brooklyn.

If you'd like to try the original, One Hungry Mama's version is called Roasted Poblano Cheesy Rice. (Abigail left out Stacie's roasted poblano peppers and sour cream and swapped in a can of beans, which transformed it into an incredibly simple one-dish meal.)

2 cups cooked brown rice

One 16-ounce container low-fat cottage
    cheese

One 15-ounce can black beans, rinsed and
    drained

Salt and pepper

½ to 1 cup shredded Cheddar cheese

Sliced avocado, chopped tomato, chopped
    red onion, and salsa, for serving

**Preheat oven to 350°F, and grease an 8-inch square baking dish.**

1. Combine the rice, cottage cheese, beans, and salt and pepper to taste in a medium bowl. Pour the mixture into the prepared baking dish.

2. Bake the rice and beans for 20 minutes, then sprinkle the Cheddar cheese on top of the casserole. Bake until the cheese is melted and bubbling, 5 to 10 minutes.

3. Serve with the avocado, tomato, onion, and salsa.

> MAKE BABY FOOD: The basic, pre-baked mixture of rice, beans, and cottage cheese is terrific for babies—puree, mash it up with a fork, or serve as-is. If your baby can handle the texture of melted Cheddar, go for the complete dish. And don't forget the avocado and tomato!

## PUMP IT

I may not be a WOHM, but hoo-boy, did I do a lot of pumping. You'll read all about that in the next chapter. All my pumping took place in the privacy of my bedroom, and because I set my own schedule I didn't have to accommodate anyone else (but Harry, of course). My mom-testers, though, know all the ins and outs of pumping at work:

**"I sneak the two sessions I need in between the classes I teach. I eat my snacks or lunch during those times, and I also catch up on phone calls or emails."** —Jesse Z., mom of two, Los Angeles, CA

**"At the beginning of the day I look at my calendar and figure out the best schedule, depending on meetings, what time the baby had woken up and nursed, and what time I was going to be home.** My work life isn't so regular that the schedule is the same every day, but if I plan ahead each day it works better than always feeling like the next session is going to sneak up inconveniently. **And here's a tip for pumping during lunch: make sure you're all set up— napkin, silverware, whatever, before you start!"**—Lauren A., mom of one, Los Angeles, CA

**"I blocked time off on my Outlook calendar so people wouldn't schedule meetings without asking me. And I have a Flickr site loaded with pictures of my daughter—I would keep those up when I pumped, to help my output."** —Kati L., mom of one, Durham, NC

**"I carried two sets of pumping supplies with me. I would use one in the morning and the other in the afternoon.** In the evening I brought both home and threw them in the dishwasher (I actually had four or five sets in total, so there was always a dry set ready to go the next day)." — Jennifer H., mom of two, Maplewood, NJ

**"Instead of buying expensive 'hands-free' pumping bras, I cut holes in some old sports bras and used those."** —Yelena B., mom of two, Houston, TX
*Note from Debbie: I did this too! It totally works, and it wasn't like those sports bras were seeing much use anyway.*

**"Keep in mind what time people take for other personal reasons at work—cigarette breaks, coffee and gab breaks, solitaire, or Facebook time—you've just got to stake your claim on your time and your space and go for it. No apologies. It's way more worthwhile than playing Minesweeper or keeping up on celebrity gossip."** —Heather B., mom of two, Westmont, IL

**"I failed miserably at this. My tip would be to drop it if it isn't working for you.** My daughter was thriving on formula and wasn't getting sick, so it wasn't worth it. Even with a boss who would have happily made whatever arrangements necessary, I really struggled with the logistics of pumping at work." —Heather M., mom of one, Los Gatos, CA

# BETH'S EASY WHITE BEAN STEW

**Serves 4**

**Cooking time: 30 minutes (20 minutes active)**

When Beth P., a Los Angeles–based mom of one, sent me this recipe, a quick read told me it was a winner. In fact, I tweaked it for my own tastes and wrote about it on One Hungry Mama, the blog I mentioned on page 240. It's gloriously adaptable—use different beans, different greens, even different canned tomatoes. Swap ½ teaspoon smoked paprika for the ham, and you've got a vegetarian version.

Beth adapted it from Epicurious, using less oil and her favorite greens, and loved the result. "I made it a *ton* last winter because it's so quick and easy yet really delicious," she said.

1 tablespoon olive oil

2 garlic cloves, minced

One 14.5-ounce can diced tomatoes, with juice

1¾ cups low-sodium chicken broth

Two 15-ounce cans cannellini beans, rinsed and drained

½ pound ham, Canadian bacon, or turkey bacon, diced

Black pepper

½ pound greens, leaves only, roughly chopped (I like the pre-chopped bags of mixed greens—collard, mustard, turnip—but Swiss chard or kale are good too)

1. Heat the olive oil in a large, heavy pot over medium heat, then add the garlic and cook just until fragrant, about 1 minute.

2. Add the tomatoes with juice, chicken broth, beans, ham, and black pepper to taste, and bring to a simmer.

3. Add the greens and cook until tender, 8 to 10 minutes, depending on which greens you're using.

MAKING BABY FOOD: Puree the mixture and it's perfect for new eaters. If you cut the greens small enough, this is fine as finger food.

· · · · · · · · · · · · · · · · · · · · · · · · · · · · · · · ·

# KATI'S QUICKIE BLACK BEANS WITH RICE

**Serves 4**

**Cooking time: 20 minutes (15 minutes active)**

I know, there are other recipes in this very book for black beans with rice. But sometimes you just can't plan ahead enough for dried beans. Consider this one the last-minute, sanity-preserving version. It comes from Kati L. of Durham, NC, who explained her inspiration: "I try to prepare food that my daughter is capable of eating (even if she rejects it). Life's too short to cook food that she can't eat right now."

2 tablespoons olive oil

1 small onion, chopped

1 cup chopped green and red bell pepper
   (half a large pepper each)

One 14.5-ounce can diced tomatoes, with
   juice

Cumin, ground ancho chile, cayenne, and salt
   and pepper to taste
   *A note from Debbie: Everywhere else in the
   book I've given you specific amounts for
   spices, but Kati addresses the "to taste"*

*instructions below and it makes perfect sense
for this recipe.*

One 15-ounce can black beans, drained

1 cup frozen corn kernels, not thawed

Cooked rice, basmati if you've got it, a boil-in
   bag if that's easier

Shredded Cheddar cheese, chopped
   avocado, sour cream, and hot sauce or
   salsa, for serving

1. Heat the olive oil in a large skillet over medium-high heat. When it shimmers, add the onions and cook, 1 to 2 minutes. Add the bell peppers. At this point, put a toddler on your hip or a baby in your sling, because you are one-handed all the way from here!

2. Add the tomatoes with their juices and season to taste. (My daughter likes a ton of cumin, a generous amount of ancho chile, and a dash of cayenne. Ancho doesn't have a lot of heat, but it's just interesting enough for her.) Stir it all together and tell your child about each ingredient.

3. Add the black beans and the corn. Reduce heat to medium and simmer, stirring occasionally, about 5 minutes. Read your toddler a book on the kitchen floor.

4. Put a small serving of rice with some of the bean mixture on top in the freezer to cool down for your toddler. Put him/her in the high chair with a sippy cup of milk or water and a small handful of Cheddar. Serve yourself, grab the kid's bowl from the freezer, and sit down to a fast, easy, cheap, and healthful dinner.

MAKE BABY FOOD: Kati addressed it beautifully in her instructions, don't you think? I'll just add that you can easily puree this for a very early eater. And if you're using it, avocado is a terrific first food.

## SKIP MEALS? NU-UH.

Tell me if this sounds familiar: You wake up to your baby's cries. Change her, feed her, dress her. Dress yourself. Maybe put on a little makeup. Dash out the door with baby, diaper bag, and briefcase hanging off your body, and get baby to daycare. Hit the office just as your boss is starting the morning meeting. Blink once or twice and it's lunchtime, when you're due to pump . . . What's missing from this schedule? That's right, *your* meal. Use these tips from my mom-testers, and that never has to happen again.

"I'm not much of a breakfast eater, but my fastest breakfast is one I think of as the genius cop-out. **I drink my coffee with a lot of skim milk, and I add a packet of Carnation Instant Breakfast.** It's almost like a mocha." —Heather B., mom of two, Westmont, IL

"My breakfast philosophy is this: **Prep as much as possible the week or day before, and eat as you get ready and then in the car if necessary.** My breakfast is typically a hard-boiled egg, bagel, baked oatmeal (the recipe I tested for this book!), and either iced coffee or tea. I boil three eggs on Sunday and the other two on Wednesday (to make one for each day). I toss them all in a Tupperware container and take one out each morning. I eat it as I walk around the house getting ready. I prep the oatmeal the night before by putting all the dry ingredients in a bowl. In the morning I preheat the oven immediately after waking, mix in the milk and water and put it in the oven. It's usually done right before the baby wakes up." —Monica W., mom of one, St. Louis, MO

"**My daughter and I have yogurt and fruit together pretty much every morning.** I have muesli in mine, and she likes to eat the raisins. We sit on the kitchen floor together and eat. Sometimes I put blueberries in hers and she eats it with a spoon. This is her big opportunity every day to practice with the spoon, so it's a big deal for her. This little bit of time is quality time for us, and a good daily reminder to be patient and cherish the in-between moments." —Heather M., mom of one, Los Gatos, CA

"**A big pan of steel-cut oats made on Sunday lasts us through the week.** When I'm assembling lunches, I put some in a container with some brown sugar and eat it when I get to work." —Alexandra S., mom of two, Baltimore, MD

"**For lunch at work, I use the microwave. One of my faves is a leftover baked potato** (I bake a couple extra with the previous night's dinner just to have them on hand). I cut it in half and mash slightly, then microwave until mostly warm. Then I add some thawed frozen peas, chopped Kalamata olives, and a handful of shredded cheese. Nuke until the cheese melts, then top with sour cream or Greek yogurt (and chopped scallion or chive if I'm particularly ambitious)." —Amanda G., mom of two, North Brunswick, NJ

"**I put leftovers in portion-size containers as I clear the table after dinner, and throw some fruit in my lunch bag.** I find it a lot less stressful when I have everything ready the night before—it reduces the hassle of getting ready in the morning. I also keep granola bars and easy-to-eat fruit like bananas and apples for snacking throughout the day." —Yelena B., mom of two, Houston, TX

"One practical tip is to **have nice tableware to eat from at work**—a bowl, plate, and real fork/knife/spoon—so you're not constantly eating out of (and heating food in) plastic crap. Same thing with having some nice stuff to transport food in, like an insulated bag or a Mr. Bento. And a nice water bottle or special tall water glass, since drinking enough water is a tough thing to keep up with at work, especially while pumping. These are just nice quality-of-life enhancers!" —Jody B., mom of two, Boston, MA

· · · · · · · · · · · · · · · · · · · · · · · · · · · · · · · · · · · · · · · ·

# AMY'S BOLIVIAN WEEKNIGHT QUINOA

**Serves 4 to 6**

**Cooking time: 25 minutes (15 minutes active)**

Remember Amy, my student with the amazing mix of ethnic influences? The woman who gave me the Thai Omelet recipe on page 236? Her next contribution is a little something she picked up in Bolivia. "This is how I use up any leftover cooked vegetables I have lying around," she told me. "I like to top each serving with two eggs, sunny-side up." That ooey-gooey egg yolk runs into the quinoa in the most satisfying way.

2 cups quinoa, rinsed

1 tablespoon olive oil

1 medium onion, chopped

2 cups chopped cooked vegetables
   (mushrooms, string beans, tomatoes, etc.)

Salt and pepper

½ to 1 cup grated Parmesan cheese, to taste

8 to 12 fried eggs, optional

1.  Combine the quinoa and 4 cups water in a saucepan and bring to a boil. Reduce heat to low, and cook, covered, 12 to 15 minutes. Remove from heat and let sit, untouched, 5 minutes, then fluff with a fork and transfer to a large bowl.

2.  Meanwhile, heat the olive oil in a skillet over medium heat. When it shimmers, add the onion and cook until softened, about 5 minutes. Add the rest of the cooked vegetables and cook until heated through. Season with salt and pepper to taste.

3.  Add the vegetables to the quinoa and stir, adding up to 1 cup of Parmesan cheese. Top each serving with 2 fried eggs, if you like.

MAKE BABY FOOD: This will work pureed (add a splash of broth or milk), mashed with a fork, or served as-is. If you're using eggs, make sure they're fully cooked for baby's portion.

· · · · · · · · · · · · · · · · · · · · · · · · · · · · · · · · · · · · · ·

# JODY'S SPAGHETTI WITH GARLIC AND SHRIMP

**Serves 4 to 6**

**Cooking time: 30 minutes (15 minutes active)**

"My kids will lick their plates for this," said my artist friend Jody. "Trader Joe's frozen wild blue shrimp are perfect—best to get shrimp with the tail on but shell off. You can also make this with nearly any seafood, the classic being clams."

| | |
|---|---|
| 1 pound spaghetti | Splash of white wine or vermouth, optional |
| ¼ cup olive oil | Half a lemon |
| 3 or 4 garlic cloves, minced | Salt and pepper |
| Shrimp | ¼ cup finely chopped parsley |

1. Bring a large pot of salted water to a boil (covered to speed things up). Add the spaghetti and cook according to package directions.

2. Meanwhile, heat the olive oil in a skillet large enough to eventually hold the pasta over medium heat. When it shimmers, add the garlic and cook until fragrant, about 1 minute.

3. Add shrimp and cook until just pink on one side, about 1 minute. Turn the shrimp over, add a splash of white wine or vermouth, if using, and cook, 1 to 2 minutes.

4. Squeeze the lemon half over the shrimp mixture, season with salt and pepper to taste, then stir in the chopped parsley.

5. Reserve a few tablespoons of the cooking water before draining the spaghetti, then add the spaghetti to the skillet. Toss to coat with sauce, adding some of the pasta cooking water to give body to the sauce.

> MAKE BABY FOOD: Shellfish is one of the more allergenic foods, so if you've got food allergies in your immediate family don't give this to babies under a year old. Allergy-free? Puree with some of the pasta cooking water, or cut up the spaghetti and the shrimp for finger food. Leave out the wine or vermouth if you're at all nervous about alcohol.

## COMMUTING IS NOT ABOUT TRAVEL

When Harry was a baby, I was soooo jealous of Stephen's commute. He had a half-hour completely to himself! Twice a day! His subway ride was usually spent listening to music on his iPod and tuning out everything else—heaven for a sleep-deprived, stretched-too-thin new dad. Turns out my mom-testers put their commutes to similarly good use:

**"I drink my coffee during my commute to work, and I talk to my husband on my commute home.** That way I can deal with getting the kids ready in the morning without having to spill coffee all over myself, and getting dinner on the table when I come home without my husband's play-by-play of his day." —Jesse Z., mom of two, Los Angeles, CA

**"I relax**—it's the only time of the day that is guaranteed to be mine. I listen to music or catch up on the news, and try to tell the non-stop to-do list running through my head to take a break." —Alexandra S., mom of two, Baltimore, MD

"I make the most of my commute by sometimes not making the most of it! **I gave myself permission to listen to the country music station rather than NPR if I need downtime.** And I got a really good hands-free earpiece for my phone so that I can talk to friends in the car, since that time often gets squeezed out otherwise." —Lauren A., mom of one, Los Angeles, CA

"I like to get **audiobooks** for the long drive, since I have no time to read books. I also negotiated a somewhat flexible schedule, so I can **wait until after the rush hour to drive into work.**" —Heather M., mom of one, Los Gatos, CA

"I take the time to **zone out and stare into space** during my short commute, especially on my way home. That way when I get there, I've had a few minutes to think about nothing and relax a bit before walking in." —Abigail K., mom of two, New York, NY

**"I slept on the bus.** Best use of time ever." —Amanda G., mom of two, North Brunswick, NJ

# JODY'S CHEATER'S POT PIE

**Serves 4 to 6**

**Cooking time: 1 hour (20 minutes active)**

"Chicken pot pie is pretty much my favorite comfort food, so even though I was a little horrified at the thought of cooking with canned soup, I love that I have an easy, healthy version to cook for my family when I don't have a lot of time. I also appreciate that this can be made with ingredients I can stock in the freezer and pantry in advance, so I can make it at a moment's notice (the worst moments of being a WOH parent are arriving home without a clue of what you're going to make for dinner, and it's 6 o'clock)."

Don't you love my friend Jody right now? I adore my own pot pie recipe, but I admit it's complicated—that's why it's in the Nap-Friendly Cooking chapter (on page 50).

**Jody adds:** "The frozen vegetables will cause the soup to get quite liquidy during cooking, like pot pie consistency liquidy, without adding any water."

Two 6-ounce boneless, skinless chicken breasts

1 medium Yukon gold potato, peeled and chopped

2 cans reduced-sodium condensed cream of chicken soup

1 pound frozen mixed vegetables

½ cup water, optional (use if you like a thinner sauce)

1 unbaked pie crust, either storebought or homemade (not pie shells)

**Preheat oven to 375°F. Grease a 9 x 13-inch baking dish.**

1. Cook the chicken breasts and the potato in salted boiling water, about 12 minutes, then drain and cut or shred the chicken into appropriately sized pieces (it's OK if the chicken's a little underdone, since it will finish cooking in the oven).

2. In a large bowl, mix the chicken, potato, soup, vegetables, and water, if using. Spread the mixture into the prepared baking dish.

3. Top the chicken mixture with the pie crust, then crimp the edges to seal and prick the top a few times with a fork. Bake until crust is golden brown, 30 to 40 minutes.

MAKE BABY FOOD: Puree the chicken and vegetables, or serve along with some crust as finger food.

## JESSE'S SLOW-COOKER CRANBERRY CHICKEN

**Serves 4**

**Cooking time: 2 to 6 hours (10 minutes active)**

Jesse Z. is what I call a "friend in the computer." Though we've been online pals for years, we've never met in person—she lives in Los Angeles, where she and her husband are raising a family of boys (the third of whom is gestating as I write this). Jesse's an International Board Certified Lactation Consultant, so she knows a thing or two about juggling babies and work. She is also something of a slow-cooker devotee. "My current favorite recipe is cranberry chicken," she told me. "I serve it with couscous, which only takes 5 minutes to make. Voilà . . . dinner!"

4 to 6 bone-in chicken pieces

½ bottle of Catalina dressing

1 can whole berry cranberry sauce

1 packet onion soup mix (reduced sodium, if possible)

1. Put the chicken into the insert of your slow cooker. Mix the remaining ingredients together and pour over the chicken.

2. Cook on LOW for 5 to 6 hours or HIGH for 2 to 3 hours.

MAKE BABY FOOD: Chicken in a sweet and tangy sauce? Babies love stuff like this—puree some with water and couscous (if you're taking Jesse's menu suggestion), or tear into pieces for finger food.

# YELENA'S NAVY MACARONI

**Serves 4**

**Cooking time: 45 minutes (30 minutes active)**

Yelena B., a mom of two in Houston, shared a little personal history along with her recipe: "This is our family's easiest dinner recipe. We call it 'Navy Macaroni'—I have no idea why! I'm originally from the former Soviet Union, and one of the meals from my childhood is this dish of macaroni sprinkled with ground meat—I'm not sure where it originated, but we had it a lot when I was little. Our family's version involves shredded veggies. It's an easy, delicious, and nutritionally sound dish."

8 ounces macaroni

1 pound ground beef or turkey

2 to 3 cups shredded vegetables of your
  choice
  *Try eggplant, zucchini, carrot, mushrooms—
  anything you have available.*

1 cup milk

Several tablespoons flour

Salt and pepper

1½ to 2 cups shredded cheese
  *Cheddar, mozzarella, Gruyère—anything that
  melts nicely will work here.*

**Preheat oven to 350°F, and grease a 9 x 13-inch baking dish.**

1. Cook the macaroni in a pot of boiling salted water according to package directions, then drain.

2. While macaroni is cooking, cook the ground meat in a large skillet until browned, then drain and transfer to a large bowl. Add the macaroni and shredded vegetables.

3. Put the milk in a small bowl, and whisk in flour by the tablespoon until it's the consistency of Alfredo sauce. Add salt and pepper to taste. Add the sauce to the macaroni mixture and stir.

4. Transfer to the prepared baking dish, sprinkle with shredded cheese, and bake until cheese is bubbling, 15 to 20 minutes.

MAKE BABY FOOD: If your baby is on finger foods, this mixture should be just fine. If you're not there yet, add a little more milk and puree.

# KAREN'S FAST AND SPICY MEAT SAUCE

**Serves 6 to 8**

**Cooking time: 40 minutes (25 minutes active)**

I don't just turn to friends for recipes—I hit up my family too. Karen, my brother David's wife, can juggle with the best of them. Seriously, the woman cannot be rattled. When she's stressed, she turns to this quickie recipe.

"A bagged salad with some cut-up carrots, cuke, and tomato makes this a balanced meal," she said. "Depending on how saucy you like your pasta, there may be leftover sauce, which can be frozen or left in the fridge for another day. I've even used the leftovers as a base for a new sauce—just add another can of crushed tomatoes and a half-pound of browned meat."

2 tablespoons olive oil

2 or 3 garlic cloves, minced

2 medium zucchini, chopped

Two 28-ounce cans crushed tomatoes

A pinch or two each of dried basil, parsley, and oregano

1 teaspoon sugar, optional

Hot sauce (we like a spicy sauce, and we use Frank's Red Hot)

1 pound ground beef, browned and drained
*See Karen's ingenious idea for pre-cooking meat on page 233.*

1 pound spaghetti

1.  Bring a large pot of salted water to a boil. While you wait, heat the olive oil in a saucepan over medium heat. When it shimmers, add the garlic and cook, 1 to 2 minutes. Add the zucchini, and cook until softened, 3 to 5 minutes.

2.  Add the tomatoes and the dried herbs, as much or as little as you like of each. Add the sugar, if using. When sauce starts to boil, add a splash or two of the hot sauce (use more if you like it spicy).

3.  Once you're happy with the flavor of the sauce, add the ground beef. Reduce heat and simmer, covered, while pasta cooks.

4.  Cook pasta according to package directions. Drain and serve with sauce.

MAKE BABY FOOD: There's nothing here a baby can't have, as long as he's OK with a bit of spice. Either puree some sauce and spaghetti, or cut it up and let baby feed himself.

## WHAT'S THE BABY EATING?

One big worry about being a working mom is that you're away for substantial chunks of your baby's day, which means you don't necessarily know how well your baby's eating. Did she drink that whole bottle? Did she like the mashed banana? Here are some tips for dealing with the uncertainty:

"**I request that my nanny write down everything that the kids eat during the day,** so that when I get home I can see what they ate and ask her any questions I might have." —Jesse Z., mom of two, Los Angeles, CA

"Because the baby responds differently to different people, **I have to trust our nanny** when she says that my daughter seemed to want more bottles when I wasn't there, or whatever. Since she's gaining weight and seeming healthy, we just relax and trust that it's all working fine. **With solids, I think it's helpful to be clear about who is responsible for what—introducing new foods, cleaning up, making food, etc.**" —Lauren A., mom of one, Los Angeles, CA

"We made sure our childcare provider understood what we were doing with our son, such as feeding on demand instead of a set schedule, that breastmilk was not to be microwaved because it kills antibodies, etc. **Open communication is always the key.**" —Yelena B., mom of two, Houston, TX

• • • • • • • • • • • • • • • • • • • • • • • • • • • • • • • • • • • •

# AMY'S SLOW-COOKER THAI BRISKET

**Serves 6 to 8**

**Cooking time: 8 to 10 hours (15 minutes active)**

Amy, my Thai-Jewish student, returns with a recipe that's a little of both. I can't think of anything more Jewish than braised brisket, but Amy gives it a Thai twist that's irresistible. And she lets it simmer all day in the slow cooker, which you know I love.

A note from Amy on ingredients: "If you can't find mushroom soy sauce, I've swapped in regular soy and an extra splash of vinegar, and I've even used teriyaki sauce!"

3 to 4 pounds brisket

½ cup Thai mushroom soy sauce

½ cup Thai oyster sauce

½ cup water

¼ cup black vinegar or rice vinegar

1 tablespoon honey

4 garlic cloves, peeled and smashed

A handful of chopped cilantro stems

1 cup straw mushrooms or sliced button mushrooms

Cooked white rice, preferably jasmine

Hot sauce and chopped cilantro, for serving

6 to 8 fried eggs, optional

1. Combine the brisket, soy sauce, oyster sauce, water, vinegar, honey, garlic, and cilantro stems in the slow cooker in the morning and cook on LOW until you get home, 8 to 10 hours, or 4 to 5 hours on HIGH.

2. Shred the meat, serve over rice, and garnish with hot sauce and cilantro. Top with a fried egg, if you like.

> MAKE BABY FOOD: Brisket cooked until it's falling-apart soft is great for babies—either puree with rice and broth (since the sauce may be too salty) or cut into small pieces for finger food. Due to botulism concerns, swap sugar for the honey if you'll be serving it to a baby who's less than one year old.

# CHAPTER 8

# UN-RECIPES FOR PARTNERS WHO CAN'T COOK

Not long after I began teaching my cooking class, I received an email from a mom who needed help:

*I have a 21-month-old and another due in August, and my husband, while a great dad, is also a stereotypical Irish man in that he's never learned to cook. He's keen to help, though, particularly in the weeks after the new baby is born, so I would love it if you could address some simple recipes that he might be able to throw together for those first weeks.*
*—Emily O., Brooklyn, NY*

I feel Emily's pain, don't you? I mean, I'm lucky enough to be married to a guy who took a cooking class long before he met me and not because he thought it was a good way to meet chicks, but my capable, well-intentioned husband floundered as much as I did in Harry's early days. Heck, Stephen was sleep-deprived too—no wonder he couldn't come up with anything more complicated than pasta with a defrosted batch of Little Gram's Sauce (page 177). (Not that I'm complaining! That sauce is so good I'd eat it every day. Seriously.) Plus, his paternity leave was all of one week. He'd come home exhausted, anxious to spend some time with his newborn son, not at the stove.

So if your beloved doesn't know his or her way around the kitchen, feeding the grownups—not to mention a toddler—once your newborn arrives can really pose a challenge.

In this chapter you'll find ideas so simple, so 1-2-3, that I'm pretty sure even a "stereotypical Irish man" can handle them. Some of them, like the Grilled Chicken Pesto Heroes on page 279, call for absolutely no cooking at all—they're so easy, I almost didn't feel right calling them "recipes." Quite a few of them begin with good-quality prepared foods—check out the Ravioli Lasagna on page 270. You might use a food processor, which is vastly easier than chopping with a knife (Gazpacho with Honeydew and Peppadew, page 263), and in a little more than half the recipes you'll turn on a burner or the oven—but it will be for something so straightforward, anyone can do it. After all, we're talking about kitchen triage here, the need to feed hungry people who are operating on very little sleep and are 100 percent responsible for the life of a helpless, teeny, adorable human being.

. . . . . . . . . . . . . . . . . . . . . . . . . . . . . . . . . . . . . . . . . . . . . . . . . . . . . . .

### MAKE IT EASY

I'm guessing that if your partner isn't used to cooking, he or she may not be used to shopping, or possibly even cleaning, either. And I know how quickly I got frustrated when I thought Stephen was doing it wrong—whatever "it" was. Take a deep breath, remember that this might be a very big deal for your partner, and be grateful. As you'll learn in the toddler years, lavish praise goes a long way toward encouraging a particular behavior.

• Is your partner new to shopping? Write your list in aisle order, to make things easier to find. Specify quantity, size, and even brand names if you have particular loyalties. If there are brands you absolutely *don't* want, you might want to spell that out too.

• Unless the money saved makes a huge difference in your life, don't worry about using coupons right now.

- Remind your partner of some basic rules for food shopping: Never shop hungry. Fill most of your cart from the outer perimeter of the store, where the freshest, least-processed foods are. Read the back and sides of packages, not the front (where the marketing copy is): If there are ingredients you don't recognize or can't pronounce, put it back on the shelf.

- Before shopping, decide on a maximum number for impulse buys—it's really easy to spend money without thinking.

- Is your partner new to cleaning the kitchen? Don't expect it to come out the way you want. As long as things are reasonably neat and not covered in grime (and you didn't have to do the work), you're golden.

- If you're persnickety about how your dishwasher is loaded, you can either hold on to that particular duty or take lots of deep, calming breaths. It's tempting to think that a detailed chart might help, but I assure you, it won't.

- Make it clear which sponge is for dishwashing and which is for wiping down counters, and do the same for any other similar-but-different cleaning implements.

. . . . . . . . . . . . . . . . . . . . . . . . . . . . . . . . . . . . . . . . . . . . . . . . . . . . . . . .

Now, please turn the book over to the loved one who will be doing the cooking. I have a few simple things to say before we get started.

. . . . . . . . . . . . . . . . . . . . . . . . . . . . . . . . . . . . . . . . . . . . . . . . . . . . . . . .

### TOTAL, 100 PERCENT NOVICE COOK? START HERE

- First, let me say that it's a wonderful thing you're doing, cooking for the mother of your child. You're scoring spousal points as well as karmic ones.

- Before you even set foot in the kitchen, read the recipe in full. Twice, maybe. You don't want to be surprised that something needs an hour to chill, know what I mean?

- If the instructions say to preheat the oven, that means turning it on a good 20 minutes before you plan to put food inside. The cooking time will be off considerably if food goes into a cold oven.

- Next, measure out your ingredients, and line them up (in order of use) wherever you'll be cooking. This is called a mise en place, and it's the best way I know to make sure you're not out of salt when you're halfway through a recipe.

- Now, make sure the pans, spoons, racks, etc., you'll need are clean and ready.

- Be mindful of the chance for cross-contamination, which is when juices from raw protein mingle with other ingredients—or the equipment that touches them. There aren't many recipes in this chapter that even call for raw meat, poultry, or fish, but when you're making the ones that do, wash your hands and your knife with soap and hot water before moving on to other ingredients; use a separate cutting board (or scrub it in between, if you'd rather use just one); and never return cooked protein to the same plate that held it raw, or use the same utensils. Clean the counter well too.

- Plan ahead. The cooking times provided here are approximate—they're based on my own experience as well as the experiences of the parents who tested the recipes. If you're truly a newbie, I'd expect things to take a good 25 to 50 percent longer. Be sure to give yourself enough time. And use a timer. It's way too easy to forget you've got something cooking, especially when you're sleep-deprived.

- Salt is your friend. If you're not satisfied with the way something tastes, an additional pinch of salt is often the answer—unless, of course, the problem is that your food is too salty already, in which case you're pretty stuck. To play it safe, start out with what feels like too little salt, and build from there. Unless you're dealing with raw protein, it's fine to taste as you go.

- Cut yourself some slack. Don't expect the results to be suitable for the cover of *Bon Appétit*. They'll taste good, and that's what counts.

- Don't be afraid to write in the book! Take notes on what you did and how it turned out; you'll have a point of reference for next time.

- And my last piece of advice: Trust yourself. You can do this. Who knows, maybe you'll even have some fun.

## CRIB NOTES

- Even if your kitchen experience has been limited to pouring yourself a bowl of cereal, you can make these recipes. I promise. If you have any questions, you can always email me at *parentsneedtoeattoo@gmail.com*.

- Many of the recipes in this chapter offer multiple variations, so once you discover that you can, in fact, follow instructions and produce something delicious, you'll have several different flavor combos to make the same way.

- Prepared food is not the enemy. In fact I'm a fan, when chosen wisely; check out the list on page 13 if you don't believe me. All I ask is that you read first the ingredients list, then the nutrition facts statement.

- Don't be afraid to buy pre-cut fruits and vegetables, if it means you'll get dinner on the table.

- Once you've mastered the recipes in this chapter, check out Chapter 3, "Quick Suppers." You're ready for something a bit more complicated, Grasshopper.

• • • • • • • • • • • • • • • • • • • • • • • • • • • • • • • • • • • • • • • • • • • •

# BAKED STUFFED POTATOES

**Serves 4, and doubles well**

**Cooking time: 1½ hours (15 minutes active)**

The beauty of this recipe is its variability. Really, you should consider it more of a basic technique than an actual recipe—I've given you some flavor combos to try, but feel free to ransack your pantry and fridge for possibilities. Generally, you'll want to have some kind of cheese along with at least one other savory element.

Some "ifs":

If you're really hungry, bake an extra potato and add the insides to the filling mixture—it'll bulk the recipe up into more substantial servings. Toss (or nibble on) the skin from that extra tater.

If you're in a rush, you can shave about 45 minutes off the cooking time by doing the initial bake in the microwave (times vary depending on the strength of the microwave oven, so you'll have to either check the instruction booklet or ask your partner), then transferring the potatoes to the oven for 10 minutes to crisp the skins. Proceed from Step 3.

And if you're looking to save some calories, either reduced-fat sour cream or fat-free Greek-style yogurt works well here, as does light butter, 1 percent milk, and turkey bacon. Don't skimp on the cheese, though—if you use a top-quality cheese (the kind you buy at the cheese shop, not the supermarket) the flavor will be so full that you can use less.

4 large baking potatoes (use russets—the     ½ cup sour cream
    kind you picture when you think "potato")     ½ cup milk
4 tablespoons butter

**Add-ins:**

### CHICKEN AND BROCCOLI

1 cup chopped cooked chicken

1½ cups frozen chopped broccoli, thawed
*If you're comfortable cutting up and steaming fresh broccoli, by all means do so here.*

1¼ cups shredded Cheddar cheese, divided

1 teaspoon salt

### BLUE CHEESE AND BACON

1¼ cups crumbled blue cheese, divided

4 strips cooked bacon, crumbled
*If you'd rather not cook bacon yourself, it's fine to use the pre-cooked variety for this. You'll find it near the uncooked bacon in the supermarket.*

3 tablespoons chopped chives or scallions, optional

### GREEK-STYLE

2 cups frozen chopped spinach, thawed and squeezed to remove as much liquid as possible

1¼ cups crumbled feta, divided

1 scallion (white and pale green parts), chopped

¼ cup chopped fresh dill, optional

½ teaspoon salt

### BUTTERNUT AND GRUYÈRE

½ pound butternut squash, peeled and chopped
*Save time and effort: Buy peeled-and-cut squash from the produce department.*

1 tablespoon olive oil

½ teaspoon salt

Freshly ground pepper

2 tablespoons chopped fresh sage, optional

¼ cups shredded Gruyère cheese, divided

**Preheat oven to 425°F.**

1. Scrub the potatoes and prick several times with a fork. Put the potatoes directly on the oven rack and bake until soft when pierced with a fork, about 1 hour. Leave the oven on.

**NOTE:** If you're making the Butternut and Gruyère version, roast the squash while you're baking the potatoes: Grease or line a baking sheet. Combine the squash pieces, olive oil, salt, and pepper to taste in a mixing bowl. Spread on the prepared baking sheet. If the pieces are large they could take 45 minutes to an hour to cook, but if they're 1 inch or smaller you shouldn't need more than 30 minutes for this. When they're fork-tender, set aside to cool. Mash along with the potatoes in Step 4.

2. Cool potatoes 10 minutes, then slice in half lengthwise (you may want to hold them with a kitchen towel to protect your hand—they'll still be pretty hot). Scoop out the insides with a spoon, leaving a thin layer of potato behind so you don't tear the skin. Transfer the insides to a large bowl, and set the skins aside for now.

3. Add the butter, sour cream, and milk to the bowl, and mash with a potato masher.

4. Stir in your add-ins, reserving ¼ cup of the cheese. Scoop the stuffing into the reserved skins, and place them into a baking dish just large enough to hold everything. Sprinkle the tops with the reserved cheese.

5. Bake for 25 to 30 minutes, until the potatoes are heated through and the cheese is lightly browned.

MAKE BABY FOOD: The basic filling is great for babies, as are all the add-ins listed. If you like, instead of using a potato shell, put some of your filling into a greased ramekin and bake alongside the potatoes. If your baby is still on purees, whir some of the filling with a little broth or even water in a food processor to thin it.

**MAMA SAID**
"Oh. My. God. These were unreal delicious. Seriously the best comfort food I've had in, um, ever? Wow. All five of us loved them—the baby ate two entire potatoes (small ones), and the preschoolers were big fans too. No leftovers! I made a double batch, and made both the Greek-style and the butternut and Gruyère fillings." —Sarah B., mom of three, Canterbury, CT

# GAZPACHO WITH HONEYDEW AND PEPPADEW

**Serves 4 to 6**

**Cooking time: 4 to 6 hours (15 to 20 minutes active)**

On its own, this gazpacho is perfect for a light lunch—stir in some sour cream or plain yogurt to make it a little heartier. At dinnertime, serve alongside crusty bread, a hunk of cheese, and some dried sausage.

There is a bit of knife work involved in this one, but you don't have to be precise. You just need to roughly chop the ingredients so they can fit in the food processor.

The recipe's nice zip comes from Peppadews, small, spicy-sweet, pickled peppers. They're sold in jars in the pickle section of the supermarket, and often on the olive bar.

1 large English cucumber (often labeled "seedless"), halved lengthwise and chopped into 1-inch pieces

2 red bell peppers, cored and chopped into 1-inch pieces

8 Peppadew peppers, drained

3 large ripe tomatoes, cored, seeded, and chopped into 1-inch pieces
*To core and seed a tomato, cut it in half through the equator. Use a paring knife to cut out the stem end, then give both halves a gentle squeeze (over a bowl or the garbage disposal) and the seeds should squirt right out. If they don't, just use a finger to scoop them out.*

1 small red onion, peeled and chopped into 1-inch pieces

3 or 4 garlic cloves, peeled and smashed
*This gets more garlicky the longer it sits, so if you're not a huge fan of the stuff, go with the lesser amount.*

½ a honeydew melon, seeded, peeled, and chopped into 1-inch pieces
*If you're not comfortable cutting your own melon, it's totally fine to buy it ready-to-go.*

One 46-ounce bottle of low-sodium vegetable juice

Good-quality extra-virgin olive oil

Sherry vinegar

Salt and pepper

1. Pulse each type of vegetable and the honeydew separately in a food processor. After each ingredient is chopped into small, uniform pieces, transfer to a large serving bowl and move on to the next vegetable; if you pulse them all at once, you'll end up with a mushy mess. (You can put the Peppadews in with the bell peppers, and toss the garlic in with the red onion.)

2. After you process all of the vegetables and stir them together in the bowl, add a few glugs each of the olive oil and sherry vinegar, and season with salt and pepper—keep tasting it until you're happy with the balance of flavors.

3. Stir to combine, then cover and refrigerate for several hours, stirring occasionally. This is much, much better after it's had a nice long rest.

MAKE BABY FOOD: If your baby's had raw tomatoes, he should be fine with this. Sometimes babies get confused by differing textures, though, so the liquid/solid combo might throw him—I'd fully puree his portion.

**MAMA SAID**
"I just love a good gazpacho, so I was really excited to try this recipe. But we don't have a food processor or even a blender. I pulled out my immersion blender and realized that there is a chopping attachment that I had never even used! It did the trick nicely. The Peppadews add a really nice flavor to this soup. It turned out delicious!" —Lee P., mom of two, Pittsburgh, PA

· · · · · · · · · · · · · · · · · · · · · · · · · · · · · · · · · · · · · · · · · · · · ·

# THE QUESADILLA VARIATIONS

**Serves as many as you like**
**Cooking time: 15 to 30 minutes (5 to 15 minutes active)**

There is absolutely no authenticity on this page. None. What there is, is a variety of formulas for ridiculously tasty, and ridiculously easy, combinations of tortillas, cheese, and stuff.

The key here—the thing that makes these quesadillas so easy, so doable by even the newest kitchen hand—is that they're baked. No need to stand in front of a stove, patiently making them one by one in a frying pan, all the time wondering if you're doing it right. It's quick, it's painless, and it's skill-free.

You'll need 2 tortillas per quesadilla. I prefer the small corn ones, but flour tortillas work here too. For a small tortilla, use about 1 ounce of cheese per quesadilla, a few tablespoons of filling, and about a tablespoon of whatever spread you use. Figure on 2 to 4 tablespoons salsa or dipping sauce per quesadilla. Larger tortillas will require larger quantities, across the board.

For dinner, Stephen and I will each eat two quesadillas made from small corn tortillas, and one each if it's a larger, burrito-sized flour tortilla. Add a simple green salad, and you've got a perfect light dinner.

## THE BASIC

Tortillas

Your choice of the following:

Drained and rinsed canned black beans or pinto beans, chopped scallions, sliced mushrooms, defrosted frozen corn kernels, chopped green chiles or roasted peppers, sliced black olives, or shredded chicken, pork, or beef

Shredded Cheddar or Jack cheese

Prepared salsa, for dipping

## PESTO-CAPRESE

Tortillas

Prepared pesto sauce, either storebought or homemade (like the ones on pages 267 to 269)

Tomatoes, thinly sliced

Shredded mozzarella cheese

Best-quality jarred tomato sauce, warmed, for dipping
 *When I say "best-quality," I mean one that only includes ingredients you would use if you were making it yourself. No multi-syllabic words you don't recognize, nothing with "-ose" on the end.*

## MANGO-CHEDDAR

Tortillas

Prepared mango chutney
 *If you like chutneys, go ahead and experiment with different kinds. Almost all of them pair nicely with melted cheese and tamarind chutney!*

Shredded sharp cheese (I like Cheddar or Manchego)

Prepared tamarind chutney, for dipping

## FRENCH ONION

Tortillas

Caramelized onions
 *This is a great way to use the leftovers from Overnight French Onion Chicken on page 151.*

Shredded Gruyère or Jarlsberg cheese

Sour cream, for dipping

## ASIAN

Tortillas (flour is best here)

Prepared hoisin sauce

Chopped scallions, green parts only

Chopped broccoli, either cooked or thawed from frozen

Shredded sharp Cheddar or Monterey Jack, or a combination

Sriracha or Chinese plum sauce, for dipping

## CUBANO

Tortillas

Yellow mustard

Roast pork, chopped

Sliced ham, chopped

Dill pickles, chopped

Sliced Swiss cheese

Prepared mojo sauce, for dipping (look for it in the Latin foods aisle)

**Preheat oven to 350°F.**

1. Coat a baking sheet, as well as one side of each tortilla, with nonstick spray or brush lightly with olive oil. Arrange tortillas flat on the sheet, oil side down with a bit of space in between. This will be the bottom of the quesadilla.

2. If you're using a spread, put that on the tortillas, then scatter or lay your filling on top of that, and finally top with the shredded cheese.

3. Cover each quesadilla with a second tortilla and press together lightly. Spray or brush tops with oil

4. Bake 4 to 5 minutes, then remove sheet from the oven and carefully flip the quesadillas with a spatula. Use two spatulas if you're having trouble. Return to the oven and bake until cheese is melted and tortilla is browned and crisp, 4 to 5 minutes.

5. Cut into quarters (I use a pizza cutter) and serve with dipping sauce.

MAKE BABY FOOD: Obviously, the baby-friendliness of your quesadilla will depend upon what you put into it. That said, the only ingredients on this page that might give one pause are the sriracha (hot!) and the pesto (made with nuts, which are of concern only if there are food allergies in your immediate family). At the very least, you can reserve the individual ingredients for your baby to eat as finger food. If you're going to serve baby the cooked quesadilla, please make sure it's cooled quite a bit first—melted cheese can get pretty molten.

**MAMA SAID**

"We tried the quesadillas last night, the Mango-Cheddar variation—it was deeeeeelicious! I did a plain cheese quesadilla for the kids, which is always a hit. My favorite part of these quesadillas was the fact that they were baked. I've never baked quesadillas before, and these turned out great and were super easy." —Jesse Z., mom of two, Los Angeles, CA

"I made the French Onion quesadillas with Jarlsberg, cut them into 6 pieces each, and served the triangles for a party appetizer. They were a smash hit—I only got one or two pieces before they were all gone." —Heather B., mom of two, Westmont, IL

• • • • • • • • • • • • • • • • • • • • • • • • • • • • • • • • • • • • • • • • • • •

## THE PESTO VARIATIONS

**Basic formula makes about 1½ cups**

**Cooking time: 10 minutes**

I love pesto. Adore it. Would eat it with a spoon. And yet somehow I managed to marry a man who just doesn't like pesto—he finds the basil overwhelming. But when Harry first started eating solids, he got a taste of the stuff somewhere and went nuts for it. For months, if we added pesto to a new food, he'd gobble it up. It was my secret weapon. At the time, the American Academy of Pediatricians was still advising all parents to withhold nuts until babies were well into toddlerhood,* so I'd reserve some of the basil-garlic-oil combination before adding pine nuts. Nowadays Harry won't touch the stuff, so I'm back to using traditional pesto only as an ingredient in other recipes (like the Turkey Pesto Meatballs on page 284). But I haven't stopped making it—I've just changed things up a bit. By varying the herbs and the nuts used, and sometimes even the cheese, you can make a pesto that would make a *nonna*'s head spin.

**NOTE:** All of these variations use unsalted nuts. I prefer them toasted—it accentuates the flavor of the nut. Many stores, including Trader Joe's, sell a variety of nuts already toasted.

---

\* In 2008, the AAP changed that recommendation: Now, if your immediate family is free of food allergies, it's fine to jump in sooner.

## YOU'VE MADE PESTO, NOW HERE'S HOW TO USE IT

- On pasta (duh): Toss about a tablespoon at a time with cooked pasta, adding a splash or two of pasta cooking water, until you're happy with the consistency.
- On sandwiches, like the Grilled Chicken Pesto Heroes on page 279. Or make a Caprese Sandwich: Italian bread, pesto, thickly sliced tomatoes, fresh mozzarella. Toasted, if you like.
- On pizza, instead of or in addition to tomato sauce.
- Stirred into a bowl of vegetable or bean soup just before serving—yes, even canned soup.
- Thinned with more oil, as a sauce for simply cooked fish or shrimp.
- In meatloaf or meatballs, like the Turkey Pesto Meatballs on page 284.
- On fish fillets: Place a fillet on a large piece of aluminum foil and smear some pesto on top. Fold foil over the fish and seal edges, leaving some breathing room inside. Bake fish in a preheated 350°F oven for 10 to 12 minutes if it's on the thin side, 12 to 15 minutes if it's an inch thick or greater. Fish is done when it's opaque throughout—stick a small knife into the thickest part and peek.
- As a salad dressing, thinned with oil and vinegar.

### BASIL PESTO

2 cups basil leaves

½ cup grated Parmesan

¼ cup pine nuts, toasted

2 garlic cloves, peeled and smashed

Good-quality extra-virgin olive oil

Salt and pepper

### PARSLEY PISTACHIO PESTO

2 cups flat-leaf parsley leaves

½ cup grated Pecorino or Parmesan cheese

¼ cup shelled pistachios

2 garlic cloves, peeled and smashed

Good-quality extra-virgin olive oil

Salt and pepper

### SPANAKOPITA PESTO

2 cups baby spinach

½ cup feta cheese

¼ cup fresh dill

¼ cup walnuts, toasted

2 scallions (white and green parts), roughly chopped

Good-quality extra-virgin olive oil

Salt and pepper

## MINT HAZELNUT PESTO

2 cups mint leaves

½ cup flat-leaf parsley leaves

½ cup grated Parmesan cheese

¼ cup hazelnuts, skinned

2 garlic cloves, peeled and smashed

Splash of hazelnut or walnut oil, optional

2 to 3 tablespoons lemon juice, or to taste

Good-quality extra-virgin olive oil

Salt and pepper

## MIX-IT-UP PESTO

1 cup basil, parsley, or cilantro leaves, or a
combination

2 tablespoons mint, sage, tarragon, or thyme
leaves

2 tablespoons rosemary or oregano leaves

½ cup grated Parmesan cheese

¼ cup pine nuts, walnuts, or toasted almonds

2 garlic cloves, peeled and smashed

Good-quality extra-virgin olive oil

Salt and pepper

1.  Put everything except the oil, salt, and pepper into a food processor. Process until it's
    a finely-chopped, dry-looking paste.

2.  With the processor running, pour the oil slowly through the feed tube until you're
    happy with the consistency. I like mine to be pretty thick, almost like cream cheese,
    but if you prefer yours more like heavy cream that's good too—just add more oil.
    Season with salt and pepper.

**NOTE:** Store unused sauce, topped with a thin layer of oil, in an airtight container in the
fridge. It should stay good for a week or two. Or skip the cheese and freeze in an ice-
cube tray. Once frozen solid, pop out and store in an airtight container. When ready to
use, thaw and stir in the cheese.

> MAKE BABY FOOD: In terms of consistency, pesto's pretty terrific for babies. If
> there are food allergies in your immediate family, save the nuts for last, reserving
> a few tablespoons of the sauce for baby before you add them.

MAMA SAID

"I made the pesto yesterday. So easy that even I couldn't mess it up! And so quick that it can
be made even when everyone is awake." —Abigail A., mom of two, New York, NY

# RAVIOLI LASAGNA

**Serves 6 to 8**

**Cooking time: 45 minutes (15 minutes active)**

There are dozens of versions of this recipe floating out there in the world—no surprise, given how simple it is. The barest-bones version has only three ingredients: frozen cheese ravioli, jarred pasta sauce, and mozzarella cheese. But if you'd like to have a little more fun with it, I've included some variations.

*If you live near an Italian neighborhood, you'll probably find frozen ravioli with dozens of different fillings. Why not experiment with flavor combos?*

### THE BASIC

3 cups prepared pasta sauce
**Little Gram's Sauce from page 177 works well here, but any good-quality jarred sauce would be fine too.**

One large package frozen cheese ravioli (about 25 ounces)

3 cups shredded mozzarella cheese

### MUSHROOM-SPINACH

3 cups prepared pasta sauce

One large package frozen mushroom ravioli (about 25 ounces)

2 cups frozen chopped spinach, thawed and squeezed to remove as much liquid as possible

*I buy my frozen spinach in bags, so I can take out as much as I need without defrosting an entire block.*

3 cups shredded mozzarella cheese

### TRADITIONAL BEEF

3 cups prepared pasta sauce

One large package frozen beef ravioli (about 25 ounces)

2 cups ricotta cheese

3 cups shredded mozzarella cheese

### SOUTHWESTERN BEEF

Two 10-ounce cans enchilada sauce

1 cup salsa

One large package frozen beef ravioli (about 25 ounces)

2 cups frozen corn kernels, thawed

3 cups shredded Cheddar or Monterey Jack cheese

**Preheat oven to 375°F. Coat a 9 x 13-inch baking dish with cooking spray.**

1. Cover the bottom of the dish with a thin layer of sauce. (If you're making the Southwestern Beef version, stir together the enchilada sauce and the salsa in a bowl first, then use that.) Arrange half of the ravioli in 1 layer over the sauce. If you're using either vegetables or ricotta cheese, layer them on top. Cover with about half of the remaining sauce and half of the shredded cheese. Arrange the remaining ravioli over the cheese, then top with the remaining sauce and shredded cheese.

2. Bake until the cheese is browned and the edges of the dish are bubbling, 25 to 30 minutes.

> MAKE BABY FOOD: All these variations are fine for babies, either pureed or as finger foods. At the very least, the ravioli filling is bound to be the right consistency, and you can always reserve some uncooked cheese.

**MAMA SAID**
"It was excellent, and the perfect meal for a busy night. My husband loved it and emailed me the next day to thank me for the yummy lunch the leftovers made. By accident, I bought two packages of refrigerated ravioli instead of frozen ravioli, but it worked just fine." —Aileen W., mom of one, Westerville, OH

# EMBARRASSINGLY EASY TAPENADE PASTA

**Serves 4 to 6**

**Cooking time: 30 minutes (5 minutes active)**

Tapenade is a Mediterranean paste made from olives, capers, and anchovies; it's available jarred in most large supermarkets, often in the "gourmet" section. Since quality varies widely and it's such a key component of this dish, I'd recommend tasting it before you use it here. If you don't like it straight from the jar, you probably won't like it on pasta, either!

One 14.5- to 16-ounce box of whole-wheat or whole-grain pasta

2 tablespoons pine nuts

½ cup prepared olive tapenade

Juice of ½ lemon (about 1½ tablespoons)

Grated Parmesan cheese, for serving

1. Bring a large pot of salted water to a boil (covered to speed things up).

2. When the water boils, add the pasta and cook according to package directions. Just before the end of cooking time, scoop out about ½ cup of the cooking water and set aside.

3. While the pasta is boiling, toast the pine nuts. The easiest way is to bake them in the toaster oven at 300°F for about 3 minutes. Keep a close eye on them so they don't burn. If you don't have a toaster oven, put them in a small, dry skillet and toast over medium heat, shaking the pan frequently, until browned, 3 to 5 minutes.

4. Drain the pasta and toss with the tapenade, lemon juice, and toasted pine nuts. If the pasta looks dry, add some of the pasta cooking water.

5. Serve topped with the Parmesan cheese.

> MAKE BABY FOOD: You might be surprised by how much your baby likes tapenade. Don't be afraid to let him try it! If there are food allergies in your immediate family, hold off on the pine nuts until your pediatrician gives the thumbs-up.

**MAMA SAID**

"It was so easy to make! I was able to take care of the kiddo, start a load of laundry and even make her lunch for the next day all while 'cooking' the dish. I appreciated the even easier clean-up!" —Sarah B., mom of one, Nashville, TN

# LINGUINE WITH PECORINO, LEMON, AND MINT

**Serves 4 to 6**

**Cooking time: 30 minutes (10 minutes active)**

In terms of flavor, this recipe is a lot like Angel Hair Pasta with Garlic and Lemon-Parmesan Breadcrumbs (page 40). But for as easy as that recipe is, this one's even easier. You barely even need a knife.

One 14.5- to 16-ounce box whole-wheat or whole-grain linguine

2 tablespoons olive oil

½ cup grated Pecorino cheese
*If Pecorino is excessively pricey in your area, a good-quality Parmesan (no green canisters, please) or Grana Padano would also work well.*

Grated zest of 1 lemon (Use a grater with fine holes or a Microplane, and grate the yellow rind only—leave the bitter white pith behind.)

Large handful of mint leaves, roughly chopped

Freshly ground pepper

1. Bring a large pot of salted water to a boil (covered to speed things up).

2. When the water boils, add the linguine and cook according to package directions. Toward the end of cooking time, scoop out about ½ cup of the cooking water and set aside. Drain the pasta and transfer to a large bowl.

3. Add the other ingredients and toss to combine. If it seems too dry, add some of the reserved cooking water.

MAKE BABY FOOD: If your baby's cool with the acidity in lemons, cut up the linguine and you're good to go.

**MAMA SAID**
"My husband and I both loved it. My preschooler thought it was horrible, but ate plain pasta and Pecorino. And my little one liked it fine." —Ann S., mom of two, Lebanon, NH

# HERBED PANZANELLA

**Serves 4**

**Cooking time: 40 minutes to 1 hour (25 minutes active)**

Panzanella is an Italian salad made with stale bread. Traditionally, the bread chunks get a quick dunk in cold water before going into the salad, but I like my bread to still have some chew to it—for me, the juices of the tomatoes and the dressing ingredients soften it plenty.

The ingredients list may look long, but it really doesn't take much effort to toss this together—the majority of the list never touches a knife.

⅓ cup good-quality extra-virgin olive oil

¼ cup balsamic vinegar

1 small garlic clove, peeled and smashed

Salt and pepper
*If you really don't want to cook, not even to make dressing, it's fine to use a good-quality bottled Italian dressing—and by "good-quality," I mean one with ingredients you recognize, not a string of multi-syllabic mumbo-jumbo.*

1 large loaf of 1- or 2-day-old country bread, torn into bite-size pieces (you should wind up with 5 or 6 cups)

1 English cucumber (often labeled "seedless"), quartered lengthwise and cut into chunks

1 pound ripe tomatoes, cut into bite-sized chunks
*The tomatoes really matter here, both for their juiciness and for their flavor. If it's not tomato season, use two pints of grape tomatoes cut in half or, if your store carries them, Campari tomatoes, which are a relatively new, extremely sweet variety sold year-round.*

Half of a medium red onion, thinly sliced
*If you don't like raw onions in your salad, soak them in a small bowl of ice water for about 10 minutes—it softens the bite considerably.*

½ cup pitted Kalamata olives
*Buy them already pitted!*

8 ounces cooked chicken, cubed, or 8 ounces fresh mozzarella or feta cheese, chopped

¾ cup flat-leaf parsley leaves, left whole

¾ cup basil leaves, torn

## OPTIONAL ADD-INS

Canned chickpeas or cannellini beans, drained and rinsed

Hard-boiled eggs, quartered

Canned light tuna in oil, drained then chunked with a fork

Anchovies

Artichoke hearts, marinated or not, drained

Capers, drained and rinsed

Pepperoncini, drained and chopped

Roasted red peppers, jarred or homemade, chopped

Leftover grilled vegetables, chopped

½ cup fresh mint leaves, left whole

1. Combine the olive oil, vinegar, smashed garlic, and salt and pepper to taste in a small airtight container and shake well. Let it sit while you tear the bread and chop the vegetables.

2. Combine all the remaining ingredients in a large salad bowl.

3. Remove and discard the garlic clove from the dressing. Cover and shake the dressing one more time, then pour over the salad. Toss to combine, then let, salad sit for at least 15 minutes and up to 2 hours. The longer the salad sits, the more juices the bread will soak up. If you think of it, give the salad a toss every few minutes.

> MAKE BABY FOOD: That juicy, softened bread is a very nice texture for early eaters. As for the rest of the ingredients: They're all fair game, but make sure your baby is comfortable with the acidity of raw tomatoes.

**MAMA SAID**
"The panzanella was delicious! My husband, my sister, and I all loved it, the preschoolers loved the veggie/cheese/olive part, and the baby loved the bread. I made it with fresh mozzarella and none of the optional ingredients this time, and served it with corn on the cob for a pretty lovely meal. Cooking was super easy, and perfect for doing with the kids—my two- and four-year-olds were totally engrossed with tearing up the bread, and the baby just gnawed on a chunk of it." —Sarah B., mom of three, Canterbury, CT

# A MEZZE FEAST

**Serves as many as you like**

**Cooking time: 10 minutes**

A mezze spread is a salad bar with a Middle Eastern twist. And I'll let you in on a secret: You can get some excellent prepared Middle Eastern salads in the supermarket. We really like the Sabra brand, for example. If you're lucky enough to live near a neighborhood with good Greek or Arabic shops, your only limit is your appetite.

In terms of quantities, you'll see I've left that up to you—it will depend on how many of the prepared dishes you include and how hungry you are.

*Feeling ambitious? Try the Quickie Hummus on page 339. If not, here's an easy trick for making store-bought hummus look homemade: Drizzle some flavorful olive oil on top, and sprinkle with a bit of paprika.*

### MOROCCAN CARROT SALAD

1 pound carrots, shredded
*If you're not thrilled about wielding a food processor or box grater, buy the pre-shredded kind.*

1½ tablespoons olive oil

Juice of ½ a lemon (about 1½ tablespoons)

½ teaspoon honey

½ teaspoon ground cumin

1. Put all the ingredients in a medium bowl, toss well, and set aside to let the flavors meld. Then prepare the other ingredients as listed below.

Hummus

Baba ghanoush

Tabbouleh

Stuffed grape leaves

Kalamata or other black olives in brine

Feta cheese

Flavorful olive oil

Dried oregano

Sliced cucumber (figure one-quarter to one-half cucumber per adult)

Grape tomatoes, or larger tomatoes cut into wedges (figure 6 to 8 grape tomatoes, or half a large tomato, per adult)

Pita, white or whole wheat (figure 1 whole pita per adult)

Moroccan carrot salad

1. Arrange the components in small bowls or platters. Drizzle olive oil over the feta, and sprinkle with the oregano.

2. Warm the pita in the microwave (depending on how many you're heating, it should take somewhere between 20 seconds and 1 minute). Cut into wedges.

> MAKE BABY FOOD: There's quite a bit on this list that's good for babies: Hummus, of course, and baba ghanoush, perhaps the stuffing from the grape leaves, the olives, a bit of the feta (not too much, since it can be quite salty), peeled cucumber, halved grape tomatoes (if your baby's OK with the acidity), and pita. No carrot salad, though, since babies under one year old can't have honey.

**MAMA SAID**
**"Thumbs up on the Mezze Feast! We found out our daughter loves baba gano . . . OK, I can't spell, but I like anything quick. Introduced something to our lunch boxes, which is great."**
**—Rachel M., mom of one, Tucson, AZ**

• • • • • • • • • • • • • • • • • • • • • • • • • • • • • • • • • • • • • • • •

# GREEK PITA POCKETS

**Serves 2 and multiplies well**
**Cooking time: 10 to 20 minutes**

Fast, fresh, and undeniably delicious, these salad-stuffed sandwiches take just minutes to assemble.

2 cooked chicken breasts, chopped
  *Use leftover chicken, or buy it already cooked, either grilled or rotisserie (I especially like lemon-pepper seasoned for this). If you're vegetarian or kosher, several of my mom-testers reported that Quorn "chicken" cutlets worked well here.*

1 small head romaine lettuce, chopped

1 cup grape tomatoes, halved if they're large, or 1 large tomato, chopped

Half a large English cucumber (often labeled "seedless"), quartered lengthwise and chopped

¼ cup Kalamata or other black olives in brine, pitted and halved
  *Buy them already pitted! And please, not the canned variety. They have so little flavor.*

4 ounces feta cheese, crumbled

2 tablespoons flavorful extra-virgin olive oil

1 tablespoon red wine vinegar

Juice of ½ lemon (about 1½ tablespoons)

¼ teaspoon dried oregano

Salt and pepper

2 pitas with pockets, white or whole wheat

1. Combine the chicken, lettuce, tomatoes, cucumber, olives, and feta cheese in a large salad bowl.

2. Combine the olive oil, vinegar, lemon juice, oregano, and a pinch each of salt and pepper in a small airtight container. Seal and shake well. Drizzle the dressing over the salad, and toss again.

3. Warm the pitas in the microwave—10 or 20 seconds should do it—and cut each in half.

4. Fill each pita half with salad, and serve. You may have more salad than will fit; if that's the case, warm a third pita and fill it, or just eat the salad with a fork.

MAKE BABY FOOD: Salad is tricky—often babies don't seem to know what to do with lettuce. But you can easily serve components of the salad as finger foods: tiny bits of chicken, peeled bits of cucumber, olives. Feta can be quite salty, so don't let your baby go to town on it (use your best judgment).

**MAMA SAID**
"This was a surprisingly delicious, fresh meal! I would not have thought to make it myself and am so glad for this 'staple' recipe. I am not a fan of grape tomatoes or cucumber and only included them to follow the rules. Boy, am I glad I did! They added freshness to the dish. At first bite, my husband and I thought it was just OK. By the middle of the pita we were preparing for seconds. Light and fresh—a new addition to our recipe rotation."
—Sarah B., mom of one, Nashville, TN

# GRILLED CHICKEN PESTO HEROES

**Serves 4**

**Cooking time: 10 minutes**

If you use all store-bought ingredients for this one, the only time you'll even need a knife is to cut open the rolls—unless you want to get fancy and slice the chicken breasts, but that's not strictly necessary. This sandwich is wonderful with almost any of the pesto variations on page 267.

Serve this with a green salad or heck, even potato chips (the baked kind to keep things virtuous), and dinner's ready.

½ cup prepared or homemade pesto (pages 267–269)

4 long Italian or French rolls, split lengthwise

4 grilled chicken breasts, whole or sliced
*If you're buying these pre-made, feel free to experiment with flavors. Anything that's remotely Mediterranean would work well here—balsamic, herbed, you get the idea.*

8 thin slices provolone or mozzarella cheese, optional

4 to 8 roasted red pepper halves, from a jar, drained and patted dry (the amount needed will depend on how big they are)

4 leaves romaine or other sturdy, crisp lettuce

1.  Spread 2 tablespoons pesto on the bottom half of each roll.

2.  Layer with the grilled chicken, cheese, if using, roasted peppers, and lettuce, and top with the other half of the roll.

*If you feel like getting fancy, after you lay the cheese on top of the chicken, stick the open-faced sandwich halves in the broiler for 30 seconds to a minute, until the cheese melts. Watch closely to make sure the bread doesn't burn. Then add the remaining ingredients and go.*

> MAKE BABY FOOD: All of this is fair game as finger foods. One big caveat: If anyone in your immediate family has food allergies, consult your pediatrician before feeding your baby pesto—almost every variety has nuts of some kind.

**MAMA SAID**

**"Yummy! My bar for these recipes has been 'Could my little brother make this?' He is a confirmed bachelor and eats Jack in the Box five nights out of seven. I think this one would pass the test." —Christy W., mom of three, Austin, TX**

• • • • • • • • • • • • • • • • • • • • • • • • • • • • • • • • • • •

# NOT-QUITE-TEXAS OVERNIGHT BRISKET

**Serves 8 to 10**

**Cooking time: 10 to 12¼ hours (15 minutes active)**

This recipe makes a barbecue-style brisket, not a Jewish-style braised one. It came to me via Cate O'Malley, who writes a wonderful food blog called Sweetnicks. The instructions are ridiculously simple: The night before you want to eat it, you put a big ol' brisket in a baking dish, season it with salt and pepper, maybe a little garlic or onion powder, and stick it in the oven. Go to bed. Wake up. Eat.

Well, maybe you don't want to eat brisket for breakfast. The idea here is that dinner's done waaaay ahead of time, and the kitchen gets heated up while nobody's in it—it's a perfect way to make brisket during the summer. You stick the cooked meat in the fridge, go about the day's business, and come home to a wonderful, easy-to-reheat dinner. I like to serve it with coleslaw and barbecue sauce on toasted whole-wheat buns. Yowza.

One thing to note: Normally, I trim my brisket of any big hunks of fat before cooking. Do that here and you'll wind up with meat so carbonized it's difficult to eat. Don't ask me how I know this. Just go with me, and don't trim the fat.

One 4- to 5-pound brisket, untrimmed
Salt and pepper
Garlic powder, optional

Onion powder, optional
Whole-wheat buns, your favorite barbecue
    sauce, coleslaw, and pickles, for serving

**Preheat oven to 225°F.**

1. Rub liberal amounts of salt (1 teaspoon or more), pepper, and the optional seasonings all over the brisket and set it fatty side up in a baking dish or roasting pan large enough to hold the meat comfortably.

2. Bake, uncovered, 10 to 12 hours. The brisket is done when a fork slides in and out easily—you're looking for meat so tender you don't need a knife.

3. Remove the brisket from the pan and let rest 10 to 15 minutes, then cut off any large gobs of fat (this will be challenging to do without sticking little bits into your mouth—that crusty fat is mighty tasty—so I won't tell if you don't). Slice the meat across the

grain, as thin or as thick as you like—but know that the thinner you get, the more likely it is to fall apart as you go.

*You see the way the brisket sorta has stripes running along its length? You want to cut across those stripes—that's cutting "across the grain."*

4. Transfer the cut meat to an airtight container and refrigerate.

5. There are two ways to reheat: Drizzle some barbecue sauce over the meat and reheat in the microwave as you would any kind of leftovers. Or put the meat into the (now clean) baking dish, pour some barbecue sauce over it, cover tightly with foil, and bake at 350°F for 20 to 30 minutes.

6. Serve on buns, with additional barbecue sauce, coleslaw, and pickles.

**NOTE:** The meat, sliced and unsauced, freezes beautifully. Wrap tightly in heavy-duty aluminum foil, and defrost in the fridge overnight or the microwave (remove foil first, obviously). Reheat as directed above.

> MAKE BABY FOOD: Brisket can be difficult for little ones to chew—either cut it into very small pieces or into one long strip, which will be good for gnawing more than eating. You could also puree it with water or broth and a bit of barbecue sauce.

**MAMA SAID**
"Awesome! I have always been intimidated by roasting meats like brisket. This was so easy it was ridiculous. If you can turn on an oven, you can make this. I had a sandwich for dinner tonight—brisket, barbecue sauce, and coleslaw on a bulkie. Holy deliciousness, Batman! Plus, this brisket recipe includes a bonus for lucky dogs . . . our Lady was thrilled with the fatty bits!" —Jess K., mom of two, Boston, MA

. . . . . . . . . . . . . . . . . . . . . . . . . . . . . . . . . . . . . . . . . .

# PEPPER-CRUSTED TUNA STEAK

**Serves 2, and doubles well**

**Cooking time: 10 minutes**

I know, I know, cooking fish is intimidating. But I learned this recipe from an old friend, a guy who could only cook two things: Pizza made with a Boboli crust, and this. Trust me, you can handle it.

Serve these tuna steaks with steamed broccoli (if you're nervous about using a knife, buy the pre-cut kind, or even frozen) and brown rice—boil-in bags or pre-cooked products make that part super-easy.

*Tuna steaks are relatively high in mercury, so the FDA recommends that pregnant or nursing women and children eat no more than six ounces per week. In other words: Don't make this every day. Fresh tuna costs so much who can afford to, anyway?*

| | |
|---|---|
| 2 tablespoons black peppercorns | Two 6-ounce tuna steaks, each about 1¼-inch |
| ½ teaspoon salt | thick |
| 2 tablespoons olive or vegetable oil, divided | Lemon wedges, for serving |

1. Put the peppercorns into a resealable bag and place on a cutting board. Use the bottom of a heavy pot or a rolling pin to crush them into small pieces—you may need to give them a couple of really good whacks to get things going. Pour the cracked pepper onto a plate and mix in the salt.

2. Rub a bit of the oil onto both sides of the tuna steaks (less than 1 tablespoon total), and press them gently into the pepper-salt mixture. Flip and press the other side. You're not looking for a perfect coating here—too much pepper would be unpleasant—and you'll likely have some leftover seasoning, which you should discard.

3. Heat the remaining oil in a large nonstick skillet over medium-high heat. When the oil shimmers, add the tuna. (Stand back—the oil might splatter.) Cook for 2 to 3 minutes per side, until it's golden on the outside but still almost raw in the center—it'll keep cooking for a bit after you take it out of the pan.

*Classically, tuna is served quite rare. If you'd like your fish a little more cooked (which I do), add an additional minute or two per side. Also, if your tuna steaks are thicker or thinner than 1¼ inches, you'll need to adjust the cooking time by about 1 minute per side.*

4. Serve with lemon wedges.

> MAKE BABY FOOD: Fish is terrific for babies, but thanks to the mercury in tuna steak this should be considered an occasional meal. Before dunking in the pepper-salt mixture, cut off a small piece from one of the steaks. Cook that little chunk until it's just cooked through, and it's perfect for a baby.

**MAMA SAID**
"This was a good dish and extremely fast. My preschooler 'helped,' which was fine because this was such a quick recipe. I served it with roasted asparagus and frozen quinoa from Trader Joe's, so the whole meal took about 30 minutes to make, which was the best part."
—Jennifer N., mom of two, Philadelphia, PA

# SPAGHETTI WITH TURKEY-PESTO MEATBALLS

**Serves 4, with leftovers**

**Cooking time: 45 minutes (15 minutes active)**

Now, this recipe requires a bit more work than most of the others in this chapter—but there's no cutting, and no meticulous timing. You *can* do this, I guarantee. And as a bonus for making the effort, you'll get enough meatballs for several meals! They make amazing heroes too.

3 cups homemade or best-quality storebought pasta sauce
*Little Gram's Sauce (page 177) is perfect here.*

*If you've made a batch from one of the recipes on pages 267–269 you're good to go, but storebought works equally well.*

1½ pounds ground turkey
*If you're buying the pre-packaged kind, which comes in a 1.3-pound container, that amount is just fine.*

1¼ cups plain dried breadcrumbs

½ cup pesto

2 eggs, lightly beaten

1 teaspoon salt

One 14.5- to 16-ounce box whole-wheat or whole-grain spaghetti

Grated Parmesan cheese, for serving

**Preheat the oven to 350°F. Grease a 9 x 13-inch rectangular baking dish.**

1. Spread half of the pasta sauce in the bottom of the baking dish and set aside.

2. Bring a large pot of salted water to a boil (covered to speed things up). Turn the faucet on, just a trickle—you'll see why in a minute.

3. Use your (clean) hands to gently combine the turkey, breadcrumbs, pesto, eggs, and salt in a large bowl—don't squish too vigorously or the meatballs will be dense.

4. Moisten your hands (aha! the faucet is already on, no need to get meatball mixture all over the handles), and shape the mixture into about 50 walnut-sized meatballs, using about a tablespoon for each. Arrange them in a single layer in the baking dish as you go. You may need to re-moisten your hands several times during the process. When all the meatballs are formed, wash your hands well with soap and hot water.

5. Spoon the remaining sauce over the meatballs, cover the dish with foil, and bake until the meatballs are cooked through (no longer pink in the center), about 20 minutes.

6.  By now the water is probably boiling. Add the spaghetti and cook according to the package directions.

7.  Serve the spaghetti with the meatballs and sauce, and top with the grated Parmesan.

**NOTE:** These meatballs freeze nicely. Let them cool, then pack them into an airtight container (like a resealable freezer bag) and you're good to go. If you like, freeze single-meal portions in individual packages. Don't stress about including enough sauce for future meals; you can easily augment with jarred. Defrost in the refrigerator for 24 hours, in the microwave, or by simmering, covered, in additional sauce for 20 minutes.

MAKE BABY FOOD: If your family has no food allergies, these meatballs make wonderful finger food—with or without the tomato sauce. If there *are* allergies, speak to your pediatrician before serving, since pesto is made with pine nuts. Cut the spaghetti into small pieces. You can also puree the entire thing with a splash of the pasta cooking water or a little more sauce.

**MAMA SAID**
"My kitchen-challenged husband made this one solo, sans oversight, and it came out perfectly. As easy as making matzoh balls from the Manischewitz mix, he tells me! We ate half and froze the rest for another night." —Beth J., mom of one, Washington, DC

# CHAPTER 9

# GALACTA-WHATS?
# RECIPES TO SUPPORT
# BREASTFEEDING

My breasts and I have a rocky relationship. When I was fat I had quite a pair of bazooms, as my *bubbe* would say, but they didn't get a whole lot of play. And by that I mean: Nobody wanted to play with them. Then I lost 100 pounds, and 85 of them came from my chest. What was left resembled a pair of deflated water balloons, and I obsessed over my sad, floppy bosom to a ridiculous degree. I even considered surgery to give me some of the perk I never had. (My therapist shut down that conversation with a single sentence: "OK, but before you do it, let's talk about why you feel the need to be perfect.") But Stephen loved all of me, and I learned to accept them.

And then came pregnancy. My deflated water balloons were refilling, and fast!

During the second trimester, when I was clearly pregnant but not yet assuming whale proportions, I felt as sexy as I ever have. By the time I gave birth I was absolutely thrilled with the state of my breasts. I had no idea what was in store.

Harry was born at 37 weeks exactly, not early enough to be considered premature, but early enough to have two problems common to near-term babies: jaundice and a poor suck. Later I learned that they're intertwined—my boy was yellow because he wasn't getting enough from my breasts.

The pediatrician kept Harry in the hospital for an extra night. I'm pretty sure that was the worst night of my life—leaving the hospital without my newborn was heart-wrenching enough, but knowing that they would be feeding him formula sent me over the edge. I'd been a bit brainwashed, you see. I'd come to believe that formula would somehow hurt my baby (breast is best!), and that introducing a bottle in the first days would put him off breastfeeding forever. I know: It's a hospital. They wouldn't knowingly do anything to *hurt* my baby. But the postpartum hormones pushed that reassuring thought aside right quick. The hospital sent me home with a flimsy little manual pump and instructions to use it every three hours, both to extract colostrum (the highly concentrated, initial milk that would help Harry get over his jaundice) and to stimulate my milk production. Result: less than a teaspoon of colostrum after four pumping sessions, sore wrists from working the pump, and nipples so raw I was afraid to let Harry anywhere near them.

And so began my seven weeks of breastfeeding hell. I warn you, this story isn't pretty. But it's also *extremely* atypical—please don't assume this might happen to you.

My bazooms were certainly getting play now, though not the kind I had wanted way back in the day! Instead they were receiving attention from a bevy of lactation consultants.

I wound up seeing four of these wonderful women, each one devoted to helping mothers breastfeed their babies, before I finally found the specialist who held the answers for our particular set of problems. The first lactation consultant was new to the job and, apparently, clueless. The second advised bacitracin for my nipples, but didn't offer much help for Harry's latch. LC number three solved my pumping problems (with a hospital-grade pump and the right size breast shields) and determined that I had supply problems as well, but still couldn't fix Harry's issues. Fourth was a phone consult with an MD/LC, who put me on a crazy pumping regimen to increase my supply: 7 to 10 minutes every *hour*. Can you imagine being hooked up to a milking machine for 7 to 10 minutes every hour, on top of caring for a newborn?

At Harry's two-week checkup, his pediatrician was thrilled with my boy's progress but distressed by mine. As she put it, women who have been told to follow regimens that don't let them take care of *themselves* almost always decide to give up on nursing, since the stress and frustration are so great. She suggested I call Freda, the woman who ultimately saved my breasts—and my sanity.

Freda Rosenfeld, IBCLC (International Board Certified Lactation Consultant), is a straight-talking, quirky goddess. With techniques like the Jim Carrey (an exercise for Harry's mouth, which made his tiny face look as rubbery as the comedian's) and full support for formula supplementation (she assured me formula wouldn't kill my kid, and that like breastmilk, formula is *food*), she soon had Harry well-fed, satisfied, and nursing like he'd been doing it all his life—without causing me pain. And for my supply issues, she introduced me to a word, and a world, which would become quite familiar: *galactagogue.*

Galactagogues promote the production and flow of milk. Freda had an impressive arsenal of galactagogues for me to try, some herbal, many of them specific ingredients. For me, a combination of things worked: cups of raspberry leaf and nettle tea plus loads of oatmeal, barley, and almonds. It was a challenge to my sleep-deprived brain, figuring out ways to work barley into my diet (oatmeal and almonds were easy), but I did it.

It took five more weeks, weeks in which I wondered daily why exactly I was putting myself through this, but Freda and her lactogenic ingredients did finally solve my supply issues. I still gave Harry formula occasionally, but it was more about convenience than necessity. By now you've probably realized that as much as I thought I'd be an earth mother—nursing-till-kindergarten, co-sleeping, sling-wearing—none of those things actually worked out. When Harry self-weaned at ten months I was wistful, but relieved. And the day we returned that rental hospital pump I felt like a prisoner wrongly accused and suddenly released.

So now my breasts are fully mine again. We're still not the best of friends (when I look in the mirror, I often sing, "Do your boobs hang low/Do they wobble to and fro . . ."), but they did their job and I'm proud of them. You go, girls!

I realize that my case is a little extreme. If you're reading this and you're currently pregnant with your first, *please* don't be scared—the vast majority of my friends had nothing even close to my particular set of challenges. Most of them managed to get their babies nursing happily before they ever left the hospital. On the other hand, it can't hurt to have expert help lined up, just in case. Ask your mom friends to recommend a lactation consultant or two now. While breastfeeding is completely natural, as everyone says, it isn't always easy—and there's no way to know ahead of time if you'll have trouble. No mom friends to ask? The International Lactation Consultant Association has a searchable database on their website, www.ilca.org.

. . . . . . . . . . . . . . . . . . . . . . . . . . . . . . . . . . . . . . . . . . . . . . . . . . . . . . .

### NUTRITIONAL NEEDS WHILE NURSING

I'm no expert on the dietary needs of a nursing mom. Luckily, I know someone who is: Lara Field, MS, RD, CSP (that's Master of Science, Registered Dietitian, Certified Specialist in Pediatric nutrition), founder of Chicago-based pediatric nutrition counseling center FEED: Forming Early Eating Decisions and author of this book's foreword. Lara was pregnant with her second child while she was reading over the manuscript, so this was all very front-of-mind for her. Here's what she'd tell any new mom who walked in her door:

- Your body needs about 500 more calories a day to support your breastfeeding—a little less if you're overweight (in addition to baby weight) or not physically active.

- A handful of specific nutrients are important in lactation:

  - **PROTEIN:** Your body needs around 70 grams of protein per day. Skim milk is an excellent source, since it also provides calcium, another nutrient nursing moms need. Look for milk or calcium-fortified milk replacements with at least 5 grams of protein per 8 ounces, and try to drink three to four glasses a day.

  - **CALCIUM:** Another reason why skim milk is so terrific for nursing moms. In our lives, there are two times women lose the most calcium: during pregnancy and lactation. The way our bodies are programmed, your baby will get the necessary calcium from your breastmilk—even if it comes from your own bones. If you're nursing, it's critical that you get an adequate supply of at least 1,000 milligrams per day. Good sources are dairy products or alternative dairy products like soy, almond, or hemp milk, or even a calcium supplement; three glasses of milk plus an ounce of cheese will cover you.

  - **VITAMIN C:** Aim for around 65 milligrams per day. You'll find it in citrus fruits, tomatoes, leafy greens, strawberries, kiwi, broccoli, green peppers, and other green and yellow vegetables. For example, one cup of strawberries packs 84 milligrams of vitamin C.

  - **VITAMIN A:** Lactation requires about 1,200 micrograms of vitamin A per day. Munch ½ cup of baby carrots and you're covered and then some—it's got a whopping 3,516 micrograms. Other good sources include kale, spinach, egg yolks, and fortified milk.

  - **VITAMIN E:** The goal here is 9 milligrams per day. Almonds are a spectacular source: 1 ounce, about 23 almonds, has 7.4 milligrams. That plus 1 tablespoon of vegetable oil over the course of the day, and you're there.

- Continue taking your prenatal multivitamin, as well as an omega-3 DHA supplement, which is essential for your baby's brain and eye development.

- Moms need fluids to ensure an adequate supply of milk. This is one of the main reasons supply diminishes—be sure to drink at least eight 8-ounce glasses per day. Make it fun; try sparkling water with a splash of juice (which is lower in calories than straight juice). Lord knows you're not getting much champagne while nursing!

- Experts say moms should continue nursing up to 12 months, or until it's no longer mutually beneficial to mom and baby. And by that they mean, if it starts interfering with your little one's normal growth and development, stop! Lara told me she's seen many children who continue to nurse well after their first birthday, and sometimes it affects their solid food consumption. They nurse so much they don't leave room for other foods, which can slow advancement. Obviously this doesn't happen with every baby, but you do want to make sure your child is learning to eat a balanced diet.

### LOOKING FOR EVEN MORE LACTOGENIC FOOD?

Check out these recipes from other chapters in the book:

**The New Mom's Pantry:**
- Mushroom Barley Soup
- Lentil and Brown Rice Soup

**Nap-Friendly Cooking:**
- Roasted Vegetable Beef Barley Soup
- Indian Spiced Black Lentil Stew

**Quick Suppers:**
- Black Bean, Corn, and Tomato Salad

**The Slow Cooker:**
- Overnight Steel-Cut Oatmeal
- Moroccan Red Lentil Stew

**Big Batch Cooking:**
- Chicken Tagine with Almonds and Apricots

**One-Handed Meals:**
- Curried Kale and Apple Empanadas
- Greek Rice Balls
- Sicilian Spinach Envelopes

**Lunchtime Pumping and Last-Minute Dinners:**
- Lauren's Carrot Soup
- Any recipe using canned beans

**Nutritious Nibbles:**
- Blueberry Oatmeal Bars
- Quickie Hummus
- Curry Roasted Chickpeas

**Easy Indulgences:**
- Jammy Oatmeal Shortbread Bars

## A CONVERSATION WITH FREDA ROSENFELD, IBCLC

As I mentioned in the introduction to this chapter, Freda Rosenfeld is my hero. She's the LC who finally fixed my nursing problems. Freda has helped thousands of new moms over the years. In a profile in the *New York Times*, she was described as "part medical professional, part therapist, and part sleuth." Precisely.

When I was working with Freda, understanding the science of breastfeeding wasn't exactly at the top of my list. But to write about galactagogues I needed to know how our bodies make milk, so I turned to my expert for help.

**Me:** Let's talk first about overall nutrition and breastfeeding.

**Freda:** There's a lot of clear evidence that people can almost starve themselves to death and they'll still have milk for their babies. We know from studies in Africa that with women who are in dire starvation situations, their nursed babies often do way better than their other children, because breastmilk is just one of these amazing things that can transcend nutrition.

But that said, what you eat can make a difference in improving your own health. Those women in Africa probably had horrible bones and other medical issues. So even though technically we would say what you eat has minimal impact on milk production, it has huge impact on the mother herself and her health, which means of course, taking care of herself and her family. For women who struggle there's clear evidence that eating healthier can make a difference.

**Me:** How does what we eat affect the baby?

**Freda:** That's a very difficult question to answer. In theory we tell people to eat everything, and we know from studies that the more varied your diet is as nursing mom, the better your child will be as an eater, because your milk picks up subtle tastes and hints of the other food. But the reality is some kids have delicate digestive systems and some foods bother them.

A general rule of thumb is, what you ate four to eight hours ago can wind up in your milk. So when we play detective, we look at what you had the meal before, combined with consistency. If you have a chocolate cookie and the baby is gassy and then the next day you have a chocolate cookie and the baby isn't gassy, obviously the cookie would not be the issue.

But I do have a few things moms should avoid. I break people's hearts every day when I tell them they can't drink juice. It concentrates the acidity of the fruit, and that acidity is passed into the milk and gives babies tummy aches. It's also a waste of calories for the mother.

Moms should also avoid any family-known allergens. Right now I'm working with a mother whose husband is highly allergic to shrimp, so I told her not to have shrimp.

Aside from that, if babies display discomfort, then we would start looking through foods that can be bothering them. There are some foods that tend to be more allergic than others, like dairy. It's the most common food sensitivity and allergen in the world. So, if your baby's very gassy or is having mucusy bowel movements or is having infant acne with digestive discomfort, there's a good chance your baby is sensitive to dairy. I'll take that mom off dairy and see if the baby's discomfort goes away.

**Me:** Now let's talk about specific foods that can help with supply. Oatmeal is a biggie. It helped me.

**Freda:** I cannot find any research to support it, and yet it's in many cultures. But the bottom line is oatmeal is a very, very, very strong source of B vitamins, which helps increase supply.

In fact, any whole grain is higher in B vitamins than white bread is. So when a nursing mom chooses to have more whole grains, she's going to get more B vitamins, which should help.

Also people who take brewer's yeast find an increase in milk production. What's so fantastic about brewer's yeast? It's got a lot of B vitamins in it. And beer is a variation of brewer's yeast. Brewer's yeast and beer really do work.

**Me:** What about alcohol? Is it OK for a nursing mom to drink beer?

**Freda:** That's one of my favorite questions, because it's not so black and white. Let's start with the bad. I've seen fetal alcohol syndrome. It's a very sad, depressing thing, but it's really rare. One not-quite-full glass of wine or half a beer each day has really not been proven to be dangerous to babies, but more than that is.

So once you drink more than that one glass of wine, that half to one glass of beer, you really need to pump and dump.

**Me:** So let's say you're having one glass of wine or beer a day, does the baby get any of that?

**Freda:** So very minimal. It's not like you drink it and it goes right to your breastmilk—and the same thing for medications that people take. It first goes into your blood system and you utilize it. And *then* it goes to your milk, takes four to six hours to get there, and by then most of the alcohol has worn out. It's the same as when we tell moms to take pain medication because they had a C-section. By the time it gets to your milk, the baby's getting a minute quantity.

**Me:** You had me on a tea of raspberry leaf and nettles.

**Freda:** That's right. That tea really helps. The herbalist Susun Weed has a book called *Wise Woman Herbal for the Childbearing Years,* and she highly recommends raspberry and nettles. Now, the raspberry leaf is a leaf tea, not the raspberries themselves. But nettles are a plant that grows, so cooking with nettles can help too.

**Me:** Any other foods that help with supply and breastfeeding in general?

**Freda:** I'm surprised you didn't ask about almonds! I again cannot find a single research article, though I've not searched high and low. I'm not exaggerating to tell you I've had clients from literally all over the world, from Africa, from South America, from Tahiti, from Alaska, grandmothers the world over say to eat almonds. I'm sorry, that's just too much of a coincidence for me!

**Me:** What if your problem is oversupply? Are there foods to help reduce the amount of milk a woman produces?

**Freda:** Sage tea. Sage can slow your milk for sure.

**Me:** Would cooking with sage do that?

**Freda:** No, you'd have to eat large, large quantities.

**Me:** What's the one piece of general advice you give to moms for the first year?

**Freda:** I'm obsessive about family meals and how eating healthy now will have an impact on your child. At least once a day when she's old enough, she should be in her high chair at the table, where she'll see her parents eat. She'll learn what eating is all about, and because you don't want your kid to see you eating junk, you'll eat healthier yourself. Long-term studies show that families who eat meals together have significantly lower rates of drug use, poor school performance, and bully behavior in school. I can't stress enough how important this is.

### CRIB NOTES

- While you're nursing, you need 500 extra calories a day, max. See the sidebar on page 289 for specific nutritional advice from Lara Field, MS, RD, CSP.

- The list of lactogenic foods, for the most part, is based on ancient wisdom rather than scientific research. These are foods that new mothers have been eating for thousands of years to support their nursing: almonds, barley, beer, blackstrap molasses, buckwheat, dried fruit (apricots, dates, and figs especially), fennel, ginger, greens, honey, legumes, nutritional yeast, seeds, and whole grains (especially oats).

- Different ingredients work for different women, so if you don't see results from, say, oatmeal, try some barley recipes instead.

- The headnote to each recipe in this chapter will tell you which of its ingredients are lactogenic. Those that contain more than one or two are specifically intended to increase your supply. If you're *not* looking to boost supply, eat those dishes less frequently—a couple times a week won't hurt, but I wouldn't go daily. The rest of the recipes support breastfeeding in general, with special focus on the nutritional needs of a nursing mother.

- For even more information on galactagogues and lactogenic foods, read *Mother Food: A Breastfeeding Diet Guide with Lactogenic Foods and Herbs* by Hilary Jacobson.

# BARLEY WITH BUTTERNUT SQUASH AND FENNEL, THREE WAYS

Don't you just love a recipe that can be used in three different ways? *And* help with your milk supply? The basic recipe here gives you a lovely side dish to serve with roast chicken or beef, and the following two transform it into a pair of one-dish meals.

Barley and fennel are both considered lactogenic.

## BARLEY PILAF WITH BUTTERNUT AND FENNEL
**Serves 6 as a side dish**
**Cooking time: 1½ hours (20 to 30 minutes active)**

2 tablespoons olive oil

1 large onion, halved lengthwise and very thinly sliced

1 fennel bulb, stalks and tough core trimmed and discarded, halved lengthwise and very thinly sliced

Salt

Half of a medium-large butternut squash, peeled and chopped into ¼-inch pieces
*It's perfectly fine to buy the pre-cut kind, and just chop it down into smaller pieces.*

1 cup pearl barley, rinsed

3 cups low-sodium vegetable or chicken broth, water, or a combination

2 teaspoons rosemary, finely chopped

1. Heat the olive oil in a very large skillet over medium heat. When it shimmers, add the onion and fennel, season with salt to taste, and reduce heat to medium-low. (You barely want to hear a sizzle—the idea here is to let the vegetables cook slowly and gently.) Cook, stirring occasionally, until the vegetables are quite soft and beginning to turn golden, about 20 minutes, then stir in the squash and a little more salt. Cook, stirring occasionally, until the squash is just barely tender, 10 to 15 minutes.

2. Add the barley and cook 1 to 2 minutes, then add the liquid and the rosemary. Bring to a boil, then reduce heat and simmer, covered and undisturbed, 30 to 40 minutes. If barley is tender but a considerable amount of liquid remains, prop the lid ajar and cook until it's mostly evaporated—you're looking for a consistency just a bit dryer than risotto. Taste and adjust seasoning.

## BUTTERNUT BARLEY CASSEROLE

**Serves 4**

**Cooking time: 2 hours (30 to 40 minutes active)**
**To the Barley Pilaf with Butternut and Fennel recipe (page 294), add:**

¾ cup to 1 cup shredded Gruyère cheese
   (feel free to use more or less, depending on how much you like cheese)

**Preheat oven to 350°F. Grease a 9 x 13-inch baking dish and set aside.**

1. Follow the instructions for the barley pilaf, but instead of cooking the pilaf until all the liquid has evaporated, remove from heat when the barley is just tender but still has some bite. Pour the mixture into the prepared baking dish and if you're a real cheese lover, mix in some of the Gruyère. If you're not, skip that step and just sprinkle the cheese on top.

2. Bake until cheese is bubbling and lightly browned, 20 to 30 minutes.

## BARLEY SOUP WITH BUTTERNUT SQUASH AND FENNEL

**Serves 6**

**Cooking time: 1½ hours (20 to 30 minutes active)**

Follow the Barley Pilaf with Butternut and Fennel recipe (page 294), but add an additional quart of liquid. If you like, top each bowl with a little shredded Gruyère.

MAKE BABY FOOD: All three versions are A-OK for babies. You can puree them with a little broth or water, or serve as finger food.

**MAMA SAID**
"I added a little bit of Parmesan (because I had it, not Gruyère), and the plan was to have a little for lunch and the rest for dinner tomorrow night, but it was so good I ate most of it. So now I need to sneak out and buy more fennel and stuff for a new batch for tomorrow. I'm really impressed with this one because it's so different from anything I've cooked before and it feels so healthy and fresh." —Nicky A., mom of one, Melbourne, Australia

# BARLEY AND WHITE BEAN SOUP WITH ESCAROLE

**Serves 6**

**Cooking time: 1 hour (20 to 30 minutes active)**

I first made this soup long before Harry was born, and when it's gray and rainy outside, it's as soothing to me as my favorite slippers. The fact that it'll help with your milk production is just lucky coincidence. The leftovers will thicken considerably, to the point where you might call it a stew rather than a soup. Just add a little broth or hot water when reheating.

Barley, beans, and greens are all considered lactogenic.

Two 14- to 15-ounce cans no-salt-added
  white beans
  *It's important to use a variety with a low
  sodium content, since you'll be using some of
  the canning liquid.*

2 tablespoons olive oil

2 ounces pancetta, bacon, or turkey bacon,
  finely chopped

1 medium onion, chopped small

2 garlic cloves, minced

1 medium carrot, chopped small

1 celery rib, chopped small

1 fresh thyme sprig

1 fresh marjoram sprig

1 cup pearl barley, rinsed

One 14.5-ounce can diced tomatoes, with
  juice

Pinch of nutmeg

One 2-inch Parmesan rind, optional

4 cups low-sodium chicken or vegetable
  broth

2 cups chopped escarole leaves

Salt and pepper

Grated Parmesan cheese, good-quality
  extra-virgin olive oil, and crusty bread, for
  serving

1.  Puree 1 can of beans with its liquid in a food processor or blender, or mash in a bowl with a potato masher. Drain and rinse the other can. Set both aside.

2.  Heat the olive oil in a large, heavy pot over medium heat. When it shimmers, add the pancetta and cook until it releases some of its fat and starts to brown, 2 to 3 minutes. Add the onion and cook until translucent, 4 to 5 minutes. Add the garlic, carrot, celery, thyme, and marjoram; cook until the vegetables begin to soften, 6 to 8 minutes.

3.  Stir in the barley, tomatoes with their juice, nutmeg, reserved bean puree, and whole beans, Parmesan rind, if using, and broth. Bring to a boil, reduce the heat,

and simmer, stirring occasionally, 15 minutes. Add the escarole and salt and pepper to taste. Cook 15 to 20 minutes more. Test the barley for doneness—it should be softened but still have some texture. Remove pot from the heat and discard the herb stems.

4. Serve with grated Parmesan, and if you're feeling decadent, add a drizzle of really good extra-virgin olive oil. Use crusty bread to scoop out every last drop of soup.

MAKE BABY FOOD: Everything becomes such a lovely, soft texture in this soup. It's perfect for babies—either pureed or as finger food. If you don't puree, be careful with the escarole: too-large strips can be difficult for a new eater to chew, so make sure it's cut into small pieces.

**MAMA SAID**
**"We both really enjoyed this recipe. I'm a big fan of one dish that covers all our bases (protein, grain, vegetables). Overall the recipe was really great to make. I appreciated that I could basically throw everything in the pot and just check it every few minutes, stir, and continue playing with the baby, set the table, or whatever." —Monica W., mom of one, St. Louis, MO**

# BEEF, BEER, AND BARLEY STEW

**Serves 6 to 8**

**Cooking time: 2½ hours (30 minutes active)**

I don't like beer. I trace this aversion back to seventh grade, when my friend Emily's parents went away and her siblings threw a party. Emily's older sister bought Budweiser tallboys for everyone. You can imagine how that turned out.

Anyway, when I was having supply problems, everyone told me to just drink beer, as if it was the easiest (and most pleasant) thing in the world. As much as I love Harry, I just couldn't bring myself to do it. So instead, I worked it into this seductive beef stew. And for good measure, I threw in a few other foods that help supply: In addition to the beer, fennel, barley, and dates are all considered to be lactogenic.

1 tablespoon olive oil

1½ pounds beef stew meat, trimmed of as much fat as possible

Salt and pepper

1 cup pearl onions (frozen is fine)
*If you're a bit of a masochist use fresh pearl onions: Dunk them in boiling water to loosen the skins, then peel and proceed with the recipe.*

3 large carrots, chopped into 1-inch pieces

2 celery ribs, chopped into 1-inch pieces

1 fennel bulb, fronds trimmed, halved lengthwise and thinly sliced

2 bay leaves

2 fresh thyme sprigs

2 tablespoons tomato paste

1 cup pearl barley, rinsed

2 tablespoons balsamic vinegar

3 cups low-sodium beef broth

3 cups water

One 12-ounce bottle dark beer, such as stout

¼ cup chopped pitted dates

**Preheat oven to 325°F.**

1. Heat the oil in a large oven-safe pot or Dutch oven over medium-high heat. Pat the beef dry and season liberally with salt and pepper. When the oil shimmers, add the beef and brown on all sides, 8 to 10 minutes. Don't crowd the pot—you may need to do this in two batches. Transfer the browned beef to a clean bowl.

2. Add the onions, carrots, celery, fennel, bay leaves, and thyme sprigs to the pot. Reduce heat to low, cover, and cook, stirring occasionally, until the vegetables begin to soften, 8 to 10 minutes.

3. Stir in the tomato paste and barley and cook 1 to 2 minutes. Add the remaining ingredients, raise heat to high, and bring to a boil. When it boils, cover the pot, remove from heat, and put it in the oven.

4. Cook until the meat is fork-tender, 1½ to 2 hours. Season with salt and pepper to taste.

> MAKE BABY FOOD: The texture of this stew is wonderful for babies, either pureed with a bit of the liquid or as finger food. It's got a bottle of beer in it, yes. But it also cooks for a good long time, so approximately 90 percent of the alcohol will evaporate. Which means you're left with 10 percent of the alcohol from a single bottle of beer, divided between 6 to 8 servings. I served this to Harry with no reservations, but please take the small amount of alcohol into account before serving it to your own baby.

**MAMA SAID**
**"It was great! The flavors really blended well together (I've never made stew with dates!). I'm going to put it in a blender for my son's lunch tomorrow. Also, I think I should get extra credit for the type of beer I used: Mother's Milk. An excellent stout." —Pamela R., mom of one, Brooklyn, NY**

• • • • • • • • • • • • • • • • • • • • • • • • • • • • • • • • • • • • • • • • • • • •

# FRUIT-INFUSED BARLEY WATER, THREE WAYS

**Each recipe makes 4 to 5 cups**
**Cooking time: 2¾ hours (10 minutes active)**

Barley water has been used as a galactagogue since the days of the ancient Greeks. Nobody knows why, but simply drinking the starchy water used to simmer barley works wonders to boost supply—several of my mom-testers reported significant gains in pumping output after just a few glasses. But plain barley water isn't the most delicious thing you'll ever drink, so I added fruit and flavorings to make it something to look forward to. Serve it mixed with sparkling water or seltzer, over ice, and it'll almost feel like a cocktail.

Barley and ginger are both considered lactogenic.

### STRAWBERRY-GINGER BARLEY WATER

½ cup pearl barley, rinsed

One ¼-inch slice fresh ginger

2 cups strawberries (frozen is fine)

Sugar or honey to taste

1. Combine the barley and ginger in a large saucepan and add 8 cups of water. Bring to a boil over high heat, then reduce heat to low and gently simmer, uncovered, 30 minutes.

2. Add the strawberries and simmer 5 minutes more. Remove from heat and mash with a potato masher to break down the strawberries.

3. Strain the mixture into a pitcher. Add sugar or honey to taste—start with just a little, and add more if it needs it. Stir well. Discard the solids.

4. Refrigerate until cold and drink within a few days. Stir before serving.

## APPLE-CINNAMON BARLEY WATER

½ cup pearl barley, rinsed

1 cinnamon stick, or ½ teaspoon ground
  cinnamon

1 cup no-added-sugar applesauce

Maple syrup, to taste

1. Combine the barley and cinnamon in a large saucepan and add 8 cups of water. Bring to a boil over high heat, then reduce the heat to low and gently simmer, uncovered, 30 minutes.

2. Put the applesauce into a pitcher. Remove the pan from the heat and strain the mixture into the pitcher. Add maple syrup to taste—start with just a little, and add more if it needs it. Stir well.

**NOTE:** Reserve the solids for Cinnamon and Brown Sugar Barley Pudding, page 302.

3. Drink by the mugful while hot, or refrigerate until cold and drink within a few days. Stir before serving.

## MANGO-LIME BARLEY WATER

1 lime

½ cup pearl barley, rinsed

2 cups mango chunks (frozen is fine, just
  thaw it first)

Honey or sugar to taste

1. Wash the lime well and use a vegetable peeler to remove a 2-inch strip of rind, green part only. Combine the rind and the barley in a large saucepan and add 8 cups of water. Bring to a boil over high heat, then reduce heat to low and gently simmer, uncovered, 30 minutes.

2. Juice the lime and pour juice into a blender or food processor. Add the mango and puree it, then transfer to a pitcher. If you'd rather not have any solids at all in your drink, pass it through a strainer first.

3. Strain the barley mixture into the pitcher. Add honey to taste—start with just a little, and add more if it needs it. Stir well. Discard the solids.

4. Refrigerate until cold and drink within a few days. Stir before serving.

MAKE BABY FOOD: Due to botulism concerns, babies under one year can't have honey—but babies don't really need added sugars anyway. If you'd like to share this with your baby, reserve some of the mixture before stirring in the sweetener.

**MAMA SAID**
**"The fruit-infused barley water worked great for me. My right side was lagging in production, but after I drank the barley water for two days I pumped 5 ounces out of that side in one sitting. It also tasted really good, especially the strawberry one!" —Jenn S., mom of two, Brooklyn, NY**

# CINNAMON AND BROWN SUGAR BARLEY PUDDING

**Serves 4**

**Cooking time: 2 hours 35 minutes (35 minutes active)**

Barley's inexpensive, but it still didn't thrill me to throw away the solids from my Fruit-Infused Barley Water. Here's a great way to use the leftovers from the Apple-Cinnamon recipe.

2 cups cooked pearl barley, left over from Apple-Cinnamon Barley Water (page 301)

1 cinnamon stick (it's fine to re-use the one from the barley water) or ½ teaspoon ground cinnamon

2 cups milk, any kind

⅓ to ½ cup light brown sugar, depending on your sweet tooth

1.  Put the barley into a large saucepan—if you just finished making barley water, put it right back into the same pan, no need to rinse.

2.  Add the remaining ingredients. Cook over medium-low heat, stirring frequently, until it starts to boil. Reduce heat to low and simmer very gently, stirring frequently, until almost all the milk has been absorbed, 25 to 30 minutes.

3.  Discard the cinnamon stick, and either serve warm or pour the barley into 4 ramekins or 1 serving bowl, cover with plastic wrap, and refrigerate until cold.

MAKE BABY FOOD: The pudding is safe for babies (pureed if you like), but given the added sugar I'd reserve it for special occasions.

**MAMA SAID**

"The pudding was a big hit! My preschooler didn't like the barley water, so I figured she wouldn't want the pudding. I didn't get a bowl for her . . . and she ate all of mine!"
—Heather B., mom of two, Westmont, IL

• • • • • • • • • • • • • • • • • • • • • • • • • • • • • • • • • • • • • • •

# WHOLE-GRAIN PASTA WITH GREENS AND BEANS

**Serves 4**

**Cooking time: 30 minutes**

Whole grains, greens, and beans are all considered lactogenic foods. This comforting dish uses all three, and it has the added benefit of being ready in just about half an hour.

2 tablespoons olive oil

5 garlic cloves, finely chopped

2 bunches kale or chard, or 2 medium heads escarole, roughly chopped, washed, and drained (leave some water clinging to the leaves)

Salt and pepper

Pinch of red pepper flakes, or to taste

One 12- to 14.5-ounce box whole-wheat or whole-grain pasta, like penne

One 14- to 15-ounce can no-salt-added white beans, drained, ½ cup of the liquid reserved *It's important to use no-salt-added beans here, since you'll be using some of the canning liquid.*

Grated Parmesan cheese, for serving

1.  Bring a large pot of salted water to a boil (covered to speed things up).

2.  Meanwhile, heat the olive oil in a very large skillet over medium heat. When it shimmers, add the garlic and cook until fragrant, about 30 seconds. Add the greens by the handful, stirring and adding more as they wilt, until they're all in. Stir in salt, pepper, and red pepper flakes to taste. Reduce the heat and simmer, covered, while the water comes to a boil.

3.  Cook the pasta according to package directions. About 5 minutes before the pasta is done cooking, stir in the drained beans—not the liquid—to the greens. Simmer, covered, while the pasta finishes cooking.

4. When the pasta's ready, drain it and add to the skillet (if it's not big enough to hold everything, return the pasta to the big pot and add the greens and bean mixture). Toss to combine, adding some of the bean liquid if the mixture looks dry.

5. Serve with grated Parmesan cheese.

MAKE BABY FOOD: Skip the red pepper flakes, which will upset most babies who find one on their tongues (if your baby's OK with heat, use a dash of hot sauce instead), cut the cooked escarole into smaller pieces, and you're good to go. If you're on purees, add a little more of the bean liquid before you whir.

**MAMA SAID**
**"Super easy, delicious, and made with all things I usually have on hand. The combination of greens (I used kale), garlic, and red pepper flakes is something I literally would have eaten out of the pan on its own. Also a great and easy lunch from the leftovers." —Alana D., mom of one, Narragansett, RI**

# CURRIED LENTIL SOUP

**Serves 8 to 10**

**Cooking time: 1 hour 10 minutes (15 to 20 minutes active)**

If I were Rachael Ray, I'd call this a "stoup": in terms of thickness, it falls somewhere between a soup and a stew, and as it sits it becomes even more stew-like. If you'd like it to be a straight-on soup, add another 2 cups of liquid. For a stew, use 1 cup less than the recipe calls for.

Both lentils and greens are considered lactogenic foods.

2 tablespoons olive oil

1 large onion, chopped

3 garlic cloves, finely chopped

2 large carrots, chopped

1 sweet potato, peeled and chopped

2 tablespoons curry powder

1 teaspoon grand cumin

¼ to ½ teaspoon cayenne, or to taste

1 bay leaf

One 28-ounce can crushed tomatoes

6 cups low-sodium chicken or vegetable broth

1 pound brown lentils, sorted, rinsed, and drained

4 cups chopped greens (spinach, chard, and kale all work nicely), or 2 cups frozen chopped spinach

Salt

Plain yogurt and chopped cilantro, optional, for serving

1. Heat the oil in a large, heavy pot or Dutch oven over medium heat. When it shimmers, add the onion, garlic, carrots, and sweet potato, and cook, stirring occasionally, until the vegetables begin to soften, 5 to 8 minutes.

2. Stir in the curry powder, cumin, cayenne, and bay leaf, and cook until fragrant, 30 seconds to 1 minute. Add the tomatoes, broth, and lentils and bring to a boil. Reduce heat and simmer, covered, until the lentils are almost tender, about 40 minutes. Stir in the chopped greens and cook, covered, until lentils are fully tender, 5 to 10 minutes more.

*If your lentils were sitting in your cabinet—or on a store shelf—for a while, it may take 15 or 20 minutes longer for them to become tender.*

3. Season to taste with salt. Remove the bay leaf, and serve with plain yogurt and cilantro.

MAKE BABY FOOD: No problems here, as long as your baby likes spice. You can puree or serve the solids as finger food.

MAMA SAID

"Response: Three very happy people—four, actually, because the baby ate some of the carrots and sweet potatoes mashed up and clamored for more. And she's a very new eater, with only a handful of foods in her repertoire. One closed-mouth protester, but he's basically on hunger strike these days. The flavor was really rich, and I was surprised at how mellow it turned out to be after how fragrant and heady the sauce was." —Christy W., mom of three, Austin, TX

# SOBA NOODLE SALAD WITH TAHINI-LIME DRESSING

**Serves 4**

**Cooking time: 30 minutes (15 to 20 minutes active)**

Soba noodles are kind of like Japanese spaghetti, made from buckwheat flour. If you can't find them in the Asian foods section of your supermarket, try a natural foods store—any type of buckwheat noodle will work here. With the protein from the edamame, this is a complete, light meal. Several of my mom-testers added shredded cooked chicken to the salad, and others served it with store-bought sushi for a more substantial dinner.

Both buckwheat, the main ingredient in soba noodles, and sesame seeds, the main ingredient in tahini, are considered lactogenic.

1 large carrot, peeled and shaved into thin strips with a vegetable peeler

1 red bell pepper, thinly sliced and cut into 2-inch strips

Half a large cucumber, peeled, halved lengthwise, seeded, and shaved into thin strips with a vegetable peeler

2 scallions (whites and pale green parts), thinly sliced

1 cup grape tomatoes, halved

½ cup shelled edamame, thawed if frozen

8 ounces soba noodles

2 tablespoons tahini

1½ tablespoons reduced-sodium soy sauce

Juice of 1 lime (about 2 tablespoons)

1 tablespoon vegetable oil

2 tablespoons water

2 tablespoons chopped fresh mint leaves

1. Bring a large pot of unsalted water to a boil (covered to speed things up).

2. Meanwhile, prep all the vegetables and put them in a large salad bowl.

3. Cook the noodles according to package directions, and drain. Rinse the noodles with cold water and drain again. Add to the bowl of vegetables.

4. Combine the remaining ingredients in a small airtight container. Seal and shake well. Adjust the seasoning to taste—you may need a touch more lime juice or soy sauce. Add it to the bowl and toss to combine.

5. Serve at room temperature.

MAKE BABY FOOD: In terms of ingredients this is perfectly safe for babies. Raw vegetables can be challenging for early eaters, though, so take care when feeding this to yours. You know better than I what your child can handle, so consider each element individually before serving it. You may want to start with just the dressed noodles, cut up into small pieces, along with a handful of gently smashed edamame. For a puree, try noodles, edamame, and dressing.

**MAMA SAID**
"I really liked this dish, it made for great lunches this week. I can definitely see making up a batch to keep in the fridge and eat from one-handed during the fourth trimester—especially since the veggie chopping can be done at a different point than the other things, so it's easy to prepare in stages. I made it originally for dinner and served it with grilled salmon that I hit with salt and pepper and lime, and it made for a great meal—very satisfying flavors."
—Alana D., mom of one, Narragansett, RI

# BLUEBERRY BUCKWHEAT PANCAKES

**Makes about 24 pancakes**

**Cooking time: 30 to 45 minutes**

The first time I cooked these, Stephen proclaimed them the best pancakes I've ever made. Not bad, eh? They cook up quite thin, somewhere between a pancake and a crêpe—if you prefer a more substantial pancake, use a little less buttermilk. You'll get fewer pancakes, but they'll have a nice heft.

Buckwheat is considered a lactogenic food.

½ cup buckwheat flour

½ cup all-purpose flour

2 teaspoons baking powder

2 tablespoons sugar

½ teaspoon salt

4 tablespoons (½ stick) unsalted butter, melted

2 large eggs

1 cup buttermilk

*I use buttermilk powder, which you'll find in larger supermarkets. It stays fresh in the fridge for months. You can also make soured milk, which works just fine: Put 1 tablespoon white vinegar or lemon juice in a measuring cup, and add enough milk to make 1 cup. Let sit 10 to 15 minutes, until it curdles, then use in place of buttermilk.*

1½ cups fresh or frozen blueberries

Butter, for cooking

Pure maple syrup, for serving

1.  Combine the flours, baking powder, sugar, and salt in a small bowl.

2.  Whisk together the melted butter, eggs, and buttermilk in a large bowl. (If you're using buttermilk powder, add it to the dry ingredients and substitute 1 cup of water here.)

3.  Add the flour mixture to the butter mixture, and whisk until well combined. Let the batter stand for 5 minutes, then gently stir in the blueberries.

4.  Melt some butter on a griddle or skillet over medium heat. When it foams, spoon, ladle, or pour out the batter into 3-inch pancakes. Cook until small holes form and the batter begins to look dry, 2 to 3 minutes, then flip and cook 2 to 3 minutes more.

5.  Transfer cooked pancakes to a plate and keep in the oven (set to "warm") while you cook the rest.

6.  Serve with maple syrup.

MAKE BABY FOOD: Babies love pancakes. There's a relatively small amount of added sugar here, but if you're at all concerned feel free to use even less.

**MAMA SAID**
**"Delicious. Instead of buttermilk I did the trick with white vinegar and milk. And I froze the leftovers (separated with freezer paper) for mornings when we have to rush." —Meaghan G., mom of one, Ottawa, ON**

• • • • • • • • • • • • • • • • • • • • • • • • • • • • • • • • • • • • • • • • • • • • • •

# ALMOND-BUCKWHEAT BISCUITS

**Makes about 30 cookies**
**Cooking time: 40 minutes (20 minutes active)**

Delicate, subtle, and crumbly, this is a cookie unlike anything you've tasted before. I adapted this recipe from one by Melissa Clark, a food columnist for the *New York Times*. The buckwheat flour gives the cookies a sandy, almost gritty texture that I really like. The butter flavor shines through, and the almonds play an understated supporting role. On first bite, you may shrug and think they're no big deal. And then you'll find yourself sneaking back into the kitchen for just one more . . . Seriously, the first time I made these, I had to pack them up and distribute among my neighbors to avoid eating every last one.

As for their galactagoguish attributes, both buckwheat and almonds can help with supply.

⅓ cup blanched almonds (slivered, whole, sliced—all will work)
⅔ cup sugar, divided
1 cup buckwheat flour
⅔ cup all-purpose flour
½ teaspoon salt
½ teaspoon baking powder
1 cup (2 sticks) cold unsalted butter, cut into pieces
2 large egg yolks, beaten

**Preheat oven to 325°F, and set the racks in the upper and lower thirds of the oven. Grease or line two baking sheets.**

1. Combine the almonds and ⅓ cup sugar in a food processor. Pulse once or twice, then process until the almonds are the texture of sand. Add the remaining sugar

and the rest of the dry ingredients, and pulse a few times to mix. Add the butter, and pulse 15 to 20 times, until you see pea-sized pieces. Add the egg yolks and pulse 10 to 12 times more, or until the dough just comes together. Transfer the dough to a medium bowl, and stir gently with a spatula until all the flour is absorbed. The dough will be crumbly.

2. Working with 1 tablespoon of dough at a time, shape dough into balls with your hands or a large cookie scoop, and arrange the balls 1½ inches apart on the prepared baking sheets. Make a criss-cross pattern with a fork to flatten a bit. (No need to go too nuts with this—it's mostly for cosmetic purposes.)

3. Bake the biscuits until golden around the edges, 15 to 20 minutes. Cool on the sheets for 2 to 3 minutes before removing to cool completely on a wire rack.

MAKE BABY FOOD: If there are no nut allergies in your immediate family, technically these are fine for babies. But I have two concerns: The added sugar, and the texture of the baked cookie. They're quite dry and crumbly, and may give a baby trouble.

**MAMA SAID**
"You are right about the buckwheat biscuits—don't seem like much, but addictive. My husband rarely eats sweets and the first words out of his mouth were, 'You baked up a batch of crack in there!' as he grabbed another cookie. So crumbly and fine. And so nice to have a lactation cookie that's not oatmeal-laden, like every other one I've tried. These are helping me sail through the feeding aspect of the six-month growth spurt with ease. If only the sleeping part went so easily!" —Heather B., mom of two, Westmont, IL

# BUCKWHEAT CARROT MUFFINS

**Makes 24 full-sized or 48 mini-muffins**

**Cooking time: 45 minutes (20 minutes active)**

I'm not gonna lie: These are health-bomb-type muffins. Definitely not decadent. And they're not especially pretty, either. But the buckwheat brings a subtle nuttiness, and the applesauce and raisins keep things sweet without much added sugar. This recipe makes a whole bunch, so throw a bagful in the freezer and you'll have an easy on-the-go breakfast whenever you need it.

Oh, and they're vegan too. See, I told you they were healthy.

Buckwheat and flaxseeds are considered to be lactogenic.

2½ cups buckwheat flour

½ cup all-purpose flour

¼ cup ground flaxseeds

2 teaspoons baking powder

1 teaspoon baking soda

½ teaspoon salt

2 teaspoons cinnamon

1 teaspoon ground ginger

½ teaspoon ground cloves, optional

2 cups no-sugar-added applesauce

½ cup brown sugar (dark or light)

¼ cup vegetable oil

2 teaspoons vanilla extract

1½ cups grated carrots (about 2 large carrots)

½ cup raisins

**Preheat oven to 375°F. Grease or line enough muffin tins to make 24 full-sized or 48 mini-muffins.**

1. Whisk together the buckwheat flour, all-purpose flour, ground flaxseeds, baking powder, baking soda, salt, and spices in a medium bowl.

2. Stir together the applesauce, sugar, oil, vanilla, carrots, and raisins in a large bowl with a wooden spoon or spatula. Pour the dry ingredients into the wet and gently mix together, until just combined.

3. Spoon the batter into the prepared muffin tins, filling each to the top. Bake mini-muffins for 15 minutes, and full-sized ones for 25 minutes.

4. Flip the muffins out of the tins and cool on a wire rack.

MAKE BABY FOOD: Half a cup of added sugar divided among 24 big muffins is 1 teaspoon per—and a mini-muffin's only got ½ teaspoon. There's nothing here a baby can't have, so if you're OK with a bit of sugar these can be a very healthy introduction to baked goods.

**MAMA SAID**

"I made your muffins last night. They were delicious. I love super-healthy muffins like these—they are the perfect snack for me to take to work. I had one this morning with a cup of 'nursing support' tea. I think next time I will add chunks of apple to the recipe." —Pamela R., mom of one, Brooklyn, NY

# SESAME-GINGER SHORTBREAD

**Makes 24 cookies**

**Cooking time: 35 to 40 minutes (10 to 15 minutes active)**

I think of these cookies as a stealth galactagogue—you'll want to eat them because they taste so good, and the nursing benefits will just be a pleasant bonus. They're the perfect accompaniment to a nice hot cup of tea.

Sesame seeds, the main ingredient in tahini, are considered lactogenic, as is ginger.

3 cups all-purpose flour

1 tablespoon ground ginger
*If you like things gingery, feel free to add another teaspoon or two.*

12 tablespoons (1½ sticks) unsalted butter, softened

⅔ cup tahini

⅔ cup sugar

2 tablespoons sesame seeds

**Preheat oven to 325°F. Grease two 8- or 9-inch round cake pans and set aside.**

1. Whisk together the flour and ginger in a small bowl.

2. In a large mixing bowl with an electric mixer or in the bowl of a standing mixer fitted with the paddle attachment, beat the butter, tahini, and sugar on medium speed, until mixture becomes pale and quite fluffy, 5 to 8 minutes.

3. Fold in the flour mixture by hand, until you no longer see patches of flour.

4. Divide the dough in half and put one half into each of the prepared baking pans. Use your hands to spread it out until it covers the pan. Do your best to keep the thickness even.

5. Sprinkle 1 tablespoon sesame seeds onto each pan, and press gently.

6. Bake the shortbreads until pale golden, 20 to 25 minutes. Cool in pans for 10 minutes.

7. Run an offset spatula or small knife around the edge of 1 pan to loosen the shortbread, then cover with a plate and flip over; the shortbread should come out easily. Invert shortbread on a cutting board, so the sesame-side is facing up. Use a pizza cutter or sharp knife to cut into 12 wedges, then carefully transfer to a wire rack to cool fully—when warm, these cookies are quite delicate. Repeat with the other pan.

MAKE BABY FOOD: Sorry, too much added sugar. But if your baby's watching you eat one with a gotta-try-that look on his face, the ingredients are perfectly safe—a taste is just fine.

**MAMA SAID**
"The texture of these cookies is fantastic! Light and flaky, and not heavy or greasy at all like other homemade shortbreads I've had. I like the nuttiness that the tahini imparted. Making the recipe was really easy and really fast. My little one was playing in the next room, but I could have easily done this with him hanging out with me." —Sarah T., mom of one, Denver, CO

# BAKED OATMEAL WITH APPLES, ALMONDS, AND BROWN SUGAR

**Serves 2 to 3**

**Cooking time: 45 minutes (15 minutes active)**

Baked oatmeal has a different consistency than the stove-top version, though the flavor is similar. It's got a mix of textures—there's a slightly firmer, almost crusty top, and then a meltingly soft interior. Cooking with milk also makes it more substantial, more filling, and more nutritious.

Oats, dried fruit, and almonds are all considered galactagogues.

**NOTE:** If your mornings are too hectic for cooking, do most of the work the night before: Mix the dry ingredients and leave them covered on the counter, and mix the wet ingredients and refrigerate. Prep the apples, sprinkle with lemon juice to prevent browning, and refrigerate. Then in the morning, all you have to do is combine everything and bake.

2 cups milk, whole or low-fat

1 cup water

1 teaspoon vanilla extract

1 teaspoon almond extract, optional

¼ cup dark brown sugar

1½ cups rolled oats

½ cup chopped dried fruit
*Dates, figs, and apricots are considered the most helpful as galactagogues.*

½ cup slivered almonds

1 teaspoon cinnamon

2 small apples, peeled, cored, and sliced
*This works equally well with peaches (frozen or fresh), pears, and any other relatively firm fruit you can think of.*

**Preheat oven to 350°F. Grease a 7 x 11-inch rectangular baking dish and set aside.**

1. Combine the milk, water, vanilla, almond extract, if using, and sugar in a medium bowl. Combine the oats, dried fruit, almonds, and cinnamon in a large bowl. Stir the wet ingredients into the dry, then pour the mixture into the prepared baking dish.

2. Top with the sliced apples and bake until apples are soft and all the liquid is absorbed, 30 to 40 minutes. Serve with additional milk.

MAKE BABY FOOD: If there are no food allergies in your immediate family, this should be fine for baby—just chop the almond slivers before mixing them in, to avoid any risk of choking. The recipe calls for added sugar, but you can leave it out and sprinkle a bit on the grown-ups' servings at the table.

**MAMA SAID**

"The oatmeal was probably the best oatmeal I've ever had. I'm a regular oatmeal eater, but usually I just heat it up, add a little dried fruit and brown sugar, and I'm done with it. I had to substitute almond milk for the cow's milk since my daughter's not down with milk protein. As for supply, I've had really good output recently. I had this for breakfast two days this week and my own oatmeal for breakfast once more, and had to stop pumping after 15 minutes because one bottle was full. Normally I pump for 20 minutes before that happens."
—Monica W., mom of one, St. Louis, MO

# ALMOND BUTTER BANANA OATMEAL COOKIES

**Makes about 24 cookies**

**Cooking time: 40 minutes (20 minutes active)**

They might not sound like much, but these cookies rival the chocolate chip ones in Chapter 11 for sheer deliciousness. The almond butter adds a subtle, mellow flavor, and given that the recipe has only two tablespoons of butter, these are fairly healthy as cookies go. Heck, I'd eat them for breakfast.

Several of my mom-testers noted the lack of chocolate in this recipe. Feel free to add a handful or two of chips!

Both almonds and oats are considered lactogenic.

1 cup all-purpose flour

½ teaspoon baking powder

½ teaspoon baking soda

¼ teaspoon salt

½ cup brown sugar

½ cup granulated sugar

2 tablespoons butter, at room temperature

1 large egg

½ cup almond butter

¼ cup mashed banana (from 1 smallish, very ripe banana)

1½ cups rolled oats (not instant)

**Preheat oven to 350°F, and set racks in upper and lower thirds of oven. Grease or line two baking sheets.**

1.  Whisk together the flour, baking powder, baking soda, and salt in a medium bowl.

2.  In a large bowl with a hand-held mixer or in the bowl of a stand mixer fitted with the paddle attachment, beat together the sugars and butter on medium speed, 2 to 3 minutes. Add the egg and mix until combined, then add the almond butter and mashed banana, and mix until well combined.

3.  Add the dry ingredients to the almond butter mixture and mix on low speed. Stir in the oats, either on low speed or by hand.

4.  Drop tablespoons of dough, about 1 inch apart, onto prepared baking sheets, flattening each slightly with moistened fingers.

5.  Bake until just golden around the edges, 10 to 12 minutes, rotating sheets halfway though to ensure even baking. Cool on a wire rack.

MAKE BABY FOOD: If you have no concerns about nut allergies, these are safe for babies used to finger foods—though given the added sugar, definitely not for every day.

**MAMA SAID**
"I think that they really did help my supply. My baby is six months old now and I felt full (and even leaked a few times!) for the first time since the fourth trimester." —Heather B., mom of two, Westmont, IL

• • • • • • • • • • • • • • • • • • • • • • • • • • • • • • • • • • • • • • • • • • •

# GALACTIC GRANOLA SQUARES

**Makes 16 squares**

**Cooking time: 50 minutes (30 minutes active)**

They won't launch you into outer space, but these chewy bars may just send your milk supply soaring. They use a whopping nine ingredients considered lactogenic: oats, almonds, three types of seeds, honey, blackstrap molasses, nutritional yeast, and dried fruit.

2 cups rolled oats (not instant)

1 cup sliced almonds

½ cup ground flaxseeds

½ cup raw sunflower or pumpkin seeds

¼ cup sesame seeds

½ cup honey
  *To make it easier to get honey or molasses out of the measuring cup, coat it lightly with cooking spray before you pour in the sticky stuff.*

¼ cup blackstrap molasses
  *Blackstrap molasses, sold in health food stores, is nutritionally preferred over the regular variety. But if you'd rather not make a special trip, you'll be just fine with what you find in the supermarket.*

2 tablespoons unsalted butter

2 tablespoons nutritional yeast, optional

2 teaspoons vanilla extract

1 teaspoon cinnamon

Pinch of salt

1 cup chopped dried fruit (apricots, figs, and dates, or a combination)

**Preheat oven to 350°F. Grease an 8-inch square baking dish.**

1. Combine the oats, almonds, ground flaxseeds, sunflower seeds, and sesame seeds on a rimmed baking sheet. Bake, stirring occasionally, until lightly browned, 10 to 15 minutes.

2. Meanwhile, combine the honey, molasses, butter, nutritional yeast, if using, vanilla, cinnamon, and salt in a medium saucepan over medium-low heat. Cook, stirring occasionally, until butter has melted and nutritional yeast has fully dissolved.

3. When oat mixture is done, remove it from the oven and reduce the heat to 300°F. Add the oat mixture and the dried fruit to the liquid mixture, and stir to combine. Transfer mixture to the prepared baking dish and press down, evenly distributing it in the dish. Bake until firm to the touch, 20 to 25 minutes. Cool completely, then cut into 16 squares and store in an airtight container.

MAKE BABY FOOD: Sorry, nope. This is much too difficult for a new eater to chew safely, and thanks to concerns about botulism honey isn't allowed until a baby is one year old.

**MAMA SAID**
"Fantastic. Easy to follow, and I am already thinking about other dried fruits to put in there next time (I used dried apricots). Also, the iron in the blackstrap molasses would have helped with my postpartum anemia." —Alana D., mom of one, Narragansett, RI

# CHAPTER 10
# NUTRITIOUS NIBBLES

Hello, my name is Debbie, and I'm a snackaholic.

That may sound snarky, but I'm serious.

My snack-habit is bad, I'm telling you. Bad. Just how bad? Well, when I'm at my worst—stressing over a cookbook deadline, for instance—I'll head into the kitchen a half-dozen times over two hours. Each time I'll grab a little something, starting with a virtuous clementine, then some whole-grain crackers, followed by a handful of almonds, maybe a granola bar, eventually working my way up to chocolate or a scoop of ice cream. In my twenties, I would have started with the chocolate and worked my way down the junk food ladder from there. This, dear reader, is how I came to weigh 260 pounds by the time I was 23. But with Weight Watchers, a really good therapist, and a lot of research into nutrition, I was able to get my habit under control and lose 100 pounds. The secret: not giving up snacks, but choosing healthy ones.

The thing is, unlike alcoholics or drug addicts, we snackaholics can't quit our drug of choice. Food isn't exactly something we can live without, is it? As you just read, I still snack a lot. A *lot*. I snacked my way through infertility (little-known fact: chocolate chip cookies are a fertility aid!) and packed on almost 20 pounds of no-baby weight. When I finally got pregnant I returned to Weight Watchers, assuming they could help me gain a healthy amount over the next nine months; I was terrified that I'd succumb to pregnancy cravings and regain everything. But they sent me away. Turns out Weight Watchers isn't built for pregnant women. I was advised to return postpartum, when they offer a special program for new moms.

I snacked my way through the first trimester. It seemed like the only thing that would fend off nausea was white food, administered approximately every two hours. Think mini-bagels, saltines, soft pretzels the size of my head. You know, the empty-calorie starches. I knew I wasn't doing myself any favors, but thanks to all that doughy goodness, I didn't puke once. But I don't think I ate a fruit or vegetable for the first three months of my pregnancy. Factor in the fact that first-tri exhaustion translated into zero exercise, and in just 12 weeks I gained another 11 pounds.

Here's what I wrote in my journal toward the end of that time. I warn you, it ain't pretty:

> *I feel totally fat. I lost all that weight, literally worked my ass off, and for years afterward carried around a fantasy of being one of those sexy, fit pregnant women. I thought I'd be on the treadmill three or four times a week, and people would comment on how from the back you couldn't tell I was pregnant. Instead I'm soft and flabby and full of dimply fat. I really don't enjoy looking at myself in the mirror these days, and it sucks. Why didn't I lose weight before getting pregnant? What was I thinking? I look old and dumpy and my skin is terrible. Stephen keeps saying I just look pregnant, but I wish I hadn't set myself up like this. Two weeks ago we started taking Saturday-morning belly pictures so we can track the progress, but I hate even baring that much of myself for the camera. The pics are quite depressing. Everything looks so soft and droopy.*

There is a happy ending to my sad story. By midway through the second trimester, I managed to get my snacking under control. The end of nausea helped, as did the fear of gestational diabetes. And once my belly popped, my self-image improved. I wound up feeling pretty darn sexy for the rest of the pregnancy. It was so liberating, not having to walk around with my stomach sucked in! I rocked one particular tight-fitting, low-cut, black jersey dress whenever possible. By the time Harry was born I'd gained 33 pounds—just right for a regular-sized person, but a bit much for an overweight one.

And then, breastfeeding. It helps to burn calories, that's for sure, but it also instills hunger. Sometimes, ravenous hunger. The truth is, nursing moms only need between 300 and 500 extra calories a day—the equivalent of two or three well-balanced snacks— though often our bodies seem to demand much more. As I learned years ago when losing that 100 pounds, the trick is to make smart choices, snacks that make every calorie count by providing good nutrition. Five hundred calories of cookies does taste good going down, but it won't help your milk supply or your baby.

Let's not forget: What you eat, your baby eats. Nutrition matters just as much as it did while you were pregnant. That's where this chapter comes in. I developed many of the recipes here while I was nursing Harry, and by the time he self-weaned at 10 months, I'd lost those 33 pounds. I'm not saying it's *because* of these recipes, but having healthy snacks at the ready made everything much easier.

Of course, there was still the matter of the no-baby weight I gained before I got pregnant. I'm pleased to report that, thanks to Weight Watchers, those pounds are now gone too.

- - - - - - - - - - - - - - - - - - - - - - - - - - - - - - - - - - - - - - - - - - - -

### MAKE A NURSING SNACK BASKET

While baby's eating you can be too, if you keep a stash of nutritious snacks in a basket next to your nursing chair. Any of these make great choices:

- Roasted almonds, measured out into one-ounce servings of approximately 17 almonds (it's easy to overdo it with nuts). Almonds are packed with fiber, protein, and vitamin E, as well as heart-healthy fat. And as we learned in the last chapter, they're terrific for lactation.

- Shelf-stable cheese, like Babybel. If you can juggle it *and* your baby, combine with four or five whole-grain crackers for a real nutritional punch.

- Protein bars. I ate at least one Clif bar every day while nursing newborn Harry. Read labels carefully; many brands contain so much sugar they may as well be candy. Choose one with a high fiber content to keep you feeling fuller for longer—look for a bar with more than five grams of fiber per serving.

- Whole-grain pretzels or soy crisps, for when you need a salty crunch—stick to about ½ cup.

- Whole-grain breakfast cereal, pre-measured into individual servings (about ¾ cup). Satisfies the munchies, and most are vitamin-fortified too.

- Fruit. That one should be a no-brainer—but keep in mind that you can overdo it here too, since fruit has natural sugars (which, in excess, are just as bad for your body as the processed kind). Dried fruit has the benefit of being high in iron, which nursing moms generally need, but watch out: The sugar content is concentrated so it's easy to eat too much. Stick to about 2 tablespoons.

- And don't forget water! Nursing takes it out of you, literally. You should be drinking at least two quarts a day.

## CRIB NOTES

- The recipes in this chapter are grouped by type of food—I don't know about you, but when I'm in the mood for something savory, a sweet snack just won't cut it. The chapter starts out fruity, then takes a brief detour into chocolate (you'll find a lot more in the next chapter) before heading straight into saltytown.

- Snacking is good! It can provide much-needed nutrients, keep you going when your body *really* wants sleep, and even substitute for a larger meal. The point is to snack wisely.

- An ideal snack includes protein, complex carbohydrates, and a bit of fat.

- Try to avoid snacks with considerable amounts of added sugar, like candy and cookies (sorry!). It will wreak havoc on your blood sugar levels, which is the last thing an already-exhausted person needs.

- You'll feel fuller (and consume fewer calories) if you snack on things with a high water content, like fruits or vegetables. Dry, crunchy foods like pretzels are easy to munch, sure, but you'll want to eat again an hour later.

# TWO REALLY GOOD SMOOTHIES

**Each makes 1 large smoothie, and doubles well**
**Cooking time: 5 minutes**

Got some over-ripe bananas? Cut them into chunks, put the chunks into a resealable bag, and stick the bag in the freezer. If there's yogurt in the fridge, you've got the base for a smoothie. It's a fabulous new-parent snack; you only need one hand to drink it!

### FABULOUSLY FRUITY

¾ cup nonfat or low-fat plain yogurt (use Greek yogurt for an extra boost of protein)
1 tablespoon ground flaxseeds
1 frozen banana, cut into chunks
½ cup frozen fruit (I like peaches and mango, or mixed berries—just make sure you're buying the kind that's pure fruit, no sugar added)
Skim or 1 percent milk, as needed to thin it out

### PB, B & C

¾ cup nonfat or low-fat plain yogurt (use Greek yogurt for an extra boost of protein)
1 tablespoon ground flaxseeds
1 frozen banana, cut into chunks
2 tablespoons peanut butter
A good squirt of your favorite chocolate sauce (a tablespoon or two)
Skim or 1 percent milk, as needed to thin it out

1. Place the yogurt and ground flaxseeds in the blender and blend on high speed.

2. Add the banana chunks 1 at a time through the blender's feeder cap, being sure to recover quickly each time to prevent splattering.

3. When the mixture appears relatively smooth, add the frozen fruit, in a similar manner as the banana, or add the peanut butter and chocolate sauce all at once.

4. If the mixture gets too thick, drizzle some milk through the feeder cap while the machine is running. Blend until smooth, and serve in a tall glass.

MAKE BABY FOOD: C'mon, this practically *is* baby food! If there are food allergies in your immediate family, hold off on the peanut butter version until your pediatrician gives the thumbs-up.

**MAMA SAID**

"This was really, really good! And the blender didn't even wake the baby when he was napping. I used soymilk, strawberries, and raspberries. I added protein powder, and it was very filling. Could definitely be a meal replacement. Easy and quick to make while caring for the baby." —Leya G., mom of one, Stuart, FL

· · · · · · · · · · · · · · · · · · · · · · · · · · · · · · · · · · · · · · · · · · · · · · · · · · · · · · · ·

### WHAT THE HECK IS FLAXSEED?

Throughout this chapter, you'll see recipes that call for ground flaxseeds (sometimes labeled flax meal), which has become something of a nutritionists' darling. If you're not familiar with flaxseeds, here's the scoop: They're high in fiber, omega-3 fatty acids, and phytochemicals called lignans, which are believed to fight cancer. There's no definitive recommended daily allowance yet, but most experts suggest eating about 1 tablespoon of ground flaxseeds each day. And it does need to be ground, since whole seeds are small enough to pass through you undigested, robbing your body of the chance to absorb the omega-3s. If you can swing it, buy whole seeds and grind as needed—once ground, those fatty acids oxidize relatively quickly. The pre-ground kind is still beneficial, so if grinding to order is too ambitious with a newborn attached to your body, don't let that stop you. Stored in the refrigerator, even the pre-ground should be good for months. Flaxseed oil, which contains those same omega-3s, has two counts against it: First, it doesn't have the fiber found in the seeds, and second, it oxidizes extremely quickly—even refrigerated, you'll need to use up a bottle in about six weeks.

· · · · · · · · · · · · · · · · · · · · · · · · · · · · · · · · · · · · · · · · · · · · · · · · · · · · · · · ·

# A FIZZY, FROSTY, FRUITY FREEZE

**Serves 2, and doubles well**
**Cooking time: 5 minutes**

Got some frozen bananas, but in the mood for something lighter and more refreshing than a smoothie? Try a freeze! This is one of my favorite summertime snacks. (And between you and me, a splash of rum makes this a pretty awesome cocktail—check out the advice on page 292 from lactation consultant Freda Rosenfeld on nursing moms and alcohol.)

1 cup ginger ale, diet or regular

1 frozen small banana (or ½ large banana) cut into chunks

6 to 8 frozen whole strawberries

½ cup pomegranate juice

1. Combine the ginger ale and the banana in the blender and blend on high speed

2. Add the strawberries and continue blending.

3. When the mixture thickens and slows the machine, drizzle the pomegranate juice through the blender's feeder cap.

MAKE BABY FOOD: Let's call this one an older person's drink, except as an occasional treat. Babies don't need the added sugar (or artificial sweetener) in ginger ale.

**MAMA SAID**
**"This was a really nice treat and easy to make. I'll be making this as a snack for me and the kiddo while working in the garden in the summer or before running errands. Two thumbs way up." —Monica W., mom of one, St. Louis, MO**

# BAKED APPLE COMPOTE

**Serves 4 to 8, depending on how you use it**
**Cooking time: 1 hour 15 minutes (15 minutes active)**

A compote is stewed fruit with a prettier name. It's cooked slowly so the fruit keeps its shape, and traditionally the fruit simmers in sugar syrup. This version uses dark brown sugar—I like the depth of flavor—but a relatively small amount.

When we were tweaking this recipe, several of my mom-testers were curious about serving size. They loved the compote straight up, but wondered about other ways to use it. Give these a try:

- Over pancakes, French toast, or waffles
- Stirred into oatmeal or plain yogurt
- Inside crêpes
- Over ice cream, cheesecake, or angel food cake
- With a shot of whipped or heavy cream
- With granola topping
- With latkes (it's a chunkier applesauce!)
- Alongside roast pork

4 to 5 apples, peeled, cored, and chopped into 1½-inch pieces (about 5 cups total; it's fine to use a mix of varieties)

½ cup dried cherries or cranberries

⅔ cup chopped pecans or walnuts (finely chopped if you'll be feeding to a baby)

⅓ cup packed dark brown sugar

⅓ cup water

1 teaspoon cinnamon

½ teaspoon ground ginger

Pinch of nutmeg

¼ teaspoon salt

**Preheat oven to 350°F. Grease a 2-quart casserole or baking dish.**

1. Combine all the ingredients in large bowl and stir well.

2. Pour into the prepared casserole, cover with aluminum foil, and bake 1 hour, stirring every 20 minutes. If the mixture looks too wet or you'd like a bit of browning on top, as I do, remove the foil for the last 10 minutes.

3. Serve warm or cold (see recommendations above).

MAKE BABY FOOD: Use less sugar if you'll be sharing this with a baby. The apples are a great consistency for babies, and the dried fruit plumps up nicely. If your immediate family has food allergies, leave out the nuts until your pediatrician clears you.

**MAMA SAID**

"Easy as pie! Make that . . . easy as compote! It made a healthy snack for the La Leche League Leaders pow-wow I held this morning. I used one Gala, one Pink Lady and two Mutsu apples, and I chopped and mixed everything up while the girls had breakfast; easy peasy." —Ariella M., mom of two, Brookline, NH

• • • • • • • • • • • • • • • • • • • • • • • • • • • • • • • • • • • • • • • • •

# FRUITY OATMEAL SQUARES

**Makes 24 squares**

**Cooking time: 1 hour (15 to 20 minutes active)**

The recipe below calls for blueberries, but that's totally up to you. You can swap in diced apples or pears, strawberries, heck, almost any fruit that appeals. I usually let Harry pick; his latest combination was frozen peaches and raspberries with fresh kiwi. A little odd, but we gobbled them up regardless. I've made this using a mix of fresh and dried fruit, and it was *still* fantastic, possibly even more so, thanks to the different textures.

The end result is like a coffee cake crossed with a granola bar—definitely cakey, but the oatmeal adds a nice chewiness. Among my group of 100+ mom-testers, this was far and away the most popular recipe in the chapter.

1½ cups all-purpose flour or whole-wheat pastry flour

1 teaspoon cinnamon

1 teaspoon baking soda

½ teaspoon salt

¼ cup ground flaxseeds

1 cup packed light brown sugar

½ cup granulated sugar

4 tablespoons butter (½ stick), softened

½ cup no-sugar-added applesauce—increase to ¾ cup if you're using only dried fruit

½ cup vegetable oil

2 large eggs

1 teaspoon vanilla extract

3 cups old-fashioned oats

2 cups fresh or frozen blueberries (or any fruit of your choice)

**Preheat oven to 350°F. Grease an 11 x 13-inch baking dish.**

1. Whisk together the flour, cinnamon, baking soda, salt, and ground flaxseeds in a small bowl.

2. In a large bowl, using an electric mixer on medium speed or a wooden spoon, beat together the brown sugar, granulated sugar, butter, and applesauce until well blended. Mix in the oil, eggs, and vanilla.

3. Add the flour mixture into the larger bowl and stir until just combined. Stir in the oats and fruit.

4. Spread batter evenly into the prepared pan. Bake until golden brown and a toothpick inserted in the center comes out clean, 35 to 40 minutes. Transfer the pan to a wire rack to cool completely. Cut into 24 squares.

MAKE BABY FOOD: Older babies can eat this safely—you know your child, so I'll let you be the judge of when she's ready! Nutritious as it is, the recipe does have added sugar, so you may want to hold off for a while.

MAMA SAID

"My husband and I enjoyed these as a bedtime snack and the next morning as breakfast. Since I'm nursing I have a ravenous hunger, but was pleasantly surprised that after eating a medium-sized bar at home I didn't need my usual second breakfast at work. This was a really simple recipe with fantastic results, and I appreciated how healthy it was too—oats, flaxseed, blueberries, and cinnamon!" —Anne V., mom of one, Brooklyn, NY

# CHILLED MANGO-POMEGRANATE-GINGER SOUP

**Serves 2 to 3**

**Cooking time: 5 minutes**

This quick treat was born out of a mistake. I left a pair of mangoes in the car. For two days. In July. After eating (and drinking) the result, I'm really glad I did. The ginger flavor here is quite pronounced; if you want to back off a bit, cut the amount in half.

**NOTE**: For a refreshing beverage, pour some soup into a tall glass, about half-full, and add seltzer. Or be daring and try it with sparkling wine. For a more substantial snack, add a small container of plain low-fat yogurt to the blender.

| | |
|---|---|
| 2 extremely ripe, large mangos | 1 tablespoon grated ginger |
| One 8-ounce can pineapple chunks or bits in juice (not syrup) | 1 cup pomegranate juice |

1. Peel and roughly chop the mangos (if they're super-ripe, you may be able to scoop out the flesh with a spoon).

2. Combine the mangos, pineapple, and ginger in a blender and puree.

3. With the machine running, add the pomegranate juice through the feeder cap.

4. Strain before serving, and discard the pulp.

> MAKE BABY FOOD: Stir this into yogurt, and watch baby gobble it up.

**MAMA SAID**

"I used an immersion blender; it worked like a charm for this recipe. I served it mixed with sparkling water. The ginger flavor came through really prominently, so I thought this would be great for an early pregnancy mocktail to help with morning sickness. My daughter also really liked it—I diluted hers with a bit of plain water. As an added bonus it worked great to give her the foul-tasting vitamin and iron drops she's on right now. That's a tough flavor to cover up and we've tried lots of things, but this was the most successful so far." —Beth P., mom of one, Los Angeles, CA

# FROZEN GRAPES

**Serves as many as you want**
**Cooking time: 2 hours (5 minutes active)**

Mention frozen grapes at any Weight Watchers meeting and listen to the sighs of remembered pleasure. Some members claimed to find them as satisfying (and addictive) as bon bons. Grapes' lush little insides attain a nearly creamy consistency when frozen, and the sweetness is magnified. Taste a room temperature grape for comparison, and you'll see: The frosty one is markedly closer to candy.

Red or green grapes, as many as you want

1. Line a shallow bowl or rimmed baking sheet with paper towels or a clean dishtowel.

2. Remove the grapes from the stems, then wash and dry thoroughly.

3. Pour the grapes into the prepared bowl (in a single layer, if possible) and freeze until solid, at least 2 hours. Transfer to an airtight container and store in the freezer.

> MAKE BABY FOOD: Since grapes in general are considered a choking hazard, I'd stay away from the frozen ones for baby. Even cut up, the hardness of them makes me wary.

**MAMA SAID**
"I had never tried this. Yum! Almost like a smoothie—perfect for a summer snack."
—Maggie K., mom of two, Pleasantville, NY

# COCONUTTY QUINOA BARS

**Makes 12 large bars, or 24 small squares**

**Cooking time: 45 minutes (15 minutes active)**

Quinoa makes for some quick pantry-based meals, but it's a pleasant surprise in a granola bar. It goes in dry and uncooked, and during baking something wonderful happens. Take a bite, and each little seed pops between your teeth. That crunch makes my mouth happy, and my body's happy too because quinoa's just so darn nutritious. It's a protein bar in disguise!

These bake up to be quite solid. Not break-a-tooth solid, but they're definitely not soft.

1½ cups rolled oats (not quick-cooking)

1½ cups quinoa

1 cup unsweetened shredded coconut, loosely packed
*You'll find unsweetened coconut in most health food stores, and supermarkets with a large organic section. Bob's Red Mill makes a fine version.*

½ cup sliced almonds

½ cup ground flaxseeds

1 teaspoon cinnamon

1½ cups chopped dried fruit
*I like figs and apricots, but if you want to sneak in some mini M&Ms or chocolate-covered sunflower seeds, I won't tell. Don't use plain chocolate chips, though, because the hot sugary goo will melt them on contact.*

3 tablespoons butter

⅔ cup honey

¼ cup light brown sugar

1½ teaspoons vanilla extract

¼ teaspoon salt

**Preheat oven to 350°F. Line a baking sheet with aluminum foil. Line a 9 x 13-inch baking dish with parchment paper (make sure it comes up the sides; this will make it easier to get the bars out).**

1. Combine the oats, quinoa, coconut, and almonds in the baking sheet. Bake, stirring once or twice, until golden brown, 10 to 12 minutes. Remove and lower heat to 300°F.

2. Combine the ground flaxseeds, cinnamon, and dried fruit in a large bowl, then stir in the toasted quinoa mixture.

3. Combine the butter, honey, brown sugar, vanilla, and salt in a small saucepan over medium heat. Bring to a boil and cook for 1 minute, stirring as needed. (It will bubble furiously and threaten to overflow, but stirring will calm it down.)

4. Pour the butter mixture over the toasted oats mixture, and stir well (make sure there are no dry patches). Transfer mixture to the prepared baking dish and spread evenly with a spatula or the back of a spoon. (The edges need to be at least as thick as the center, or they will burn.)

5. Bake until golden brown, 25 to 30 minutes. Cool completely in the pan before removing to a cutting board (use the overhanging parchment to help transfer), then use a large, sharp knife to cut into 12 bars or 24 squares.

6. Store, tightly wrapped, up to 2 weeks.

MAKE BABY FOOD: Sorry, not for Junior.

**MAMA SAID**
"I love these! I love the crunchiness of the quinoa and the sweetness of the coconut. I used dried cherries and they paired really well with the other ingredients. I also like that there is so little sugar." —Jessica C., mom of one, Brooklyn, NY

# CHOCOLATE-DIPPED FROZEN BANANAS

**Serves 4**

**Cooking time: 2 hours 15 minutes (15 minutes active)**

The first thing I think of when I hear the words "frozen banana" is poor nebbishy George Michael Bluth burning down the family's frozen banana stand on *Arrested Development* (which, if you haven't seen, I highly recommend watching on DVD while nursing—I tore through dozens of TV shows that way). But once I get past the giggles, things turn quite serious. Seriously delicious. Have you ever eaten a frozen banana? The creaminess is surprising—it's similar to ice cream, which is not a description I throw around lightly. When dipped in bittersweet chocolate and rolled in your favorite combination of nuts and dried fruit, frozen bananas are about as healthy a decadent treat as you're likely to find.

*Some of my favorite fruit/nut combos: sliced almonds and chopped dried cherries; salted pistachios and candied ginger; hazelnuts and figs.*

2 bananas, ripe but still firm

½ cup nuts, toasted and finely chopped (the food processor comes in handy here)

¼ cup dried fruit, finely chopped (no food processor for this, but coating a knife with

nonstick spray will help chopping go more smoothly)

Fleur de sel or other finishing salt, optional

4 ounces bittersweet chocolate, chopped

1 teaspoon flavorful extra-virgin olive oil

**Equipment needed: Some sort of stick—Popsicle, lollipop, small wooden skewers. Or use toothpicks, cut the fruit into 6 to 8 pieces each, and make banana bites.**

1. Line a baking sheet with wax paper or parchment. Cut each banana into thirds. Push a stick into the cut side of each piece, and arrange on prepared baking sheet.

2. Freeze for at least 1 hour.

3. Put chopped nuts and dried fruits onto separate small plates (unless you're combining flavors, in which case use just one). If you're using fleur de sel, stir a bit into each plate.

4. Combine the chocolate and olive oil in a small shallow bowl, and melt the chocolate in the microwave, about 20 seconds at a time, stirring in between. Stop when the chocolate is almost melted, but not quite—the stirring will finish the job.

5. Working quickly, dip the banana pieces one at a time into the melted chocolate and turn to coat. Immediately dip the banana in the nuts and dried fruits, then arrange on the baking sheet. Repeat with the remaining banana pieces. If the chocolate begins to harden before you've got them all coated, reheat in the microwave for about 10 seconds and stir.

6. When the bananas are all coated, freeze for at least 1 hour.

7. If not eating right away, transfer the dipped bananas to resealable bags and store in freezer. If you'd like a softer experience, let the chocolate-coated banana sit at room temperature for about 5 minutes before taking that first bite.

MAKE BABY FOOD: Take an additional banana and cut it into chunks or spears before freezing. Plain ol' frozen bananas make babies—especially teething ones—happy. To make what I call "banana ice cream" when Harry's clamoring for a treat, I pulse small pieces of frozen banana in the food processor until they break down, then puree fully. It looks and tastes like ice cream. For real.

**MAMA SAID**
"Awesome! I used milk chocolate, almonds, and some sea salt. Very quick, very easy, and very good." —Mary T., mom of one, Ankeny, IA

# DARK CHOCOLATE PUDDING

**Serves 4**

**Cooking time: 2½ hours (15 minutes active)**

This sweet little recipe could just as easily have fit into the next chapter, "Easy Indulgences," but I really like a bowl of pudding in the mid-afternoon. Or mid-morning. Or after dinner. Pretty much any time, really. And given the specifics of this particular recipe, pudding can be every bit as nutritious as it is indulgent. It's adapted from *Moosewood Restaurant Low-Fat Favorites*—yes, you read that right, it's *low-fat.* But if I didn't tell you, you'd never guess. It's thick and rich, yet healthy, with the milk providing much-needed calcium and protein and the cocoa/dark chocolate combo adding healthy flavonoids (all with only 3 tablespoons of added sugar!). Try the Mexican variation for kicks.

**NOTE:** You'll be at the stove, stirring, for 8 to 10 minutes, so I'd make this while baby sleeps.

3 tablespoons cornstarch

3 tablespoons sugar

2 tablespoons unsweetened cocoa powder
  (natural or Dutch-process)

Pinch of salt

2 cups 1 percent milk

1 ounce bittersweet chocolate, chopped
  (about 2 tablespoons)

1 teaspoon vanilla extract

1. Whisk together the cornstarch, sugar, cocoa powder, and salt in a small saucepan. Add the milk and cook over medium heat, stirring constantly, until the pudding comes to a boil. Lower the heat and gently simmer, stirring constantly, 3 to 4 minutes. Remove from heat.

2. Add the chopped chocolate and vanilla, and stir until the chocolate melts. Pour the hot pudding into a serving bowl or individual ramekins. Serve warm or refrigerate for about 2 hours, until set. If you want to avoid a skin on your pudding (in which case I think you're crazy), place plastic wrap directly on the pudding's surface before chilling.

*Mexican variation: Add ¼ teaspoon cinnamon and ⅛ teaspoon chili powder when you're making the cornstarch mixture, then proceed with the recipe.*

MAKE BABY FOOD: Strictly speaking, this is fine for infants. But it does have some added sugar, so you might want to enjoy it when baby's not around.

**MAMA SAID**

"This recipe is just as easy as the boxed cook-and-serve pudding, only much more delicious! It's pudding for grown-ups. Granted, standing at the stove and stirring continuously is kind of monotonous, but necessary. I made it late at night when my husband and I got a chocolate craving. Is it wrong that I had some for breakfast the next day?" —Lee P., mom of two, Pittsburgh, PA

· · · · · · · · · · · · · · · · · · · · · · · · · · · · · · · · · · · · · · · · · · · · · · · ·

# HONEYED CRACKERSNACK

**Serves 10 to 12**

**Cooking time: 40 minutes**

It's been pointed out to me that "crackersnack" might be a bit misleading, since there's popcorn, not crackers, in this snack. But I have two reasons for liking the name: 1. It's a play on Crackerjack, get it? And 2. It's as addictive as, well, crack. The specks of flaxseed mean that it's not the prettiest caramel corn you'll ever see, but it's probably the healthiest. In addition to the benefits of flax, you're getting fiber, vitamin E, and even calcium from the almonds. Plus, there's the whole-grain goodness of popcorn itself.

*If you don't have an air-popper, it's easy to make popcorn in the microwave without buying the ready-to-go bags, which have added chemicals. Just take a large brown paper lunch bag and put in about ¼ cup popcorn kernels. Fold the top over once or twice and microwave on high for 2 to 3 minutes. (Set it for 3 minutes and stand nearby; stop the machine when the popping slows to every few seconds.)*

8 cups air-popped popcorn (from about ¼ cup popcorn kernels)

¾ cup Marcona almonds (plain whole almonds would work too)

½ cup chopped dried cherries or other dried fruit

½ cup butter (1 stick), cut into chunks

½ cup honey

*Here's a tip: Grease your measuring cup before pouring in the honey (I use nonstick spray). The sticky stuff slides right out!*

¼ teaspoon salt

2 teaspoons vanilla extract

½ cup ground flaxseeds, optional

**Preheat oven to 325°F. Grease a large roasting pan.**

1. Combine the popcorn, almonds, and dried cherries in the pan.

2. Combine the butter, honey, and salt in a medium saucepan and cook over medium heat, stirring constantly, until the butter is melted. Raise the heat and bring to a boil. Boil for 1 minute, stirring constantly. Remove from heat and carefully stir in the vanilla.

3. Carefully pour the honey mixture over the popcorn mixture in the roasting pan, then sprinkle with the ground flaxseeds, if using, and stir gently to coat. Bake, stirring every 10 minutes, until deep golden all over, about 30 minutes.

4. Cool at least 5 minutes before you even think of tasting it—that goo will be *hot.* Cool completely before storing in an airtight container. It will keep at room temperature for up to 2 weeks.

MAKE BABY FOOD: Sorry, nope.

**MAMA SAID**
"It's recipes like these that make working from home a dangerous proposition. This stuff is addictive! Beyond that, it's easy to make and seems infinitely customizable. If I had this in the fourth tri there would definitely have been a big baggie of it in my nursing basket."
—Beth P., mom of one, Los Angeles, CA

# BAKED POTATO (OR SWEET POTATO) CHIPS

**Serves 2 to 4, depending on one's ability to control oneself**
**Cooking time: 35 minutes (10 minutes active)**

This is one of those Whatever Strikes Your Fancy recipes. Feel like something salty? Go with baking potatoes, and toss on whatever spice blend you like best. Something more on the sweet side, but still a bit savory? Sweet potatoes, tossed with salt (yes, salt! a little bit brings out the flavor) and spices typically used for baking. Chili powder swings both ways.

2 large baking potatoes or 2 medium sweet
    potatoes
1 tablespoon olive oil
Salt
For baking potatoes: 1 teaspoon chili powder,
    curry powder, Old Bay seasoning, or your
    favorite spice blend

For sweet potatoes: 1 teaspoon Chinese five-
    spice powder, chili powder, or cinnamon
    with a pinch of nutmeg

**Preheat oven to 425°F and set the racks in the upper and lower thirds of the oven. Line two baking sheets.**

1. Slice the potatoes crosswise into very thin rounds using a mandoline or a food processor with the slicing blade, or carefully by hand. Combine sliced potatoes, oil, salt, and your choice of spice in a gallon-sized resealable bag. Seal and toss to coat. (Depending on how many slices your potatoes yielded, you may want to do this in 2 or 3 batches, adjusting the oil and spice amounts accordingly.)

2. Arrange the potatoes in a single layer on the prepared baking sheets. Bake, switching the placement of the trays halfway through, until they're as done as you like them, 20 to 25 minutes for regular potatoes, 15 to 20 minutes for sweet potatoes (I prefer them more on the browned and crispy side, but if you take them out sooner they'll have a nice chewiness to them.) Note that the cooking time will depend on how thin you've sliced the potatoes—the thinner, the quicker.

MAKE BABY FOOD: These are good for gumming—they don't get shatteringly crisp the way fried chips do. Take them out of the oven on the early side to play it safe, and let them cool before serving.

**MAMA SAID**

"We made the baked sweet potato chips. We don't have a mandoline, so I used the thinnest slicing blade on our food processor. I thought they were great and they were a *huge* hit with my son. I loved your trick of tossing them with the oil and spices in the bag. We have done baked sweet potato fries in the past and I was always trying to toss them with the oil and spices in a bowl or on the pan and I can't believe I never thought to use a bag. So much easier! I used cinnamon with a pinch of nutmeg for our spices." —Marisa K., mom of one, East Greenwich, RI

· · · · · · · · · · · · · · · · · · · · · · · · · · · · · · · · · · · · · · · · · · ·

# QUICKIE HUMMUS

**Serves 8 to 10 as a snack, 4 to 6 as part of a meal**

**Cooking time: 5 minutes**

This ain't no traditional hummus, no sirree. I'm not a huge fan of tahini, so I generally leave it out. Instead I use a bit of yogurt, which gives the hummus a lovely, though neutral, creaminess with just a hint of tang.

One 14- to 15-ounce can chickpeas, rinsed and drained

2 tablespoons olive oil

2 tablespoons low-fat or nonfat plain yogurt

1 to 2 tablespoons lemon juice

1 large or 2 small garlic cloves, peeled and smashed

1 teaspoon ground cumin

Salt and pepper

Paprika and flavorful olive oil, for serving

**OPTIONAL ADD-INS (use one or a combination)**

A large handful of baby spinach

1 roasted red pepper from a jar, patted dry

½ cup Kalamata olives

1 head roasted garlic (in which case, leave out the raw garlic)

**TO DIP**

Pita wedges or chips, baby carrots, celery sticks, grape or cherry tomatoes, bell pepper strips, cucumber slices, jicama spears, broccoli or cauliflower florets

1. Combine the chickpeas, olive oil, yogurt, lemon juice to taste, garlic, cumin, and salt and pepper to taste in a food processor, and process until the mixture is smooth and thick.

2. Serve sprinkled with the paprika and drizzled with the flavorful olive oil.

MAKE BABY FOOD: This should be a big, nutritious hit.

**MAMA SAID**

"This was the first time I made hummus instead of picking it up, although I've been meaning to forever. My husband was shocked at how easy and fast it was! I didn't notice a huge difference from the taste of traditional hummus with the yogurt instead of tahini. The recipe was a little chunkier than I prefer, so I added another tablespoon of yogurt to smooth it out."
—Jennifer S., mom of two, San Diego, CA

# CRUNCHY CHILI SPLIT PEAS

**Serves 6 to 8**

**Cooking time: 5 hours (15 minutes active)**

These super-crunchy yellow split peas are similar conceptually to the Curry-Roasted Chickpeas that follow, but they're made differently and the flavor is quite distinct. They're equally habit-forming, though!

1 cup dried yellow split peas
2 tablespoons olive oil

1 teaspoon chili powder, or to taste
Salt

1. Soak the peas in 3 cups of water for at least 4½ and up to 6 hours. Drain and pat dry (I rub a kitchen towel through them while still in the colander).

2. Heat the oil in a very large nonstick skillet over medium-high heat. When it shimmers, add the peas (you may need to do this in 2 batches, in which case divide the oil and seasoning) and cook, stirring occasionally, until lightly browned and crunchy, 10 to 12 minutes. Add the chili powder and salt to taste, stir, and cook 1 to 2 minutes more.

3. Cool completely, then store in an airtight container for up to 1 week. The peas will lose some of their crunch after a day or 2 but will still be yummy.

MAKE BABY FOOD: I wouldn't serve this to the toothless crowd. They're all for you!

**MAMA SAID**

"I was surprised that you suggested using yellow split peas, because when we think of split peas we automatically think of green, but they are beautiful and delicious, absolutely addictive! They are so much better for us than potato chips and other salty snacks. I also like how easy it would be to change the flavors depending on your personal taste or to suit a theme dinner." —Jane B., mom of one, Pleasanton, CA

• • • • • • • • • • • • • • • • • • • • • • • • • • • • • • • • • • • • •

# CURRY ROASTED CHICKPEAS

**Serves as few as 1, as many as 4**

**Cooking time: 35 minutes**

Ad.dic.tive. That is all.

Theoretically, these flavor bombs will stay good for about a week in an airtight container (though they'll soften up a bit). But I've never had a batch last long enough to find out for sure.

2 teaspoons olive oil

2 teaspoons curry powder

One 14- to 15-ounce can chickpeas, drained, rinsed, and dried

*If you're obsessive (which I'll admit, sometimes I am), you can slip off and toss the chickpea skins. If not, don't sweat it—the chickpeas will still be delicious.*

1 teaspoon sea salt

**Preheat oven to 425°F. Line a baking sheet.**

1.  Heat the olive oil over low heat in a nonstick skillet large enough to hold the chickpeas comfortably. When it shimmers, add the curry powder. Cook, stirring with a wooden spoon, until fragrant, about 30 seconds.

2.  Add the chickpeas and the salt, and stir just long enough to coat. Remove from the heat.

3.  Arrange the chickpeas in a single layer on the prepared baking sheet and roast, shaking the pan every 10 minutes, until crisp and golden, 25 to 30 minutes.

4.  Cool completely, then store in an airtight container for up to 1 week.

## VARIATIONS

- Roast the chickpeas with oil and salt but no spices; while still hot, toss with 1 teaspoon grated lemon zest.
- Substitute Chinese five-spice powder, adobo seasoning, Old Bay seasoning, or your favorite spice mixture for the curry powder.
- Use chili powder in place of the curry, and squeeze the juice of 1 lime on the just-roasted chickpeas.

MAKE BABY FOOD: When roasted, the chickpeas become quite hard. I'd save these until your child has teeth and knows how to use them—otherwise they'd be a choking hazard.

### MAMA SAID

"This recipe was *extremely* simple to make, which was great for a busy schedule. It's nice to have a guilt-free, nutritious snack, and even better when it contains protein and can help fill in between meals." —Sarah P., mom of two, Colorado Springs, CO

# SUPER-QUICK GUACAMOLE

**Serves 2, and multiplies nicely**
**Cooking time: 5 minutes**

I'm pretty sure if you look up the word "cheat," you'll find this recipe. Not a bit of authenticity here and it even includes some semi-processed food, but for a quick, healthy snack it's tough to beat. Eat the guac with cut-up veggies or baked tortilla chips (try the ones from my Chipotle Tortilla Soup, on page 21) and it will keep you going for a few more hours.

**NOTE:** This is definitely better with fresh salsa, the kind you find in the refrigerator case. But if you're desperate, a good-quality jarred salsa will work too.

1 ripe avocado
*Know how to pit an avocado? Hold the half that includes the pit in your palm, pit facing up. Whack the pit with the blade of a big kitchen knife and twist—it comes right out. This requires some force and takes good aim, so only try it if you're fairly confident in your knife skills.*

½ cup fresh or jarred salsa
1 small garlic clove, minced, optional
Lime juice to taste

1. Scoop the avocado flesh from the peel and put into a medium bowl.

2. Add the salsa and garlic, if using, and mash with a fork until well combined.

3. Add the lime juice to taste.

MAKE BABY FOOD: Avocados, definitely. Harry ate some nearly every day for his first six months on solids. Initially I mashed them with a fork, and later I cut them into chunks for finger food. If your baby likes spice, go ahead and give her some of the prepared dish.

**MAMA SAID**
**"It doesn't get much quicker or easier, and it was delicious! Also, it made a delightful addition to a lunch wrap for a husband home sick from work." —Ariella M., mom of two, Brookline, NH**

# CHAPTER 11

## EASY INDULGENCES

So we've established that I'm a snackaholic. But I'll bet you didn't realize that within the snackaholic community, there are factions: Crunch hounds. Gooey heads. Salt fiends. Sugar whores. I'm something of a social butterfly when it comes to the snack-set, flitting from group to group, nibbling a bit here, a bit there, but when I'm super-stressed I dive head-first into the sugar bowl. For example, here's an entry I posted on my moms' message board when Harry was just shy of three months old:

> Today turned into Hell Day and it's still going—Harry hasn't slept for more than thirty consecutive minutes all day long. Even loading him into the Björn for a long walk didn't buy me more than a half-hour. At around 5:30 Stephen tried to give him a bottle of defrosted expressed breastmilk, and we discovered the hard way that my breastmilk goes rancid when frozen (excess lipase, I think, so we'll have to start scalding before storage)— Harry started screaming like someone was trying to kill him, and he still hasn't really

*calmed down. He's screaming on the boob, he's screaming in the crib, he's screaming with the vacuum cleaner on, he's just screaming. Scary, terrifying, Why Are You Torturing Me screams, the kind that make the neighbors call the police, the kind that leave his whole body heaving for long, long minutes after he calms down. I finally nursed him in the rocking chair, something I haven't done since he was two weeks old, and he fell asleep. He's in the crib now out cold, but I'm betting it won't be for long.*

What do you suppose I did after I wrote that post? That's right, I headed for the nearest cookie. No doubt about it, in my heart I'm a sugar whore. I bake for fun! I fantasize about sea salt caramels, biting into a dark, smooth chocolate shell and letting the buttery insides ooze into my mouth, little flecks of salt clinging to my lips . . .

*Oh, ahem, pardon me. Where was I?*

The truth is, sometimes I can't help it. As several studies have shown, stress chemically induces many women to eat more, especially sweets. So diving into that Häagen-Dazs is a physical response as well as an emotional one. You're a new mom. Are you under stress like I was on Hell Day? Maybe you're dealing with this parenting gig a little better than I did, but few periods in my life have been as stress-filled as the first six months of Harry's.

But sweets are a tricky thing. On the one hand, we've all heard the mantra, "everything in moderation," which reassures us that a sweet treat isn't necessarily a bad thing. But on the other hand, if you lose track of the "moderation" part and, oh I don't know, *eat a daily pint of ice cream*, that baby weight probably ain't coming off.

I realize that my whole preamble is making you wonder why this cookbook even has a chapter called "Easy Indulgences." It's because I don't believe it's possible, or advisable, to completely avoid sweets, especially when stressed. The idea, just like in the last chapter, is to be sweet smart. Make good choices. Any treat you make yourself is almost guaranteed to be better for your body (and your baby, if you're breastfeeding) than something commercially produced. It's likely to have less sugar and fat, and it will be free of preservatives or chemical additives. And since I'm a Lifetime Member of Weight Watchers, most of my treat-y recipes offer some measure of healthfulness—whole-grain flour, fruit, yogurt instead of gobs of butter . . . except, of course, for The Best Homemade Chocolate Chip Cookies in the Entire World (page 348). That recipe is just crazy good, and I don't want to live in a world without chocolate chip cookies.

So go ahead. Have a treat. We moms—especially new moms—can sometimes be too hard on ourselves. A small daily indulgence won't harm you, or your baby if you're nursing (breastmilk is naturally sweet anyway). Just stick to less-processed, more wholesome goodies, and practice portion control: Give yourself a single serving. Don't grab the cake and a fork.

## SWEETS AND BABIES

Unlike their stressed-out parents, babies don't have that *need* for sweets. They don't even know there is such a (delightful, satisfying) category of food. The longer you wait to introduce your infant to foods with added sugar, the better. I'm not saying he should go to kindergarten without knowing what a cookie is, but try to hold off until he's at least one year old. (Sad but true: My older brother took his first steps chasing a cookie used as a lure.)

Each recipe in this chapter does have instructions for feeding it to a baby, but that's only because I know that sometimes reality gets in the way of our best intentions. If you're eating a Jammy Oatmeal Shortbread Bar in junior's vicinity, he's gonna notice. And you might want to give him a taste (I know I did, with Harry). So at least you should know what's safe.

## CRIB NOTES

- Approach the recipes in this chapter as what they are: treats. As in, "I enjoy an occasional treat." Aim to make this the least-used chapter in the cookbook.

- I'm not an advocate for sneak eating, but babies model their behavior on other people, especially their parents. If your baby sees you eating a whole tray of brownies, she's going to think that's normal. Wait, it's *not* normal, right?

- Hold off on sharing sugary treats with your baby for the first year—if he doesn't know it exists, he can't clamor for it. (See the sidebar, "Sweets and Babies," opposite, for more info.)

- Not everyone is a baker. Maybe you're not so sure about this whole deal. Maybe the thought of baking a cake from scratch actually scares you a little. Well, fret not. In this chapter, I've noted the recipes that are appropriate for beginners.

- If you *are* a beginner, I'm betting you don't have a ton of baking equipment, and probably not a mixer either. But there are quite a few recipes that don't call for anything special, just a couple of bowls, some measuring cups and spoons, a spoon to mix with, and a baking sheet or two. One recipe can even be mixed with your hands!

• • • • • • • • • • • • • • • • • • • • • • • • • • • • • • • • • • • • • • • • • • •

# THE BEST HOMEMADE CHOCOLATE CHIP COOKIES IN THE ENTIRE WORLD

**Makes about 2 dozen cookies**
**Cooking time: 2 to 37 hours (40 minutes active)**

This is by far the most popular recipe on *Words to Eat By*; I get hundreds of visitors a day, just looking for these cookies. In that blog post, written when we had barely begun trying to conceive, I described it as "the cookie recipe I want to pass down to my future children." It's definitely the cookie my boy will crave—and hopefully bake himself—as an adult. Aside from Harry, this might be my finest creation.

A few things to note about this recipe: First, the cookies become incredibly good (I mean it, can't-stop-eating good) after the dough has had a good long rest in the fridge. We're talking as long as 36 hours, but if you can only wait one hour that'll still produce some very, very good cookies.

And second, since I have, let's say, self-control issues, I find it easiest to bake these in small batches. I portion the dough out into cookie balls on a lined baking sheet, then stick the sheet in the freezer. Once they're solid, the balls go into a resealable freezer bag, and I can bake as many or as few as I like. Don't ask me why, but for most people the baking time remains the same for frozen and unfrozen dough. (I must warn you: As good as this dough is raw, it's even better in the form of frozen dough-balls.)

1½ cups all-purpose flour
½ teaspoon baking soda
½ teaspoon salt
½ cup (1 stick) cold unsalted butter, cut into
    ½-inch pieces
¾ cup packed light brown sugar
½ cup granulated sugar

1½ teaspoons vanilla extract
1 large egg, at room temperature, lightly
    beaten
6 to 7 ounces good-quality bittersweet
    chocolate chunks (1 generous cup; no need
    to get crazy with the scale here—it's fine to
    just use half a 12-ounce bag)

1.  Sift together the flour, baking soda, and salt into a medium bowl.
    *No sifter? Use a regular ol' mesh strainer.*

2.  Using a standing mixer fitted with a paddle attachment or a hand mixer, beat the butter and sugars on low speed until smooth, about 3 minutes. Stop the mixer and scrape down the sides of the bowl and the paddle.

3.  Add the vanilla and egg and beat on low speed until fully incorporated, about 15 seconds. Do not overbeat. Stop the machine and scrape down the sides of the bowl and the paddle.

4.  With your mixer on low speed, add the flour mixture to the butter and egg mixture. Beat until just incorporated. Scrape down the sides of the bowl. Add the chocolate chunks and mix until they are just incorporated. If using a hand mixer (which has a weaker motor), use a wooden spoon to stir instead. Refrigerate the dough for at least 1 hour, and preferably 24 to 36 hours.

5.  Preheat oven to 350°F and set racks to lower and upper thirds of oven. Line two baking sheets.

6.  Drop dough by a tablespoon or large cookie scoop, 2 inches apart, onto the prepared baking sheets. Bake until golden brown around the edges but still soft, almost underdone-looking, in the center, 11 to 13 minutes. To ensure even baking, rotate the sheets front to back and switch racks halfway through.

7.  Remove the sheets from the oven and carefully slide the liner with cookies directly onto a work surface. When the cookies are set (after about 3 minutes), transfer to a rack. Cool at least 5 minutes before serving or 20 minutes before storing in an airtight container for up to 3 days.

> MAKE BABY FOOD: Though in terms of ingredients they're perfectly safe, I'd only give these cookies to a baby on *very* special occasions.

**MAMA SAID**
"I like that I was able to make them in two shifts, so I could prepare the dough one evening and then bake them the next. This works really well for a working-mom schedule. The cookies are soooo good. They remind me of the chocolate chip cookies I used to make with my mom, so I will save this recipe to use with my daughter when she's older." —Heather M., mom of one, Los Gatos, CA

# FLOURLESS HONEY-ROASTED PEANUT BUTTER CHOCOLATE CHIP COOKIES

**Makes about 36 cookies**

**Cooking time: 30 minutes (15 minutes active)**

**BEGINNER**

After a particularly frustrating day, when nothing but baking (and, um, eating) could assuage my disappointment, I came up with this one-bowl (and no mixer) cookie recipe. It has only seven ingredients, and it satisfies both sweet *and* salty cravings thanks to a generous helping of chopped honey-roasted peanuts. It's flourless, which is a bonus for our gluten-free friends. And its major ingredient is peanut butter with a minor in dark chocolate, so I can almost convince myself these cookies are healthy. Not low-fat, certainly, but full of nutrition—at least as far as cookies go.

One 16-ounce jar natural creamy peanut
    butter
1½ cups lightly packed light brown sugar
2 eggs, lightly beaten
2 teaspoons baking soda

1 teaspoon vanilla extract
1 cup good-quality dark chocolate chips
1 cup honey-roasted peanuts, roughly
    chopped

**Preheat oven to 350°F. Line two baking sheets.**

1. Combine the peanut butter, brown sugar, eggs, baking soda, and vanilla in a large bowl (I find it easiest to begin with a whisk, then switch to a wooden spoon). Add the chocolate chips and peanuts and stir to combine.

2. Use a large cookie scoop to portion out balls of the dough and place them, 1½ inches apart, on the prepared cookie sheets. (You can also use moistened hands to form the balls, taking about a tablespoon at a time.) These cookies don't spread much, so flatten the balls slightly with your fingers.

3. Bake until the cookies are puffed and golden brown, about 12 minutes, rotating the baking sheets in the oven halfway through. Cool on baking sheets for at least 5 minutes before transferring to a rack to cool completely. Store in an airtight container for up to 3 days.

MAKE BABY FOOD: Between the small amount of honey in the peanuts—
off-limits for the under-one set due to botulism concerns—and the relatively
large amount of sugar in the recipe, I'd avoid feeding these to infants.

**MAMA SAID**

"This recipe was great all around! I put the baby to bed and started working on the recipe.
She woke up about 45 minutes into it, but this was simple enough that I could just leave it,
go get her and rock her back to bed, and resume making the cookies. Wonderful. On top of
tasting great and being easy to make, I took half of the dough and stuffed it back into the
empty peanut butter jar. A day or two later I took the jar out of the refrigerator and made a
dozen more cookies—a huge time saver." —Monica W., mom of one, St. Louis, MO

• • • • • • • • • • • • • • • • • • • • • • • • • • • • • • • • • • • • • • • •

# THE BROWNIE VARIATIONS

**Makes 12**

**Cooking time: 45 minutes (15 to 20 minutes active)**

**BEGINNER**

If you're like me, a fudgy brownie-lover (as opposed to a cakey brownie-lover), these
pups will knock your socks off. I learned to make the basic recipe at Sage American
Kitchen in Long Island City, Queens, a café and takeout shop where I worked back-of-
the-house, when I still fantasized about owning my own shop. Leslie Nilsson, the owner,
graciously gave permission for me to include it here. The two variations, spicy Aztec
Brownies and Mint Brownies, are my own adaptations to her foundation.

## SAGE'S FUDGY BROWNIES

6 ounces semisweet chocolate, chopped

¼ cup chocolate syrup

½ cup (1 stick) unsalted butter, softened
*Make sure your butter is good and soft before you start, or you'll have trouble getting the ingredients to combine smoothly.*

2 eggs, lightly beaten

1 teaspoon vanilla extract

¾ cup sugar

½ cup all-purpose flour

Pinch of salt

**Preheat oven to 350°F. Grease an 8-inch square baking dish.**

1.  Put the chocolate in a large, heavy saucepan over very low heat, stirring constantly until chocolate has melted. Remove from heat. Or microwave the chocolate in a large microwave-proof bowl in 30-second increments, stirring in between, until the chocolate has nearly melted—take it out and stir well, and the residual heat will melt the remaining lumps.

    *Most chocolate recipes will have you melt the chocolate in a bowl resting on a small pot containing simmering water, but if you stir constantly and keep the heat quite low, you can skip that extra step. Of course, if you're at all nervous about this, go right ahead and simmer that water!*

2.  Stir in the chocolate syrup, then add the butter and stir with a wooden spoon or spatula until smooth. Add the eggs and vanilla and stir until well combined.

3.  Sift the sugar, flour, and salt over the chocolate mixture. Stir until just combined and pour the batter into the prepared baking dish.

    *No sifter? Use a strainer! The mesh will catch any lumps.*

4.  Bake until the top is dry and the center is set, 28 to 30 minutes. The brownies will look soft, but that's OK. Cool brownies completely before cutting into squares.

## AZTEC BROWNIES

Additional ingredients:

1 teaspoon cinnamon
½ teaspoon chili powder

*Add the spices when you sift the dry ingredients, then proceed with the recipe.*

**NOTE:** These are exceptionally good cut into 1-inch squares and frozen. I keep a stash on the freezer door for when I need a hit of intense chocolate.

## MINT BROWNIES

Additional ingredients:

¼ teaspoon mint extract, optional
One 4.67-ounce package Andes Thins
   candies, unwrapped
   *Andes Thins are an old-school candy*
   *(you'll find them in the candy aisle of any*
   *supermarket), with two layers of chocolate*
   *sandwiching a creamy mint filling.*

If you're using the mint extract, add it when you add the vanilla.

Then, at the end of Step 3, pour half of the batter into the prepared baking dish and spread to cover the bottom. Arrange the unwrapped candies in a single layer over the batter. Spoon the remaining batter over the candies and carefully spread to cover the entire dish. Bake as directed.

> MAKE BABY FOOD: Both the basic recipe and the Aztec brownies are technically safe for babies (the Andes candies will harden as they cool, which makes them a choking hazard). But . . . special occasions only.

### MAMA SAID
"I made the Aztec brownie variation and these are wonderful. I managed to make it and get it out of the oven again within a 50-minute nap. I don't think these are going to last the day!" —Nicky A., mom of one, Melbourne, Australia

. . . . . . . . . . . . . . . . . . . . . . . . . . . . . . . . . . . . . .

# AMAZON CAKE

**Serves 6 to 8**

**Cooking time: 45 minutes (10 minutes active)**

**BEGINNER**

This cake is downright miraculous. It's butter- and egg-free (yup, vegan and pareve) and it comes together in a flash. No mixer required. Versions of this recipe are all over the Internet, often called "Wacky Cake" (according to Wikipedia, it was inspired by World War II rationing), but the one that I first used came from a 2002 article in the *New York Times.*

Amazon Cake is my go-to recipe when we need a hit of chocolate. If you want to make a layer cake, it doubles beautifully. It adapts easily to cupcakes (bake for 15 to 18 minutes). And since it's egg-free, I can give Harry the bowl for licking without hesitation.

1½ cups all-purpose flour

1 cup sugar

⅓ cup unsweetened cocoa powder (I use Dutch-process cocoa for this)

1 teaspoon baking soda

½ teaspoon salt

1 cup cold water

5 tablespoons vegetable oil

1 tablespoon cider vinegar, white vinegar, or strained lemon juice

1½ teaspoons vanilla extract

Confectioners' sugar or frosting of your choice

**Preheat oven to 350°F. Grease a 9-inch round cake pan.**

1.  Whisk together the flour, sugar, cocoa powder, baking soda, and salt in a medium bowl.

2.  Whisk together the cold water, oil, vinegar, and vanilla in a large bowl.

3.  Stir the dry ingredients into the wet, just until batter is smooth. Pour into the prepared cake pan.

4.  Bake until a cake tester or toothpick inserted in the center comes out with a few moist crumbs clinging to it, 30 to 35 minutes.

5.  Cool completely on a rack before removing from pan. Serve plain, dusted with powdered sugar, or frosted.

MAKE BABY FOOD: Another one to save for special occasions. It's perfectly safe, but no baby needs cake.

**MAMA SAID**

"I! love! this cake! It is not only delicious, but it is so simple—I always feel like I'm making a mix cake because it is just as easy. I love that it is vegan because I can serve it to our little friends who are egg and dairy allergic, and I can also use it as a pareve dessert for our kosher friends." —Jesse Z., mom of two, Los Angeles, CA

. . . . . . . . . . . . . . . . . . . . . . . . . . . . . . . . . . . . . . . . . . . . . . . . .

# CHOCOLATE YOGURT LOAF

**Serves 9**

**Cooking time: 1 hour (20 minutes active)**

This little treat was inspired by my usual mid-afternoon pick-me-up when I worked in an office. If you live in New York City, you know which treat I'm talking about: It's a very dark and moist-looking loaf cake, sliced, about an inch thick, clad in plastic wrap and usually found up by the register at your neighborhood deli. It's *crazy* good. So crazy good that I knew it couldn't be virtuous, even though it has "yogurt" in the name. I decided to make it myself.

The smell while this is baking is *hypnotic*, and it tastes just as good as the ones I bought for all those years. If I didn't tell you it was dietlicious, you'd never guess.

| | |
|---|---|
| 1 cup all-purpose flour | 5 tablespoons unsalted butter, softened |
| ¼ cup unsweetened Dutch-process cocoa | ¾ cup sugar |
| ½ teaspoon baking soda | 1 large egg |
| ½ teaspoon baking powder | 1 teaspoon vanilla extract |
| ½ teaspoon salt | ½ cup plain nonfat yogurt |

**Preheat oven to 350°F. Grease a loaf pan and dust it with cocoa or flour.**

1. In a small bowl, whisk together the flour, cocoa powder baking soda, baking powder, and salt.

2. Using a hand-held or stand mixer fitted with a paddle attachment, beat the butter and sugar on medium-high speed until pale yellow and fluffy, about 3 minutes. Add the egg and vanilla, and mix until well combined.

3. Add about half of the flour mixture, and mix until just combined. Add about half of the yogurt, and mix, scraping down the sides of the bowl as needed. Repeat with the remaining flour and yogurt and mix until just combined. Don't overmix or the finished loaf will be tough. This batter will be stiff but should still mix easily.

4. Spread batter evenly into the prepared loaf pan and bake on the center rack of the oven until a cake tester or toothpick inserted in the center comes out clean, 35 to 40 minutes.

5. Cool on a rack for about 10 minutes, then turn it out onto the rack to cool completely.

> MAKE BABY FOOD: I'm starting to bore myself . . . special occasions only, please.

**MAMA SAID**
"We really enjoyed this—it was tasty but not heavy. If I were more into chocolate I'd claim this is perfect for breakfast!" —Sarah D., mom of two, Olney, MD

. . . . . . . . . . . . . . . . . . . . . . . . . . . . . . . . . . . . . . . . . . .

# CHUNKY MONKEY PUDDING CAKE

**Serves 6**
**Cooking time: 1 hour (20 minutes active)**

**BEGINNER**
If you like Ben & Jerry's classic ice cream, I'm about to make you mighty happy. The appeal of this recipe (in addition to the flavor combo) is its dual textures—as it bakes, the top layer becomes cake-like, while the underneath remains pudding-like. When you pull it from the oven you might look at it and be unimpressed. But once the serving spoon breaks through the cake, you'll find a gooey, toffee-like sauce; as you serve the cake, spoon some of that glorious stuff on top. Your bowl may not be terribly pleasing to the eye, but I guarantee your mouth won't mind.

1 cup all-purpose flour

1¼ cups packed dark brown sugar, divided

1½ teaspoons baking powder

½ teaspoon salt

1 teaspoon vanilla extract

1½ tablespoons butter, melted, plus 3 tablespoons butter, cut into small pieces

½ cup milk (low-fat is fine)

3 ripe bananas, thickly sliced

¼ cup chopped toasted walnuts or pecans

¼ cup chocolate chips

1 cup boiling water

Vanilla ice cream or whipped cream, for serving

**Preheat oven to 350°F. Grease a 2-quart baking dish with high sides (a soufflé dish is perfect).**

1.  Combine the flour, ¾ cup brown sugar, baking powder, salt, vanilla extract, melted butter, and milk in a large bowl. Stir in the bananas, and spread the mixture into the prepared dish.

2.  Combine the walnuts, chocolate chips, the remaining brown sugar, and the cut-up butter in a small bowl. Don't worry about fully incorporating the butter—chunks are just fine. Sprinkle mixture over the batter.

3.  Carefully pour the boiling water over the entire dish, and bake until the top feels firm to the touch and the edges are bubbling furiously, 40 to 50 minutes.

4.  Serve hot, with vanilla ice cream or whipped cream, and the sauce spooned on top. Don't let it sit too long, or the sauce will be absorbed into the cake.

> MAKE BABY FOOD: Babies love bananas and the ingredients here are safe (provided your family has no food allergies), but this is so deliciously full of sugar I wouldn't give it to a little one. Reserve some of the ripe bananas instead.

**MAMA SAID**
"Wow, I loved this cake. It was so easy to make, I was able to do it while supervising my eight-month-old in her newfound ability to play by herself (yay!). It baked up nicely in 50 minutes, the texture and flavor were perfect, and I had to stop myself from having two pieces." —Melissa K., mom of one, Seattle, WA

• • • • • • • • • • • • • • • • • • • • • • • • • • • • • • • • • • • • • • • • • •

# BANANA-NUTELLA QUESADILLAS

**Serves 1, and multiplies well**

**Cooking time: 10 minutes**

**BEGINNER**

This one's for when you're jonesing for a treat, but don't feel like going to much trouble. You'll be eating in *minutes.*

1 teaspoon butter, softened

1 flour tortilla

1 tablespoon chocolate-hazelnut spread, such
   as Nutella

½ ripe banana, sliced in ¼-inch pieces

1. Heat a small skillet (not nonstick) over medium heat. Spread the butter on one side of the tortilla, and spread the chocolate-hazelnut spread on the other side (this is a bit messy, but it's worth it).

2. Arrange the tortilla, butter-side down, in the warm skillet. Lay the banana slices over one half of the tortilla, and fold over. Press lightly.

3. Cook the quesadilla, undisturbed, until the bottom is lightly browned, 2 to 3 minutes, then flip with a spatula. Cook another 2 to 3 minutes, until that side is browned too, then remove from heat.

4. Cut into wedges (I use a pizza cutter) and serve.

> MAKE BABY FOOD: Tortilla, yes. Banana, yes. Nutella, not so much. It's safe if your family's free of food allergies, just not particularly advisable (read the label: the first ingredient is sugar!).

**MAMA SAID**

"It's a good source of vitamins and healthy stuff, covered in just a tiny bit of indulgence. Made us all chocolatey-faced monkeys come dessert time. I'll definitely make it again. Our four-year-old loved helping to make it!" —Alexandra S., mom of two, Baltimore, MD

# THE GRANITA VARIATIONS

**Serves 6 to 8**

**Cooking time: 2 to 3 hours (15 to 20 minutes active)**

### BEGINNER

Are you familiar with the word "granita"? It's a fancy-shmancy way of saying "sorbet made without an ice cream maker." I tossed my machine a few years ago—the only way to be spontaneous about using it was to keep the darn bowl in the freezer, and it just took up too much space. So now I make granitas. The technique couldn't be simpler: Puree ripe, really ripe, super-ripe fruit. Add a bit of sugar if, God forbid, the super-ripe fruit isn't sweet enough. Add a touch of acid like citrus juice. Strain into a shallow bowl, and stick it in the freezer. Rake a fork across the top every so often, and big, frosty crystals will pile up. Put those into a bowl. Eat.

## WATERMELON-LIME GRANITA

5 cups chopped seedless watermelon

2 tablespoons to ½ cup sugar, to taste
  *Taste your watermelon—if it's really sweet, add
  2 tablespoons sugar. If it's pretty sweet, add
  ¼ cup. If it's not terribly-sweet, add a full ½ cup.*

2 tablespoons lime juice

## STRAWBERRY-BALSAMIC GRANITA

1 pound ripe strawberries, hulled and thickly
  sliced

1 tablespoon to ¼ cup sugar, to taste
  *If the strawberries are really ripe and sweet,
  you won't need more than 1 or 2 tablespoons.*

1 to 2 tablespoons balsamic vinegar, to taste

## MANGO-CHILI GRANITA

3 large, very ripe mangos, peeled, pitted, and
   roughly chopped

1 tablespoon to ¼ cup sugar, to taste
*If mangos are squishy-ripe, 1 or 2 tablespoons
will do it. Use more if they're not quite there.*

1 teaspoon chili powder

Pinch of salt

Juice of 1 lime (about 2 tablespoons)

1. Puree all the ingredients in a blender or food processor (I'd recommend a blender for the watermelon—it may leak from a food processor).

2. Strain into a metal pan or shallow bowl, and place in the freezer.

*If your freezer's as much of a booby trap as mine is, use a sealable container to prevent it from spilling everywhere. Trust me, it's no fun to clean sticky, slushy stuff from a million spilled-on freezer packages. I use a rectangular Rubbermaid container.*

3. After about 1 hour, scrape and stir the mixture with a fork. Return to the freezer for 30 minutes more, then scrape and stir again. Repeat until the mixture is fully frozen, 2 to 3 hours total.

4. To serve, rake the frozen surface with a fork—light, fluffy crystals will form. Use a spoon to scoop the crystals into small bowls.

> MAKE BABY FOOD: If you've got really ripe fruit and aren't using much sugar, this is perfect for babies. You'll know if your baby can handle the spice in the Mango-Chili version.

### MAMA SAID
"It's the middle of summer, it is hot, sticky, and there is no relief. Watermelon granita was perfect. And my daughter loved it." —Rachel M., mom of one, Tucson, AZ

# EASY GINGERSNAP PEACH CRISP

**Serves 4**

**Cooking time: 40 minutes (20 minutes active)**

**BEGINNER (Use frozen peaches)**

This is spectacular served warm with a little something cold on top: vanilla ice cream or frozen yogurt, whipped cream, crème fraîche, even plain yogurt. It's also surprisingly good eaten cold early the next morning, when standing in front of the fridge.

5 medium very ripe peaches, or 4 cups sliced frozen peaches, thawed

1 tablespoon dark brown sugar

1 tablespoon all-purpose flour

½ teaspoon cinnamon

¼ teaspoon ground ginger

15 gingersnaps, crushed
*You can do this in a mini-food processor, or just pop them into a resealable plastic bag and whack (gently) with a rolling pin or the bottom of a saucepan.*

2 tablespoons sliced almonds

2 tablespoons unsalted butter, melted

Whipped cream or vanilla ice cream, for serving

**Preheat oven to 375°F. Grease an 8-inch square baking dish.**

1. If using fresh peaches, bring a large pot of water to a boil. Place a large bowl of ice water next to the stove. Cut a shallow "X" in the bottom of each peach and drop into the boiling water, until the skins loosen, about 20 seconds. Using a slotted spoon, immediately transfer peaches to the ice water to stop the cooking, then slide off the skins. Slice peaches into a medium bowl.

2. Add the brown sugar, flour, cinnamon, and ginger, and gently stir to combine.

3. Transfer peaches to the prepared baking dish.

4. Combine the crushed gingersnaps, almonds, and melted butter (don't worry if the butter doesn't coat everything) and scatter over the peaches. Bake until the top is browned and the peaches are bubbly, about 20 minutes.

5. Serve warm with whipped cream or vanilla ice cream.

MAKE BABY FOOD: Since this is fruit-based, with little added sugar, it's fine for babies (stick with just the fruit, not the topping—the almonds can be a choking hazard). If you have food allergies in your immediate family, either leave out the almonds or don't give this to your baby at all.

**MAMA SAID**
"This peach crisp is delicious! The recipe is very straightforward. Definitely a great dessert to make when we have company." —Amber N., mom of one, Brooklyn, NY

. . . . . . . . . . . . . . . . . . . . . . . . . . . . . . . . . . . . . . . . . . .

# ROASTED PEARS À LA MODE

**Serves 8**
**Cooking time: 1 hour 10 minutes (15 minutes active)**

**BEGINNER**
These roasted pears are decadent—roasting accentuates their sweetness, crunchy pecans add textural contrast, and caramel sauce really puts this dessert over the top. But if you serve it with low-fat ice cream or frozen yogurt, this is actually quite a diet-friendly dish. Only 1 tablespoon of butter for 8 servings? A teaspoon of added sweetener? As long as you don't drown the plate in caramel, you can enjoy this *and* lose the baby weight.

8 ripe-but-firm pears, peeled, halved, and cored (a melon baller is ideal for coring)
1 tablespoon unsalted butter, melted
1 teaspoon honey or maple syrup
½ teaspoon cinnamon

¼ teaspoon salt
Vanilla ice cream or frozen yogurt, and a handful of chopped toasted pecans for serving
Prepared caramel sauce, for serving, optional

*The easiest way to toast nuts is in the toaster oven—bake at 300°F for 3 to 5 minutes (watch closely; they go from toasted to burnt in a heartbeat). If you don't have a toaster, put the nuts in a small, dry skillet and cook over medium-low heat for 3 to 5 minutes, shaking frequently.*

**Preheat oven to 450°F. Grease a large baking dish or baking sheet (large enough to hold the pear halves in a single layer).**

1. Arrange the pears on the baking sheet, cut side up.

2. Combine the butter, honey, cinnamon, and salt in a small bowl. Brush the mixture lightly onto the cut sides of the pears, then turn them over and brush the rounded sides.

3. Roast until the pears are tender, 45 to 55 minutes, flipping the pears halfway through.

4. Cool slightly, then place two pear halves on each plate and top with ice cream and chopped pecans. Drizzle with caramel sauce, if using.

> MAKE BABY FOOD: When made with maple syrup, the pears themselves are just fine for babies. (Due to botulism concerns, honey is a no-no for those under one year old.) You can puree or use as finger food. Skip the nuts, ice cream, and caramel sauce completely for infants.

**MAMA SAID**

**"We tried this recipe this afternoon and had a great time with it! The recipe was easy to follow, even while wrangling a toddler who was eager to help. She had fun 'helping' to chop the pears (with a plastic knife while I did the grown-up chopping) and measuring and stirring the ingredients to go on the pears. The pears are also nice as cold finger foods, so I may adapt them as afternoon snacks occasionally. Really great recipe if you're doing baby-led weaning—instead of half pears we cut them in half again, making long quarters. This made them easy for our daughter to manage to eat by herself." —April M., mom of one, Edinburgh, Scotland**

· · · · · · · · · · · · · · · · · · · · · · · · · · · · · · · · · · · · · · · · · · · · ·

# ROASTED PINEAPPLE

**Serves 4 to 6**

**Cooking time: 40 minutes (15 to 20 minutes active)**

**BEGINNER**

Here's a delicious and virtuous treat—it's fruit, with just a touch of butter and sugar—that is also delightfully flexible. One of my mom-testers served hers with a squeeze of lime juice, which sounds like a fantastic addition. Another ate the roasted pineapple for breakfast, topped with yogurt. And if you'd like to transform it into a dessert impressive enough for company, serve the pineapple over storebought pound cake or angel food cake and top with jarred lemon curd, vanilla ice cream, frozen yogurt, or whipped cream.

1 tablespoon unsalted butter, melted

1 tablespoon brown sugar, optional (taste the pineapple—if it's plenty sweet already, you can skip this)

1 good-sized ripe pineapple, trimmed, quartered vertically, cored, and sliced ¼-inch thick

*Buy it pre-sliced if you're not comfortable cutting up a pineapple on your own.*

10 mint leaves, thinly sliced, for serving

**Preheat oven to 425°F. Grease a baking sheet.**

1. Combine the melted butter and sugar in a bowl large enough to also hold the pineapple. Add the sliced pineapple and toss—don't worry if every piece isn't perfectly coated. Arrange pineapple in a single layer on the prepared baking sheet and roast for 15 minutes.

2. Remove sheet from oven, and increase heat to broil. Flip the pineapple slices, then broil, watching carefully, until browned and glistening, 2 to 4 minutes.

3. Serve topped with mint.

> MAKE BABY FOOD: Roasted pineapple is fine for babies, though it may be difficult to chew—be sure to cut the bits quite small, or puree. If you're afraid of that burning-tongue sensation that sometimes comes from eating pineapples, relax: Cooking should neutralize the enzyme that causes it. (To be absolutely certain, taste the roasted pineapple first!)

**MAMA SAID**
**"The pineapple was so easy and I liked that it's fruit-based and (relatively) healthy. We served it one night for dessert with some vanilla ice cream, and had the rest for breakfast the next day." —Julie O., mom of two, New Canaan, CT**

• • • • • • • • • • • • • • • • • • • • • • • • • • • • • • • • • • • • • •

# BERRY-ALMOND CLAFOUTIS

**Serves 6 to 8**

**Cooking time: 1 hour to 1 hour 15 minutes (15 to 20 minutes active)**

Clafoutis is a terrific way to use up fruit that's threatening to go mushy—it's a baked dessert of fruit surrounded by an eggy, custardy batter. The end result is something like a crêpe, something like a popover, and completely scrumptious.

If you don't have fresh fruit on hand, frozen fruit will work just fine.

3 cups mixed berries, sliced peaches, or
pitted cherries, washed and dried

¼ cup sliced almonds, toasted

*I like to do this in the toaster oven: Bake at
300°F for 3 to 5 minutes, until golden brown.
Keep a close eye so they don't burn. If you
don't have a toaster oven, toast them in a dry
skillet over medium heat, stirring frequently,
3 to 5 minutes.*

1 cup milk (low-fat is fine)

3 eggs

½ cup sugar

½ cup all-purpose flour

1 teaspoon vanilla extract

½ teaspoon almond extract, optional

⅛ teaspoon salt

Confectioners' sugar or whipped cream, for
serving

**Preheat oven to 350°F. Grease a 9- or 10-inch round baking dish or deep-dish pie pan.**

1. Pour the berries into the dish, and scatter the toasted almonds all around them.

2. Combine the milk, eggs, sugar, flour, vanilla, almond extract, if using, and salt in a
   blender and blend until smooth. Pour the batter over the berries and almonds and
   bake until puffy and golden, and a knife inserted in the center comes out clean,
   40 to 60 minutes. Note that the shape of your baking dish will affect baking time;
   the deeper and smaller in diameter the dish is, the longer it will take.

3. Cool for at least 15 minutes—the center will sink—and serve warm or at room
   temperature, dusted with confectioners sugar or with whipped cream.

> MAKE BABY FOOD: There's sugar in this one, yes. But it's so chock-full of fruit
> that I served this to Harry when he was wee, making sure that I gave him mostly
> the fruity bits. As long as there are no allergy concerns, you're good to go—just
> 1) crumble the almonds a bit to make sure they're not chokable, and 2) make
> sure the berries have cooled off, because they can be pretty molten inside.

**MAMA SAID**

**"The clafoutis is delicious and tastes much more complex than it is. I would even serve
it to guests. The texture was perfect—I used a 9-inch ceramic tart pan and baked it for
43 minutes. I used a jar of Morello cherries instead of berries, and it was très French and
really good. I think I'll have it for breakfast too." —Jennifer F., mom of one, Montreal, CA**

. . . . . . . . . . . . . . . . . . . . . . . . . . . . . . . . . . . . . . .

# BROWN SUGAR YOGURT CAKE

**Serves 6 to 8**

**Cooking time: 45 minutes (10 to 15 minutes active)**

**BEGINNER**

This cake may be as simple as can be, but the result is gorgeously moist and rich-tasting. You can top it with fresh fruit or a dusting of confectioners' sugar, if you like, or even jam. I also like to have a small slice with a cup of hot chocolate in colder weather.

The original recipe came from Chocolate and Zucchini, the food blog that first inspired me to start *Words to Eat By*. Clotilde Dusoulier, the blog's author, says that it's a classic French recipe, one of the first cakes schoolchildren learn to make on their own. Lucky them!

| | |
|---|---|
| 2 eggs | 1 tablespoon orange zest, optional |
| 1 cup plain yogurt (low-fat is fine) | 1 tablespoon Cointreau, optional |
| 1 cup dark brown sugar | 2 cups all-purpose flour |
| ⅓ cup vegetable oil | 1½ teaspoons baking powder |
| 1 teaspoon vanilla extract | ½ teaspoon baking soda |

**Preheat oven to 350°F. Grease a 9-inch round cake pan and line the bottom with parchment paper (this will help in removing the cake, but if you don't have parchment paper it's OK to skip—just grease the pan well).**

1. Stir together the eggs, yogurt, brown sugar, oil, vanilla, orange zest, and Cointreau, if using, in a large mixing bowl. Sift the flour, baking powder, and baking soda over the top and gently combine—stop when you no longer see flour.

   *No sifter? Use a strainer.*

2. Pour the batter into the prepared cake pan, and bake until the top is golden brown and a cake tester inserted in the center comes out clean, 30 to 35 minutes.

3. Cool the cake in the pan for 10 minutes, then turn it out onto a wire rack and peel off the parchment. If you'd like the pretty, rounded side to be on top, invert a plate over the cake and, grasping both the rack and the plate with the cake sandwiched between, flip the whole thing over. Remove the wire rack, and slide the cake off the plate onto it to cool fully.

MAKE BABY FOOD: Thanks to the sugar content, reserve this for special occasions.

**MAMA SAID**
"I can see why French schoolchildren learn to make this so young. It's a great, simple recipe! My three-year-old was very proud to have made this herself, with help from me. We didn't use parchment paper (just cooking spray) and the cake slid right out with no problem."
—Rebecca P., mom of two, Oakton, VA

• • • • • • • • • • • • • • • • • • • • • • • • • • • • • • • • • • • •

# JAMMY OATMEAL SHORTBREAD BARS

**Makes 12**

**Cooking time: 40 minutes (10 minutes active)**

**BEGINNER**
Yes, you read that right. These crumbly, sweet, satisfying bars come together in 10 minutes. I'm pretty sure even a baking novice can pull this one off—you can mix the dough with your hands, people!

Check out Mama Said, on the next page, to see how one inventive young man enjoyed his treat.

3½ cups rolled oats

⅔ cup packed dark brown sugar

¼ cup all-purpose flour

½ teaspoon salt

12 tablespoons (1½ sticks) butter, softened

1 teaspoon vanilla extract

½ cup raspberry jam
*I like the sweet-tart flavor of raspberry here— the shortbread is quite sweet—but if you prefer a different fruit, by all means use it.*

**Preheat oven to 350°F. Grease an 8-inch square baking dish.**

1. Combine the oats, brown sugar, flour, and salt in a large bowl, making sure to break up any large clumps of brown sugar. Use a wooden spoon or clean hands to thoroughly mix in the softened butter and vanilla.

2. Warm the jam, either in the microwave or in a small saucepan, until it's pourable. (It takes about 20 seconds on high in my microwave.)

3. Transfer just more than half the dough to the baking dish and press to cover the bottom of the pan evenly. Pour the warmed jam on top and spread it evenly across the surface (a small offset spatula is ideal for this). Top with the remaining dough and press gently, making the surface as flat and even as you can.

4. Bake until golden and firm, 20 to 30 minutes. Cool completely in the dish before cutting—it's quite delicate when warm.

> MAKE BABY FOOD: Thanks to the oatmeal, these are a bit healthier than some of the other indulgences—but they've still got added sugar, so tread carefully when deciding whether or not to let your baby taste one.

**MAMA SAID**
"I made the Jammy Oatmeal Shortbread last night. When my older son spotted it this morning in the kitchen, he asked if he could have some with breakfast. I suggested breaking it up into yogurt, but he decided to put it in his cereal with milk and liked it a lot. Whatever works!" —Abigail A., mom of two, New York, NY

# APPENDICES
## COUNTDOWN TO BABY

Pregnant? Here's a food-focused third-tri timeline to help you prepare for the first month or two at home with baby:

- **Weeks 28 to 29:** You're about to start feeling very pregnant. Now's a good time to research things like doulas, lactation consultants, pediatricians, and grocery delivery services.

- **Weeks 30 to 31:** It's a little soon to start stocking the freezer, but take the time to assess your readiness for big-batch cooking—make sure you have the equipment you'll need to prepare and freeze meals to eat once the baby's born. See page 5 for tips on the basics. Consult the pantry lists in Chapter 1, and make sure you're fully stocked with shelf-stable items.

- **Weeks 32 to 33:** The home stretch is on the horizon, but the discomfort's probably ramping up already. Even though the real sleep disturbances won't happen until the baby's outside your body, you may have trouble getting a good night's rest right now. Use whatever you have at your disposal to catch some zzzz's! If heartburn's keeping you up at night, eat dinner earlier and cut out acidic or spicy foods. Get yourself a body pillow to help you sleep on your side.

- **Weeks 34 to 35:** Nesting much? If you're not already cooking and freezing meals to get you through the first month or two, the time has definitely come. And be sure to sign up for my newsletter, at ParentsNeedtoEatToo.com. When you barely have time to think in the next few months, it will be ever so helpful to have tips and suggestions magically appear in your in-box.

- **Weeks 36 to 37:** Your baby will be considered full-term in a matter of days! At this point, you're on labor watch. Nail down the visiting schedule for out-of-town family members—do you want your mom in town for the birth, or will she be more helpful after the baby comes home? What about your in-laws? If everyone's open to it, see if you can stagger the visits so you'll have help for longer.

- **Weeks 38 to 39:** If you haven't spent much time in your hospital's neighborhood, do a little reconnaissance (online, if you're too pooped to shlep) and find out what local restaurants are a) good and b) willing to deliver. You do *not* want to count on hospital food being edible, never mind appealing.

- **Weeks 40 to 41:** Still pregnant? Sorry! But don't worry, that baby is coming out, and soon. When things do start happening, try to labor at home for as long as possible, and have something light but nourishing to eat before you leave for the hospital (think yogurt, fruit, granola)—once labor really gets going, you likely won't have the chance to eat until it's all over. Good luck!

# "NOW WHERE DID I SEE THAT?"

## Index of Sidebars

# RESOURCES

**PARENTING WEBSITES**

I'm sure you already know about all-purpose parenting sites like BabyCenter and Parents.com; here are some that offer different types of help:

- **www.healthychildren.org** A parent-oriented site from the American Academy of Pediatrics, where you'll find all their most current recommendations without the doctorese.

- **www.ilca.org** The International Lactation Consultant Association, which has a searchable database of certified consultants.

- **www.altdotlife.com** The women-centered Internet community that got me through infertility, pregnancy, the fourth trimester, and much more. Whatever's happening with your baby, odds are good that someone there has been through it too.

- **http://parents.berkeley.edu** and **www.parkslopeparents.com** The Berkeley Parents Network and Park Slope Parents are two enormous—and enormously helpful—fonts of parent-to-parent information and advice. In my area, there are also Yahoo groups devoted to parenting in specific neighborhoods—check there and you may find one for where you live too.

- **www.momsrising.org** Moms Rising is comprised of more than 1,000,000 mom-activists, fighting for everything from paid family leave to removing toxic chemicals like BPA from baby products.

### FOOD-RELATED WEBSITES

Feed yourself and your baby with help from these sites:

- **http://parentsneedtoeattoo.com** Sign up for my newsletter, get ideas and new recipes written post-book, and ask questions.

- **www.kellymom.com** An extremely thorough, evidence-based site devoted to breastfeeding. No wives' tales here, just solid information.

- **www.wholesomebabyfood.com** Tons of advice about introducing solids.

- **www.babyledweaning.com** If you'd like to skip purees entirely, this approach (in which baby feeds himself from Day One) may be for you.

- **www.feedkids.com** FEED: Forming Early Eating Decisions, the pediatric nutrition counseling center of Lara Field, MS, RD, CSP.

- **www.ewg.org** The Environmental Working Group, where you'll find a list of the "Dirty Dozen" and "Clean Fifteen" types of produce, guides to sunscreen and cosmetics, and much more.

- **www.montereybayaquarium.org/cr/seafoodwatch.aspx?c=ln** The Monterey Bay Aquarium's Seafood Watch, where you can search for sustainable fish available in your area.

- **http://stilltasty.com** Has that leftover Chicken Chili passed its use-by date? Check here to find out.

**BOOKS**

- *Wise Woman Herbal for the Childbearing Year* by Susun S. Weed

- *Mother Food: A Breastfeeding Diet Guide with Lactogenic Foods and Herbs* by Hilary Jacobson

- *Child of Mine: Feeding with Love and Good Sense* by Ellyn Satter

- *Food Fights: Winning the Nutritional Challenges of Parenthood Armed with Insight, Humor, and a Bottle of Ketchup* by Laura A. Jana, MD FAAP, and Jennifer Shu, MD FAAP

- *Not Your Mother's Slow Cooker Cookbook* by Beth Hensperger and Julie Kaufmann

- *To Buy or Not to Buy Organic: What You Need to Know to Choose the Healthiest, Safest, Most Earth-Friendly Food* by Cindy Burke

# ACKNOWLEDGMENTS

Giant, ceaseless, heartfelt thanks to:

My family—Stephen, Harry, my parents, my siblings, my in-laws—for being nothing but supportive from Day One. My wonderful agents, Anne Marie O'Farrell and Denise Marcil, for being equal parts sounding board and advocate. Everyone at Harper, in particular Amy Bendell, my wise, funny, insightful, level-headed editor; Lisa Sharkey, a woman whose vision knows no bounds; Jennifer Hart, Shelby Meizlik, Jean Marie Kelly, Maggie Oberrender, and the entire marketing and publicity team, who've entertained my pesky ideas with kindness and understanding; Kate Winslow and Lelia Mander, who took my manuscript and made it read like a book; Amanda Kain and Lisa Stokes, who made the actual book look so good my face hurts from smiling over it; and Michael Morrison, a friend since I sat on the other side of the table. Lara Field, for ensuring that everything in the book is nutritionally sound. Freda Rosenfeld, for sharing her wisdom for the book. Catherine Strohbein, for providing guidance on food safety. Lorraine Carley of the National Fire Protection Association, for providing guidance on slow-cooking in the oven. Erin McHugh, for being a never-ending font of information about the business of book-writing. And Sharon Moskal, for first suggesting that teaching new parents how to cook might be my *thing*.

Acknowledgments

This book literally would not be what it is without my mom-testers, who voluntarily cooked my rough recipes and reported back, every month for a year. The book came together with their voices, their experiences, and their suggestions:

Lauren A., Megan A., Nicky A., Paige A., Shani A., Amanda B., Chris B., Emma B., Heather B., Jane B., Jody B., Kate B., Sarah B., Susan B., Yelena B., Aimee C., Alana C., Charity C., Corrin C., Heather C., Jennifer C., Jessica C., Lisa C., Paige C., Sona C., Sonia Marie C., Amber D., Heather D., Jessica D., Sarah D., Tara D., Jennifer E., Jennifer F., Natasha F., Amanda G., Bethany G., Christine G., Darcy G., Hilary G., Leya G., Meaghan G., Christine H., Deeya H., Helen H., Jennifer H., Natalie H., Nicky H., Amy J., Anita J., Elizabeth J., Karissa J., Magda J., Abigail K., Bari K., Elizabeth K., Heather K., Jess K., Karen K., Marisa K., Melissa K., Rae K., Kati L., Meredith L., Sarah L., Amy M., April M., Ariella M., Brandi M., Heather M., Karen M., Kim M., Linda M., Rachel M., Robin M., Sandra M., Taryn M., Tracy M., Amber N., Dana N., Jennifer N., Rebecca N., Julie O., Beth P., Emily P., Kristy P., Laura P., Lee P., Madeline P., Michelle P., Rebecca P., Jen R., Maggie R., Melanie R., Pamela R., Alexandra S., Ann S., Bethany S., Carol S., Gali S., Jen S., Jenn S., Jennifer S., Laurel S., Leslie S., Rachel S., Suzanne S., Kamila T., Lisa T., Mary T., Sarah T., Adriana V., Anne V., Elisa V., Aileen W., Christy W., Deborah W., Leah W., Lia W., Martha W., Monica W., Jesse Z., and Kristina Z.

(I believe I've got you all listed there, but if I missed someone please forgive me!)

# INDEX